Prevention Practice

A Physical Therapist's Guide to Health, Fitness, and Wellness

Prevention Practice

A Physical Therapist's Guide to Health, Fitness, and Wellness

Edited by

Catherine Rush Thompson, PhD, MS, PT
Assistant Professor of Physical Therapy
Rockhurst University
Kansas City, Mo

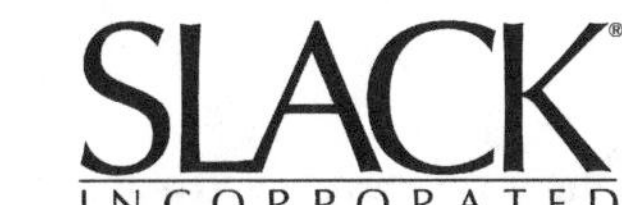

Delivering the best in health care information and education worldwide www.slackbooks.com

ISBN: 978-1-55642-617-9

Prevention Practice: A Physical Therapist's Guide to Health, Fitness, and Wellness Instructor's Manual is also available from SLACK Incorporated. Don't miss this important companion to this book. To obtain the Instructor's Manual, please visit www.efacultylounge.com.

The procedures and practices described in this book should be implemented in a manner consistent with the professional standards set for the circumstances that apply in each specific situation. Every effort has been made to confirm the accuracy of the information presented and to correctly relate generally accepted practices. The authors, editor, and publisher cannot accept responsibility for errors or exclusions or for the outcome of the material presented herein. There is no expressed or implied warranty of this book or information imparted by it. Care has been taken to ensure that drug selection and dosages are in accordance with currently accepted/recommended practice. Due to continuing research, changes in government policy and regulations, and various effects of drug reactions and interactions, it is recommended that the reader carefully review all materials and literature provided for each drug, especially those that are new or not frequently used. Any review or mention of specific companies or products is not intended as an endorsement by the author or publisher.

SLACK Incorporated uses a review process to evaluate submitted material. Prior to publication, educators or clinicians provide important feedback on the content that we publish. We welcome feedback on this work.

Published by: SLACK Incorporated
6900 Grove Road
Thorofare, NJ 08086 USA
Telephone: 856-848-1000
Fax: 856-853-5991
www.slackbooks.com

Contact SLACK Incorporated for more information about other books in this field or about the availability of our books from distributors outside the United States.

Library of Congress Cataloging-in-Publication Data

Prevention practice : a physical therapist's guide to health, fitness, and wellness / edited by Catherine Rush Thompson.
p. ; cm.
Includes bibliographical references and index.
ISBN-13: 978-1-55642-617-9 (alk. paper)
ISBN-10: 1-55642-617-8 (alk. paper)
1. Physical therapy. 2. Physical fitness. 3. Health promotion. I. Thompson, Catherine Rush, 1954-
[DNLM: 1. Physical Therapy Modalities--organization & administration. 2. Health Promotion. 3. Physical Fitness. 4. Primary Prevention--methods. 5. Primary Prevention--organization & administration. WB 460 P944 2006]

RM700.P82 2006
613.7--dc22

Printed in the United States of America.

Last digit is print number: 10 9 8 7 6 5 4 3 2

Dedication

"Imagine life as a game in which you are juggling five balls in the air.
You name them—work, family, health, friends, and spirit—
and you're keeping all of these in the air.
You will soon understand that work is a rubber ball.
If you drop it, it will bounce back.
But the other four balls—family, health, friends, and spirit—are made of glass.
If you drop one of these, they will be irrevocably scuffed, marked,
nicked, damaged, or even shattered.
They will never be the same.
You must understand that and strive for balance in your life."

~ **BRIAN DYSON**
CEO OF COCA COLA ENTERPRISES FROM 1959–1994

This book is dedicated to Ellen F. Spake, PT, PhD, a teacher, a mentor, a colleague, and a friend who has served as a professional role model in physical therapy for me and so many others. Her ability to juggle her work, her family, her health, her friends, and her spirit exemplifies the dedication and commitment that has made her the remarkable person she is. I am grateful for her continual inspiration.

Contents

Prevention Practice: A Physical Therapist's Guide to Health, Fitness, and Wellness Instructor's Manual is also available from SLACK Incorporated. Don't miss this important companion to this book. To obtain the Instructor's Manual, please visit www.efacultylounge.com.

Acknowledgments

The American Physical Therapy Association's Vision 2020 statement provided the impetus for this book, which is designed to extend the scope of preventive care through direct access:

> *By 2020, physical therapy will be provided by physical therapists who are doctors of physical therapy, recognized by consumers and other health care professionals as the practitioners of choice to whom consumers have direct access for the diagnosis of, intervention for, and for the prevention of impairments, functional limitations, and disabilities related to movement, function, and health. (HOD 06-00-24-35)*

I would personally like to thank my professional colleagues who have supported this effort and provided valuable insight regarding the growing role of preventive care in physical therapy practice. More specifically, I would like to thank those who contributed their time and effort to this book through sharing their expertise and reviewing the book's contents for accuracy and relevance. I am also indebted to family members, friends, physical therapy students, and clients who provided an incentive for developing a text promoting health, fitness, and wellness.

About the Editor

Catherine Rush Thompson, PhD, MS, PT, was born in Kansas City and attended the University of Colorado Medical Center, graduating with distinction with a BS in physical therapy. With support from the William Hillman Medical Student Fellowship, she attended and graduated with distinction from the University of Kansas Medical Center with an MS in Special Education with an emphasis on Children with Illness and Other Health Impairments. With support from the Arthur Mag Fellowship and the UMKC Community Scholars Fellowship at the University of Missouri at Kansas City, she completed her Interdisciplinary PhD, incorporating studies in physiological psychology, biochemistry, neuroscience, exercise science, and education. While her primary clinical practice focuses on pediatric physical therapy and neurological rehabilitation, she has worked in practice settings in acute care, outpatient care, long-term care, school-based therapy, home health, and private practice. Currently she is an assistant professor in the Department of Physical Therapy Education at Rockhurst University, and she presents her work at state, national, and international meetings.

Dr. Thompson's travel to over 50 countries gives her insight into global health care disparities and the need for multicultural education. Her research interests focus on pediatric growth and development, the use of motor imagery in physical therapy practice, and prevention practice across the lifespan. She hopes that this book will contribute to realizing the goals of Healthy People 2010 with physical therapists playing an integral role in prevention practice.

Contributors

Shawn T. Blakeley, PT, CWI, CEES
Interim Administrative Director
Rehabilitation Manager
CorporateCare/Urgent Care
Lenexa, Kansas

Shannon N. Buhs, PT
Physical Therapy Clinician in Women's Health
Olathe Medical Center
Olathe, Kansas

Ann Marie Decker, PT, MSA, GCS
Clinical Assistant Professor of Physical Therapy
Department of Physical Therapy Education
Rockhurst University
Kansas City, Missouri

Amy Foley, DPT, PT, MA
Assistant Professor of Physical Therapy
Department of Physical Therapy Education
Rockhurst University
Kansas City, Missouri

Paul Hansen, PhD, PT
Rehabiliation Director
Consonus Healthcare
Washington Soldiers Home
Orting, Washington

Martha Highfield, PhD, RN, AOCN
Professor of Nursing
California State University
Northridge, California

Steven G. Lesh, PhD, MPA, PT, SCS, ATC
Director of Physical Therapy Program
Associate Professor of Physical Therapy
Southwest Baptist University
Bolivar, Missouri

Gail R. Regan, PhD, PT
Assistant Professor
Psychology Department
Castleton State College
Castleton, Vermont

Preface

All parts of the body which have a function, if used in moderation and exercised in labors in which each is accustomed, become thereby healthy, well-developed, and age more slowly. But, if unused, they become liable to disease, defective in growth, and age quickly.

~HIPPOCRATES

The authors of *Prevention Practice: A Physical Therapist's Guide to Health, Fitness, and Wellness* have compiled information relevant to health, wellness, and fitness as a ready resource for physical therapists working in diverse practice settings. Written for students and clinicians, this book provides resources for screening individuals across the lifespan, identifying key risk factors for specific populations, educating clients and their families about healthy lifestyle behaviors, and developing effective interventions to promote health, fitness, and wellness. Additionally, this book provides a theoretical framework for program development, including marketing and management strategies to address both individual and community needs.

Based upon the goals outlined in Healthy People 2010, this book combines the vision of direct access for physical therapists with the overarching goals of national health care: to increase the quality and years of healthy life and to eliminate health disparities among various populations. Recognizing the cost effectiveness of preventive care, physical therapists have joined other professionals in an expanded role in health promotion and wellness, complementing evidence-based physical therapy management of medical conditions.

The intent of this book is to introduce key concepts of health, fitness, and wellness for both healthy populations and those with impairments affecting their quality of life. Additional resources are offered throughout the book to link the reader to the vast array of information designed to promote health, fitness, and wellness for healthy, at-risk, and special needs populations.

Chapter 1

Prevention Practice: A Holistic Perspective for Physical Therapy

Catherine Rush Thompson, PhD, MS, PT

"The Doctor of the future will give no medicine, but will interest his patient in the care of the human frame, in diet, and in the cause and prevention of disease."

~THOMAS EDISON

Health

The word *health* is derived from the Old English term *hal*, meaning sound, or whole. Health is essentially the purpose of medicine, the promotion and restoration of wholeness. While health is broadly defined by the *Webster Dictionary* as "the state of being healthy, happy, and prosperous," the World Health Organization defines health as "a state of complete physical, mental and social well-being, and not merely the absence of disease or infirmity."[1] Defined in the *Community Health and Education and Promotion Manual*, health is a more dynamic process, "a quality of life involving dynamic interaction and independence among an individual's physical well-being, his [her] mental and emotional reactions, and the social complex in which he [she] exists."[2] Finally, "spiritual health" or "the passion one has to fulfill a need" or personal goal is yet another aspect of health that should be recognized by health professionals.[3] In all of these definitions of health, there are physical, mental, social, and spiritual components—key factors for the comprehensive health examination.

Medical professionals have experienced a shift in their health care paradigm perspective from one emphasizing illness to one stressing health, function, quality of life, and well-being. This shift in health care has resulted in a surge in prevention practice designed to reduce disease through helping people modify their lifestyle behaviors to optimize health. *Optimal health* is defined as a balance of physical, mental, and social health.[4] Lifestyle changes promoting optimal health can be facilitated through a combination of efforts that (1) enhance self-awareness and knowledge of healthy habits, (2) change behaviors that interfere with good health, and (3) create environments that support good health practices.[5] The importance of supportive environments for producing lasting change cannot be overemphasized.

Poor health may include physical ailments causing acute or chronic disabilities as well as mental health issues that limit independent functioning. Poor health has a significant impact on the individual, the family, the community, and society at large. Depending on the severity of illness, the individual may lose functional independence and the opportunity to fulfill a role in the home and community. Family members also lose the support of those who are ill and often must adjust their roles and goals to meet the needs of someone who is disabled. Society also suffers from injury and disease that may be preventable. In a recent study, the National Academy of Sciences found that musculoskeletal disabilities in the workplace cost the United States more than $1 trillion per year in total costs.[6,7] Effective prevention of musculoskeletal disabilities through active intervention is not only

TABLE 1-1

BEHAVIORAL RISK FACTOR SURVEILLANCE SYSTEM (1995 TO 1997)

	% of adults	Mean Number of Days (of the Past 30 Days)						
		Not good physical health	Not good mental health	Healthy days*	Activity limitation	Pain	Sad, blue, depressed	Anxious
ACTIVITY								
No activity limitation	81	1.7	2.3	26.2	0.7	1.1	2.4	4.5
Difficulty walking	1.2	10.8	3.7	17.8	6.3	11.8	5.1	6.5
PATHOLOGICAL CONDITIONS								
Musculoskeletal conditions	*7.8*							
Back or neck problems	3.2	10.2	6.1	16.9	7.1	13.5	7.0	10.0
Fracture/joint injury	1.7	8.9	3.9	18.9	5.8	11.8	4.8	7.4
Arthritis/Rheumatism	2.9	10.2	4.0	18.1	4.7	13.4	5.4	7.9
Cardiopulmonary conditions	*3.0*							
High blood pressure	0.2	9.9	6.3	14.8	7.5	7.4	8.8	7.7
Heart problem	1.5	11.2	4.5	17.1	6.7	7.4	5.5	7.2
Lung or breathing problem	1.3	10.1	5.2	16.9	6.4	6.2	6.0	9.0
Neurological conditions	*1.4*							
Depression, anxiety, or other emotional problem	0.4	9.8	15.7	9.0	13.1	7.2	18.6	19.0
Stroke	0.3	12.6	4.1	17.0	8.0	7.1	6.7	8.1
Eye problem or visual impairment	0.6	5.8	4.2	21.8	2.9	4.1	5.1	5.4
Hearing impairment	0.1	4.2	2.0	23.9	2.6	4.1	3.1	5.5
Other conditions	*3.9*							
Cancer	0.3	16.4	9.3	10.8	12.9	12.1	10.0	11.1
Diabetes	0.4	13.1	7.0	14.5	9.8	8.7	9.4	9.4
Other health conditions	3.2	9.2	6.7	17.9	6.8	8.7	6.6	9.5

*On the average, Americans said they felt unhealthy (physically or mentally) about 6 days per month and felt "healthy and full of energy "about 19 days per month. Individuals aged 18 to 24 years experienced more mental health problems than other populations. Older adults experienced more unhealthy physical health days" and more "activity limitation" than other populations. Those with chronic diseases/disabilities and lower incomes reported fewer healthy days. Native Americans and Alaskans reported the highest number of unhealthy days.

Adapted from Centers of Disease Control and Prevention. Measuring healthy days. Population assessment of health-related quality of life. 2000. Available at: http://www.cdc.gov/hrqol/activitylimit.htm and http://www.cdc.gov/hrqol/findings.htm. Accessed October 15, 2005.

possible but results in a significant cost savings for employers while reducing employee disability.[7]

A rising trend in poor health reported in the United States indicates an immediate need for preventive care in order to reduce medical conditions that lead to disability. Between 1993 and 2002, the National Center for Chronic Disease Prevention and Health Promotion conducted a health-related quality-of-life surveillance survey of 1,291,986 American adults to examine self-rated health and its impact on the quality of life for this sample.[8] When asked questions about their mental and physical health, 4.1% reported poor health in 2001 (up from 3.5% in 1993), and 22.1% reported excellent health in 2001 (down from 25.3% in 1993). A mean number of 5.5 "unhealthy" days were reported for the preceding 30 days. Also, these individuals experienced activity limitations in their work, their leisure activities, or other normal daily activities an average of 2 days during the preceding 30 days in 2001, as compared to only 1.6 days in 1993.[8] These data suggest a trend toward increasingly limited activity and poor health over the last decade. Table 1-1 lists results from a separate survey of behavioral risk factors conducted by the Centers for Disease Control from and Prevention 1995 to 1997.

These survey results provide details about the types of conditions affecting mental health, physical health, activity limitation, and emotions. Additional data related to health-related quality of life are located on the Centers for Disease Control and Prevention website.[8]

When an individual reports poor health, it is likely that work productivity in all arenas of that person's life is reduced. Poor health affects personal satisfaction, the ability to meet family needs and personal responsibilities, and the perpetual demands in the workplace. Poor health is not only financially costly, but also takes a toll on emotional, psychological, and social well-being of all affected.

According to the National Center for Chronic Disease Prevention and Health Promotion, a variety of unhealthy lifestyle behaviors commonly developed early in life often lead to disability, chronic disease, and ultimately, premature death. These lifestyle behaviors include well-known risk factors for heart disease and diabetes, including smoking and other forms of tobacco abuse, eating high-fat and low-fiber diets, maintaining a sedentary lifestyle, and engaging in alcohol and drug abuse. Other factors carrying similar risks include lack of preventive medical screenings and engaging in violent behaviors or behaviors leading to unintentional injuries, such as driving under the influence of drugs or alcohol. While some of these lifestyle behaviors are contingent upon personal choices, others may be dependent upon accessible and affordable health education and health care.[9]

A study conducted by the Centers for Disease Control and Prevention determined that depression, anxiety, and other emotional problems were a leading cause of limited activity, as measured in a quality-of-life profile.[8] Mental health issues were followed by cancer, diabetes, stroke, high blood pressure, back and neck problems, other impairments, heart problems, walking problems, and joint problems.[8] All of these conditions can be positively affected by health promotion activities and a healthy lifestyle.

Wellness

Wellness is often used synonymously with health; however, wellness is a more comprehensive construct. According to the National Wellness Institute, "wellness is an active process of becoming aware of and making choices toward a more successful existence."[10] In other words, wellness is an active, lifelong process of becoming aware of choices and making decisions toward a more balanced and fulfilling life. Wellness involves choices about one's life and the priorities that determine one's lifestyle. Wellness integrates mental, social, occupational, emotional, spiritual, and physical dimensions of one's life and reflects how one feels about life as well as one's ability to function effectively.

Dimensions of Wellness

According to the Systems Theory of Wellness, the multiple dimensions of wellness are essential sub-elements of a larger system, yet these dimensions function independently as their own sub-elements.[11] When one dimension of wellness is disrupted, such as when an individual gets injured in an accident, other dimensions of wellness reciprocally interrelated to that dimension are also disrupted, requiring adaptation of the whole individual. When an individual has emotional problems, these problems affect the mental, social, occupational, spiritual, and physical dimensions of that person.

Corbin, Lindsey, and Welk, prominent educators in the field of exercise and health promotion, describe the six dimensions of wellness outlined by the National Wellness Institute. These descriptions include examples of physical wellness, spiritual wellness, social wellness, psychological wellness, emotional wellness, and intellectual wellness[12]:

- *Physical wellness* is the positive perception and expectation of health. Physical wellness includes the ability to effectively meet daily demands at work and to use free time. A person with a positive perception and expectation of health may be more likely to embrace healthy lifestyle behaviors that prevent injury and illness.
- *Spiritual wellness* is the belief in a unifying force between the mind and body. Spiritual wellness includes a person's ability to establish values and act on a system of beliefs as well as to establish and carry out meaningful and constructive lifetime goals. Those individuals with a strong belief system may be more likely to carry out goals that keep both the mind and body healthy.
- *Social wellness* is the perception of having support available from family or friends in times of need and the perception of being a valued support provider. Social wellness includes a person's ability to successfully interact with others and to establish meaningful relationships that enhance the quality of life for all people involved in the interaction, including oneself. Social support is a valuable asset for health and wellness, as well as recovery from illness and injury.

- *Psychological wellness* is a general perception that one will experience positive outcomes to the events and circumstances in life. This perception suggests a positive attitude or outlook about life. The intangible qualities of optimism, determination, and hope are vital in preventive practice and positively dealing with life problems.
- *Emotional wellness* is the progression of a secure self-identity and a positive sense of self-regard, both of which are facets of self-esteem. Emotional wellness includes the ability to cope with daily circumstances and to deal with personal feelings in a positive, optimistic, and constructive manner. A person who dwells on negative emotions and who has a negative self-esteem does not reap the benefits of a positive self-attitude. It is important for a physical therapist to consider that ill or injured individuals are at risk for lower self-esteem as they lose functional abilities and, potentially, their significant roles in life.
- *Intellectual wellness* is the perception of being internally energized by an optimal amount of intellectually stimulating activity. This type of intellectual stimulation must be sufficient to challenge intellectual abilities but not so overwhelming that there is no time for mental repose. Both intellectual overload and intellectual underload can adversely affect health. Intellectual wellness includes a person's ability to learn and to use information to enhance the quality of daily living and optimal functioning.

Howard Clinebell, a theologian, offers an even more comprehensive perspective of wellness with his seven dimensions of wellness.[13] His dimensions are more encompassing of the environment and a world-perspective. The definitions of his seven dimensions of wellness include spiritual well-being, mental well-being, physical well-being, relationship well-being, work well-being, play well-being, and the well-being of our world:

- The *Spiritual Well-Being Dimension* incorporates healthy religious beliefs, practices, values, and institutions that energize and enrich all aspects of our lives. This dimension of well-being addresses an individual's need for purpose, guidance, meaning, and values. The ill person who has healthy religious or spiritual beliefs and values has a sense of personal value and spiritual security.
- The *Mental Well-Being Dimension* represents the profound interdependence of the mind and body that manifests itself in our mental and physical health. Mental well-being incorporates problem solving, creativity, clarity in thinking, service, and productivity. Those who are given the opportunity to creatively problem solve and provide services to others are believed to have an improved mental well-being.
- The *Physical Well-Being Dimension* reflects the body's health. Physical well-being is evidenced by the ability to experience sensations without pain, to effectively function with adequate energy, to be responsible for self-care, and to nurture others. Many pathologies and injuries significantly affect this dimension, particularly those presenting with pain.
- The *Relationship Well-Being Dimension* represents the most important factor for our healing and general wellness. This dimension incorporates the need for nurturing and love, for giving and receiving, for empowering others, and for creating interpersonal bonds. On a larger scale, this well-being relates to peaceful coexistence with others.
- The *Work Well-Being Dimension* satisfies the thirst for purpose. This dimension of wellness addresses the need for fulfilling a purpose in one's vocation. Self-worth, satisfaction, and personal fulfillment are all related to the individual's ability to serve the community in a meaningful way.
- The *Play Well-Being Dimension* acknowledges that play provides the individual with laughter, cheer, energy, and balance. It is the ability to successfully play that provides the needed healing and revitalization to meet the demands of the other dimensions. Allowing time for this important dimension is a high priority for overall well-being, as noted in the following quote by Kahil Gibran: "In the sweetness of friendship let there be laughter, and sharing of pleasures. For in the dew of little things the heart finds its morning and is refreshed."[14]
- The *Well-Being of Our World Dimension* reflects an individual's perspective on living in a healthy environment and protecting natural resources. This final dimension incorporates a broad overview of the world. Wellness in this dimension includes responsibility, justice, an earth-caring lifestyle, a desire of well-being for all, adequate health care, dependence on others in the community, political participation, and the recognition of institutions as potential resources for meeting needs beyond the self.

These seven dimensions are more holistic and provide a framework for exploring various aspects of health and wellness, including the multifaceted individual and perspectives of the world.

TABLE 1-2

WELLNESS GRID: PRIORITIES FOR YOUR WELL-BEING

	Highest Priority	Second Priority	Third Priority
Spiritual well-being			
Mental well-being			
Physical well-being			
Relationship well-being			
Work well-being			
Play well-being			
World well-being			

Premature Death **High Level of Wellness**

Disability Symptoms Signs ☐ Awareness Education Growth

Neutral point

(No discernible illness or wellness)

Figure 1-1. Travis' Illness-Wellness Continuum. (Adapted from Wellness Associates. Illness-wellness continuum. Available at: http://www.thewellspring.com/Pubs/iw_cont.html. Accessed October 15, 2005.)

While the health care provider is often trained to provide education focusing on the physical dimensions of wellness, a more comprehensive or holistic perspective enables these professionals to make appropriate referrals to address other dimensions of well-being. Those in poor health benefit from additional resources, such as educational materials, support groups, or referrals to professionals with expert knowledge. The wellness grid shown in Table 1-2 can be used by health care professionals to help their clients identify the dimensions of their lives needing priority and additional resources.

MODELS OF WELLNESS

Various theorists have developed models and simplified descriptions of the multi-dimensional aspects of wellness. In addition to providing a framework for identifying clients' needs, these models of wellness offer insight for the management of illness and prevention practice.

As early as 1972, John W. Travis[15] developed a continuum of wellness illustrating the impact of wellness on health and premature death (Figure 1-1). According to this model, signs and symptoms of pathology and, ultimately, disability precede premature death.

Medical testing such as blood tests, vital signs, and imaging studies generally detect *signs* (ie, physiological and anatomical markers of pathology or illness). *Symptoms* of pathology are sensations or changes in bodily function experienced by a client or patient. The individual often discerns symptoms of pathology or the awareness of illness after pathophysiological changes have taken place at the subcellular and cellular level. *Disability*, or the inability to engage in gainful activity or work, often results from chronic or long-term illness and has a significant impact on an individual's well-being.[16] Acute illness and injury can also be significantly disabling and may lead to premature death if not managed properly. According to the Social Security Administration, disability is "an inability to engage in any substantial gainful activity by reason of any medically determinable physical or mental impairment which can be expected to result in death or has lasted or can be expected to last for a continuous period of not less than 12 months."[17] Chronic disability significantly affects multiple dimensions of wellness, including mental well-being, physical well-being, work well-being, and relationship well-being.

Travis' wellness model is helpful in recognizing the point where prevention practice may affect health and wellness. While health care intervention often initiates when an individual presents with

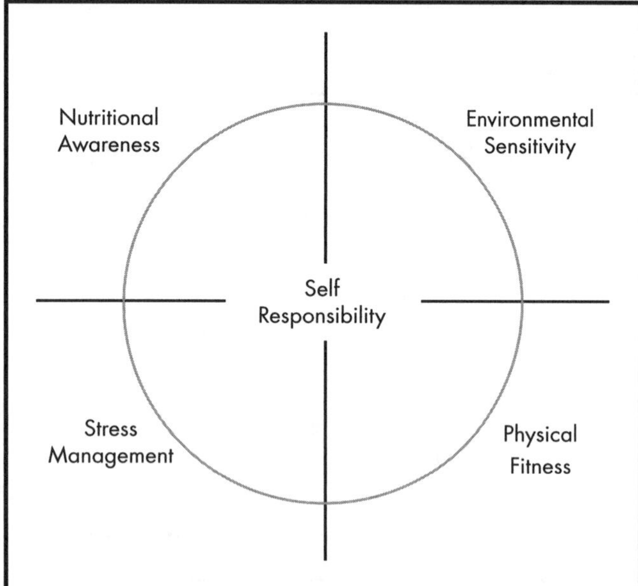

Figure 1-2. Ardell's Model of Wellness (1977). (Adapted from Ardell D. *14 Days to Wellness: The Easy, Effective, and Fun Way to Optimum Health.* New York, NY: New World Library; 1999.)

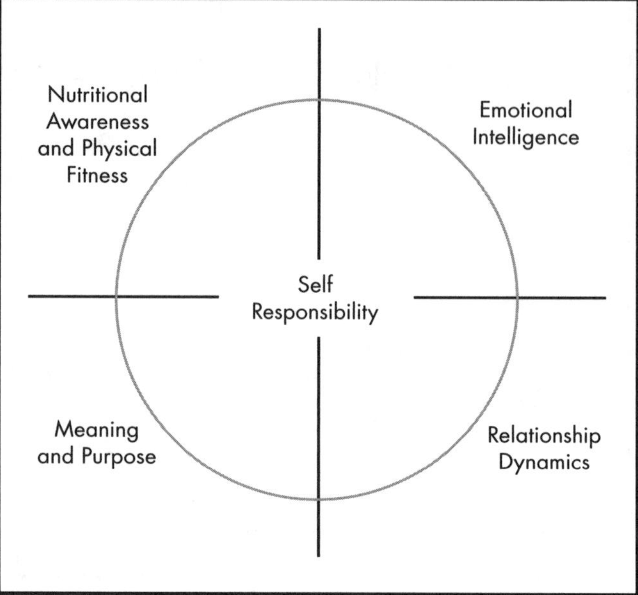

Figure 1-3. Ardell's Model of Wellness (1986). (Adapted from Ardell D. *14 Days to Wellness: The Easy, Effective, and Fun Way to Optimum Health.* New York, NY: New World Library; 1999.)

signs or symptoms of pathology, earlier intervention (emphasizing awareness and avoidance of risk factors for illness, education about healthy lifestyle behaviors, and access to up-to-date and accurate knowledge) can provide a level of wisdom that buffers many from pathology and premature death. For example, if an individual knows that a sedentary lifestyle and high-fat diet can increase the risks of heart disease, engaging in exercise and healthy nutritional habits can postpone potential illness. If an individual who is predisposed to illness has routine screenings, then these tests oftentimes can detect signs of pathology earlier in the course of disease and allow more immediate interventions. Early treatment often limits the damage caused by pathology. A wellness perspective invites the health professional to provide interventions across the spectrum of health and wellness, offering healthy individuals the awareness and knowledge to develop appropriate lifestyle behaviors. Even when an individual presents with signs and symptoms of pathology, education of secondary complications prevents further signs and symptoms leading to disability.

In 1977, Donald B. Ardell introduced a new model of wellness that placed self-responsibility at the center his wellness paradigm (Figure 1-2).[18] *Self-responsibility* was surrounded by nutritional awareness, environmental sensitivity, stress management, and physical fitness components of wellness. According to Ardell, "Wellness is first and foremost a choice to assume responsibility for the quality of your life. It begins with a conscious decision to shape a healthy lifestyle. Wellness is a mind-set, a predisposition to adopt a series of key principles in varied life areas that lead to high levels of well-being and life satisfaction."[18] Self-responsibility in assuming wellness behaviors is recognized as one, if not the most, significant factor determining health status.[18] This model emphasizing self-responsibility suggests that health professionals need to provide educational programs that not only promote health and wellness, but also relationship skills and the importance of nurturing one's well-being.

Ardell's model was revised in 1986 to incorporate additional dimensions of wellness. Today, the model includes self-responsibility (featured in the center), nutritional awareness, physical fitness, meaning/purpose, relationship dynamics, and emotional intelligence (Figure 1-3).[18] This newer model acknowledges the personal values that motivate individuals: meaning/purpose and interpersonal relationships.

In his most recent model, Ardell further developed the domains of wellness to include the *Physical Domain*, the *Mental Domain*, and the *Meaning and Purpose Domain* with 14 skill areas across these three domains (Figure 1-4).[18] Exercise, nutrition, appearance, adaptation and challenges, and lifestyle habits are included in the Physical Domain. Emotional intelligence, effective decisions, stress management, factual knowledge, and mental health are listed in the Mental Domain. Finally, meaning/purpose, relationships, humor, and play are incorporated in the domain designated as the Meaning and Purpose Domain. This model still emphasizes the role of

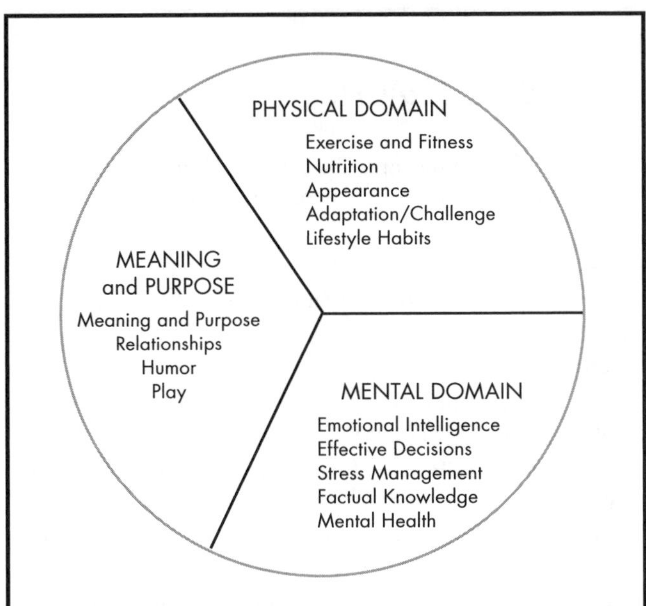

Figure 1-4. Ardell's Model in Three Domains. (Adapted from Ardell D. *14 Days to Wellness: The Easy, Effective, and Fun Way to Optimum Health.* New York, NY: New World Library; 1999.)

self-responsibility in controlling personal health and wellness. It also expands all three domains with specific skill areas that can be incorporated into prevention practice. While health care professionals might focus on the physical domain (particularly addressing exercise, nutrition, knowledge of potential impairments, functional limitations, and lifestyle behaviors influencing health), effective strategies to manage stress, receive social support, and achieve personal goals are also key components of intervention. This model suggests that humor, play, mentally challenging activities, and physically challenging activities should be incorporated into comprehensive wellness programs.

Quality of Life

Quality of life is defined in various ways, ranging from the ability to lead a normal life to the fulfillment of personal goals and self-actualization. According to the World Health Organization, quality of life is "the individuals' perceptions of their positions in life, in the context of the cultural and value systems in which they live, and in relation to their goals, expectations, standards, and concerns."[19] Quality-of-life measures emphasize health "profiles," as described by one assessment called the SF-36.[20] The SF-36 assesses eight health concepts:

1. Limitations in physical activities because of health problems
2. Limitations in social activities because of physical or emotional problems
3. Limitations in usual role activities because of physical health problems
4. Bodily pain
5. General mental health (psychological distress and well-being)
6. Limitations in usual role activities because of emotional problems
7. Vitality (energy and fatigue)
8. General health perceptions

Other measures focus on health indices that determine the *quality adjusted life years (QALY)* or a year of life adjusted for its "quality" or its "value." A year in perfect health is considered equal to 1.0 QALY. For this measure, the QALY would be discounted by each year in ill health. For example, a year during which the individual was bedridden for 6 months might have a value equal to 0.5 QALY.[21] While considering objective quality-of-life measures, the health care professional must keep in mind that multiple personal, social, and environmental factors can affect an individual's quality of life.

Holistic Health

The philosophy of holistic health care is compatible with medicine designed to restore health and wellness. The health care provider's comprehensive role in health care requires a holistic perspective of the individual seeking care. This holistic perspective looks beyond the physical functioning of the individual and recognizes the importance of multiple factors contributing to good health and optimal wellness, emphasizing the unity of mind, spirit, and body. According to the American Holistic Health Association, this expanded perspective of holistic health care considers *the whole person and the whole situation*.[22] While there are many definitions of holistic health care, the characteristics of holistic medicine that apply to a wellness practice incorporate recognizing the interdependent parts of the whole being, including the physical, mental, emotional, and spiritual aspects of the individual. This recognition of the multiple factors influencing health and wellness leads to the following[22]:

- Identifying and managing the root causes of disease processes
- Empowering the individual to manage these pathological processes
- Providing a comprehensive perspective of the individual in multiple social roles

TABLE 1-3

PRINCIPLES OF HOLISTIC MEDICAL PRACTICE

1. The goal of holistic medical practice is achieving *optimal health* for each client. Optimal health involves both a *conscious awareness* of wellness domains (social, spiritual, mental, emotional, physical, and environmental) and achieving balance in these domains.
2. Practitioners offer "holistic care," ie, care to the *entire person* (mind, body, and spirit).
3. Holistic medicine is person-centered, treating the *individual* with pathology rather than focusing on the pathology itself.
4. Practitioners help clients *take control* of their health and use their innate abilities to heal.
5. Holistic medicine involves health promotion, preventive care, and education designed to increase awareness of factors contributing to illness while emphasizing *options that optimize well-being.*
6. Holistic medicine incorporates a *variety of healing systems,* including lifestyle changes, conventional medicine (drugs and surgery), and alternative and complementary medicine, to meet each individual's unique needs.
7. The relationship of the practitioner and client focuses on the client's *autonomy and needs,* while *valuing the insights* of both parties.
8. Using *love, kindness, acceptance, grace, humor, enthusiasm, and hope,* practitioners help clients optimize their lives while managing any illness.
9. Practitioners serve as role *models of optimal care* by incorporating the principles of holistic medicine into the healing relationship shared with their clients.
10. Life experiences (birth, suffering, and dying) are viewed as *profound learning experiences* for both the client and the practitioner of holistic medicine. The quality of life is emphasized as a key component of healing.

Adapted from:
American Holistic Medicine Association. Principles of holistic medical practice. Available at: http://www.holisticmedicine.org/about/about_principles.shtml. Accessed December 16, 2006.
American Board of Holistic Medicine. Available at: http://www.holisticboard.org/aboutus.html. Accessed December 16, 2006.

According to the holistic perspective, disease or illness manifests when the individual's state of being ("the balanced state of mind, body, and spirit") is not in equilibrium.[22] Holistic health recognizes the multiple dimensions of wellness and the importance of balancing these dimensions for optimal health (Table 1-3).

Health care professionals can choose to use a more holistic approach to client management as compared to a more traditional approach; however, evidence-based practice is essential. Additional research is needed in the areas of alternative medicine to determine whether less traditional approaches are cost-effective and are the most appropriate. The holistic approach tends to be more health-oriented and teaches the patient to be responsible for one's own health. Table 1-4 illustrates the differences between traditional or conventional medicine and holistic medicine as well as strengths and weaknesses of the two approaches.[22]

Prevention Practice

Prevention practice encompasses health care designed to promote health, fitness, and wellness through education and appropriate guidance designed to prevent or delay the progression of pathology. Preventive care not only focuses on the promotion of general health in susceptible or potentially susceptible populations, but also aims to minimize the impairments and functional limitations arising from pathological conditions potentially affecting an individual's quality of life.

According to the *Guide to Physical Therapist Practice,*[23] health care professionals are involved in three types of preventive practice: primary prevention, secondary prevention, and tertiary prevention[23]:

- "*Primary prevention* is preventing a target condition in a susceptible or potentially susceptible population through specific measures, such as general health promotion efforts.
- *Secondary prevention* is decreasing the duration of illness, severity of disease, and number of sequelae (abnormalities following or resulting from disease, injury, or treatment) through early diagnosis and prompt intervention.
- *Tertiary prevention* involves limiting the degree of disability and promoting rehabilitation and restoration of function in patients with chronic or reversible disease."

TABLE 1-4

COMPARING HOLISTIC MEDICINE AND CONVENTIONAL MEDICINE

	Holistic Medicine	Conventional Medicine
Philosophy	Based on allopathic (MD), osteopathic (DO), naturopathic (ND), energy, and ethno-medicine.	Based on allopathic medicine.
Primary objective of care	To promote optimal health. To prevent and treat disease.	To cure or reduce pathology.
Diagnosis	Medical history, physical exam, laboratory data, holistic health care sheet.	Medical history, physical exam, laboratory data.
Primary method of care	Empower patients to heal themselves through health promotion and lifestyle changes.	Eliminate signs and symptoms.
Primary care treatment options	Diet, exercise, environmental measures, attitudinal, and behavioral modifications; relationship and spiritual counseling.	Medications and surgery.
Secondary care treatment options	Botanical (herbal) medicine, homeopathy, acupuncture, manual medicine, biomolecular therapies, physical therapy, medications, and surgery.	Diet, exercise, physical therapy, and stress management.
Weaknesses	Shortage of holistic physicians and training programs; time-intensive, requiring a commitment to a healing process, not a quick-fix.	Ineffective in preventing and curing chronic disease; expensive.
Strengths	Teaches patients to take responsibility for their own health, and in so doing, is cost-effective in treating both acute and chronic illness, therapeutic in preventing and treating chronic disease, and essential in creating optimal health.	Highly therapeutic in treating both acute and life-threatening illness and injuries.

Adapted from Ivker RS. Comparing holistic and conventional medicine. *Holistic Medicine: The Journal of the American Holistic Medical Association.* Winter 1999.

Examples of preventive care performed by physical therapists include screening for potential health problems and providing education or activities to promote health, fitness, and wellness. Screening activities may include identification of children with possible developmental delays, detection of ergonomic risk factors in the workplace, and recognition of factors putting older adults at risk for falls. Examples of prevention activities designed to promote general health include prepartum and postpartum exercise classes to improve women's health, exercise classes for well elders to enhance balance and flexibility, and cardiovascular conditioning activities for individuals who are at risk for obesity.

Preventive care also includes instruction to minimize or eliminate injurious forces throughout daily life. This instruction includes recommendations to optimize conditions for performance, whether the performance is related to simple activities of daily living, work activities, leisure activities, or activities related to competitive sports. With nearly 75% of the population experiencing back pain at one point in their lives and a prevalence of 15% to 30% in adults,[6,7] programs to prevent back problems through proper exercise and body mechanics are essential. Finally, individuals with chronic or progressive pathology can benefit from programs that reduce the intensity, duration, and frequency of complications arising from their conditions while improving their health and wellness. Customized exercises for individuals with musculoskeletal, neurological, cardiopulmonary, and integumentary pathologies may forestall secondary complications arising from their conditions as well as improve their overall health.

Risk Reduction

Identification of populations at risk for developing physical and mental health problems help curtail the number of people whose quality of life is diminished by preventable pathology. While many pathological conditions are genetic, some conditions are preventable. Knowing the populations at risk for a particular disease allows health care providers to target health promotion education and screening programs to populations at the greatest risk for illness. Healthy People 2010, described in Chapter 2, provides more information about specific populations at the greatest risk for particular types of pathology.

One key to achieving wellness is developing an awareness of how to achieve a balance among the various dimensions affecting health and well-being. Populations that are susceptible to illness or injury are in particular need of this awareness, accomplished through appropriate education and guidance. Risk factors that may predispose an individual to diminished well-being and health problems include physical risk factors: poor nutrition, physical inactivity, a poor physical environment, and substance abuse; psychological, spiritual, and social risk factors: low self-esteem and lacking values and a direction in one's life plan; and environmental risk factors: persons, things, or conditions that negatively influence other dimensions. By identifying and addressing these risk factors, the health professional can reduce the incidence of injury and illness.

The Physical Therapist's Role in Promoting Health and Wellness

Physical therapists are beginning to play major roles as prevention practitioners in health care. While physical therapists have traditionally been involved in the management of physical impairments and functional limitations associated with an individual's medical problems, their current role encompasses identifying risk factors and developing health promotion strategies that significantly affect health, fitness, and wellness. Physical therapists are uniquely prepared to apply their extensive knowledge for improving or adapting movements and motor tasks for more independent function. In addition, physical therapists are experts in examining and evaluating the motor capabilities, goals, and functional limitations of individuals with musculoskeletal, neurological, cardiopulmonary, integumentary, and other body system impairments. Knowledge that spans the spectrum of optimizing health and managing illness enables therapists to design customized exercises that enhance motor control, improve overall fitness, and address potential medical complications that may arise in populations at risk.

A key element of health care management is directing clients' energies toward improving capabilities for functional independence, maintaining optimal health, and fulfilling important roles in their lives. The physical therapist determines an individual's functional capabilities by examining the requisite motor skills and behaviors needed to perform tasks relevant to that individual's role in society. In one case, a physical therapist may help an elite athlete prepare for an Olympic event, ensuring that the training schedule for the athlete promotes optimal performance and prevents injury. In another case, the physical therapist may evaluate an older patient's requisite abilities for resuming multiple roles in the home, in social circles, and in the community. Function, in this respect, comprises not only the physical capabilities of the individual but also includes the psychosocial environment and well-being of the individual. Social support can contribute significantly to individual well-being. This well-being, in turn, leads to the individual's ability to develop a personal sense of meaningful living.

According to the *Guide to Physical Therapist Practice*, physical therapists "restore, maintain, and promote not only optimal physical function, but optimal wellness and fitness and optimal quality of life as it relates to movement and health."[23] The practice of physical therapy encompasses the full spectrum of health and wellness that includes preventing disease and illness as well as optimizing health. Physical therapists play a key role in providing education, guidance, consultation, and direct interventions to enable individuals to maintain physical activity for self-care, mobility, leisure skills, work, and play. According to recent statistics from the National Center for Chronic Disease Prevention and Health Promotion, nearly 6% of Americans spend 14 or more days limited in their activity.[29] This loss of functional abilities can limit an individual's independent functioning and may place a burden on others who must either care for the individual or assume the other person's roles.

Summary

Prevention practice is the holistic practice of medicine that encompasses care of the individual in the context of that person's home, work, and community. The impact of prevention practice influences not only the individual but also influences society. As members of the health-care team, physical therapists play a key role in identifying risk factors for poor health and promoting wellness through various strategies, including screening, health education to encourage self-responsibility and awareness of risk factors, and promoting healthy lifestyle behaviors. The following chapters discuss how physical therapists can identify individuals at risk and how to promote health, fitness, and wellness through a variety of evidence-based strategies.

References

1. Merriam-Webster Dictionary Online. Available at: http://www.m-w.com. Accessed December 10, 2004.
2. Wurzbach M. *Community Health Education and Promotion: A Guide to Program Design and Evaluation.* 2nd ed. Boston, Mass: Jones and Barlett; 2004.
3. Banks R. Health and the spiritual dimension: relationships and implications for professional preparation programs. *J School Health.* 1980;50(4):195–202.
4. Optimal Health Institute. What is optimal health? Available at: http://www.optimal-health.net/definition.htm. Accessed January 30, 2006.
5. Nutbeam D. Health literacy as a public health goal: a challenge for contemporary health education and communication strategies into the 21st century. *Health Promotion International.* 2000;15(3):259–267.
6. Abenhaim L, Suisa S, Rossignol M. Risk of recurrence of occupational back pain over three year follow up. *Brit J Ind Med.* 1988;45:829–833.
7. Adams MA, Mannion AF, Dolan P. Personal risk factors for first-time low back pain. *Spine.* 1999;23:2497–2505.
8. Centers for Disease Control and Prevention. Health-related quality of life. Available at: http://apps.nccd.cdc.gov/HRQOL. Accessed October 10, 2005.
9. National Center for Chronic Disease Prevention and Health Promotion. Chronic disease overview. Available at: www.cdc.gov/nccdphp. Accessed December 10, 2004.
10. National Wellness Institute. Defining wellness. Available at: http://www.nationalwellness.org/indexphp?id=3908&id_tier=81. Accessed October 15, 2005.
11. Dacher E. A systems theory approach to an expanded medical mode: a change for biomedicine. *Alternative Therapies in Health and Medicine.* 1996;1:2.
12. Corbin C, Corbin W, Lindsey R, Welk G. *Concepts of Fitness.* 11th ed. New York, NY: McGraw-Hill; 2003.
13. Clinebell H. *Anchoring Your Well-being: Christian Wholeness in a Fractured World.* Nashville, Tenn: McMillan Publishing Co; 1997.
14. Quotation Page. Quotation #31761 from Classic Quotes: Kahil Gibran. Available at: http://www.quotationspage.com/quote/31761.html. Accessed January 30, 2006.
15. Travis J, Ryan R. *Wellness Workbook: How to Achieve Enduring Health and Vitality.* 3rd ed. Berkley, Calif: Ten Speed Press; 2003.
16. Wikipedia. World Health Organization. Available at: n.wikipedia.org/wiki/World_Health_Organization. Accessed December 10, 2004.
17. Social Security Administration. What we mean by disability. Available at: http://www.ssa.gov/dibplan/dqualify4.htm. Accessed December 10, 2004.
18. Ardell D. *14 Days to Wellness: The Easy, Effective, and Fun Way to Optimum Health.* New York, NY: New World Library; 1999.
19. Scottish Executive Publications. Quality of life and well-being: measuring the benefits of culture and sport: literature review and thinkpiece. Examples of quality of life definitions. Available at: http://www.scotland.gov.uk/Publications/2006/01/13110743/11. Accessed February 6, 2006.
20. Brazier JE, Harper R, Jones NM, O'Cathain A, Thomas KJ, Usherwood T, Westlake L. Validating the SF-36 health survey questionnaire: new outcome measure for primary care. *BMJ.* 1992;305(6846):160–164.
21. Measuring Healthy Days: Population assessment of health-related quality of life. CDC. November 2000. Available at: http://www.cdc.gov/hrqol/activitylimit.htm. Accessed December 10, 2004.
22. American Holistic Medical Association. The principles of holistic medical practice. Available at: http://www.holisticmedicine.org/about/about_principles.shtml. Accessed December 10, 2004.
23. American Physical Therapy Association. *Guide to Physical Therapist Practice.* 2nd ed. Alexandria, Va: American Physical Therapy Association; 2003.

Chapter 2

HEALTHY PEOPLE 2010

Catherine Rush Thompson, PhD, MS, PT

"The greatest wealth is health."

~VIRGIL

Healthy People 2010 is a federal health promotion and disease prevention agenda developed to promote healthy lifestyles for Americans.[1] The developers of this government initiative include the Healthy People Consortium, an alliance of more than 350 national organizations; 250 public health, mental health, substance abuse and environmental agencies; and teams of experts from a variety of Federal agencies under the direction of Health and Human Services and working in conjunction with the Office of Disease Prevention and Health Promotion. The Healthy People 2010 document was developed through a broad consultation process including focus groups and representatives from varied populations, built on a foundation of scientific evidence, and designed to measure progress over time.[1]

According to its developers, the purpose of Healthy People 2010 was promoting health and preventing illness, disability, and premature death. "Healthy People 2010 was designed to achieve two overarching goals: (1) to increase the quality and years of healthy life and (2) to eliminate health disparities among various populations."[1] The importance of a national health promotion initiative such as Healthy People 2010 cannot be overstated. While individual lifestyle behaviors contribute significantly to overall health, various settings, including the home setting, the work environment, and community settings (leisure, commerce, religious, government, etc) can play key roles in health. Each setting poses various risks and opportunities for health promotion. For example, it is well known that second-hand smoke is associated with significant morbidity and mortality; communities have enacted laws to restrict exposure to second-hand smoke in public places in order to limit exposure to smoke toxins and to prevent illness.

Factors other than environmental risks play key roles in the development of pathology leading to shortened life spans. Socioeconomic status is a significant factor affecting mortality rates.[2] In one study, the highest mortality rate (adjusted for age and gender) was among poor individuals living in disadvantaged neighborhoods. When comparing populations in neighborhoods with varying socioeconomic variables, researchers found that mortality rates related to cardiovascular pathology and other disease processes decreased with increasing neighborhood socioeconomic advantage and family income in all race-gender groups.[2]

While both environmental and socioeconomic factors affect an individual's health, so do collective attitudes, beliefs, and perceptions related to health, fitness, and wellness. In one study examining factors influencing health behaviors in a rural community, researchers found that low reimbursement, poor community attitudes, personnel shortages, low educational levels, weak local economies, and large older populations were often barriers to health promotion and disease prevention services.[3] Researchers determined that the implementation of an effective health initiative requires a collaborative effort beyond the local community and health care providers. Organizations within and beyond communities trying to develop health initiatives are essential to expand and leverage facilities, acquire needed equipment, establish legitimacy, secure adequate funding, develop interpersonal connections, and expand resources. Health care providers must collaborate with philanthropists and grant writers to secure funding for health promotion activities. Political advocacy is also essential for establishing adequate national funding to support the Healthy People 2010 initiative.[4] Implementing the needed programs for a healthy nation requires effective leadership, communication, interpersonal relations, and trust building. A collective effort to promote national health should provide a positive impact on all Americans seeking a healthier lifestyle.

The vision of *Healthy People in Healthy Communities*[5] is a community-oriented planning guide based on Healthy People 2010 with the purpose of encouraging individuals to participate in achieving the overarching goals of the national initiative. This user-friendly resource was designed for individuals "regardless of age, gender, education level, income, race, ethnicity, cultural customs, language, religious beliefs, disability, sexual orientation, geographic location, or occupation to determine how to participate most effectively in improving the Nation's health." While some individuals may be more capable of affecting health care policy for communities, others may implement health care screening programs or provide health promotion activities for a specific population. As physical therapists, it is important to work in concert with others in achieving Healthy People 2010 goals. Helpful resources, such as *Healthy People in Healthy Communities*, can guide community efforts to improve national health.

Physical therapy educators have unique opportunities for offering health education in their local communities. One example of how college students can affect community health is through service learning, such as promoting healthy lifestyle behaviors and providing educational materials about healthy choices. According to one researcher, "The values, methods, and intended results of service learning are closely related to effective health promotion and disease prevention. Service learning focuses on personal and civic responsibility, thus providing students with opportunities for enhancing individual and community health. Service learning also espouses social justice and provides a vehicle for students to learn about, reflect on, and address health disparities."[6]

Healthy People 2010 provides a useful framework for improving the health of individuals, the health of communities, and the health of the nation. This health initiative in conjunction with *Healthy People in Healthy Communities*, focuses on the overriding goals of increasing the quality and years of healthy life and eliminating health disparities among various populations. These comprehensive resources can guide the development of needed health and wellness programs for underserved populations and populations at risk for injury and illness.

Goal 1: Increase Quality and Years of Healthy Life

One primary goal of Healthy People 2010 is to increase the life expectancy and improve the quality of life of all individuals. The average life expectancy at birth is currently 77 years, while it was only 47 years at the beginning of the twentieth century.[7] Life expectancy has increased for every age group over the past 100 years; however, life expectancy varies with gender (women outlive men by 6 years), race (African-American males live longer than Caucasian males), and income (those who earn less than $10,000 have diminished life expectancy compared to those who earn at least $25,000 per year).[7]

While the increased years of an individual's life may reflect improved health, increasing each person's quality of life is equally important. *Quality of life*, as described in Chapter 1, is the sense of satisfaction and happiness with one's life and environment, a broader view of health or well-being. Overall quality of life reflects health and well-being that encompasses work and leisure activities, cultural values and beliefs, rights, and aspirations. More specifically, *health-related quality of life* "reflects a personal sense of physical and mental health and the ability to react to factors in the physical and social environments."[8] Health-related quality of life is based upon one's overall perceived health and is generally rated as "poor," "fair," "good," "very good," or "excellent."[8] While this rating is subjective and individualized, it offers some measure of the multiple factors contributing to personal health. In 1996, 90% of people in the United States reported their health as "good," "very good," or "excellent." Another measure of health-related quality of life is the number of days that a person regards as "healthy."[8] *Older adults* tend to experience more *physically unhealthy* days while *younger adults* generally report more *mentally unhealthy days*.[8]

The Healthy People progress report states as follows:[1]

People in the lowest income households are five times more likely to report their health as "fair" or "poor" than people in the highest income households. A higher percentage of women report their health as "fair" or "poor" compared to men. Adults in rural areas are 36% more likely to report their health status as "fair" or "poor" than are adults in urban areas.

Not only is it important to increase the quality and years of healthy life, but it is important to identify and remedy factors that cause health disparities among various populations.

Goal 2: Eliminate Health Disparities Among Various Populations

Gender, race or ethnicity, education or income, disability, geographic location, and sexual orientation have all been factors contributing to health disparities. The second goal of Healthy People 2010 is designed to recognize these disparities and eliminate barriers to good health.

Gender differences are responsible for obvious disparities in health, such as the incidence of cervical and prostate cancer. Other differences are less obvious. Men tend to have a shorter life expectancy than women as well as higher death rates for leading causes of death. Women, on the other hand, have a greater prevalence of depression, mood disorders, anxiety, and *somatoform disorders* (physical symptoms that appear as medical condition, however are lacking any measurable pathology), while men are more likely to have substance use disorders.[9]

More recent research has focused on health disparities among Caucasians, African Americans, Hispanics, American Indians, Alaska Natives, Asians, Native Hawaiians, and Pacific Islanders.[1] While biological and sociological factors contribute to these disparities, most disparities are caused by multi-factorial interactions involving genetic variation, environmental factors, and lifestyle behaviors. National statistics collected as part of Healthy People 2010 show the following[1]:

Heart disease death rates are more than 40% higher for African-Americans than for Caucasians. The death rate for all cancers is 30% higher for African-Americans than for Caucasians; for prostate cancer, the death rate is more than double that for whites. African-American women have a higher death rate from breast cancer despite having a mammography screening rate that is nearly the same as the rate for white women. The death rate from human immunodeficiency virus (HIV)/acquired immunodeficiency syndrome (AIDS) for African-Americans is more than seven times that for whites; the rate of homicide is six times that for whites. Even though the Nation's infant mortality rate is down, the infant death rate among African-Americans is still more than double that of whites.

One study points out specific factors believed to contribute to the health disparities of African-Americans and other Americans. These contributing factors include (1) excessive cardiovascular risk factors such as high blood pressure, diabetes, obesity, physical inactivity, and psychosocial stress; (2) unfamiliarity with information linking personal risk factors to atherosclerosis and heart disease; (3) cultural factors impacting an individual's desire to seek health care; (4) economic factors limiting health care access; (5) psychosocial stress, racism, and frustration dealing with health care providers; and (6) genetic predisposition to these pathologies.[10]

The population of Hispanics is increasing in the United States, and this group is suffering from health disparities. According to national health statistics, Hispanics are at an increased risk of dying from diabetes, developing high blood pressure, and becoming obese.[1] The rate of diabetes in American Indians and Alaska Natives is twice that for Caucasians. The Pima of Arizona have one of the highest rates of diabetes in the world. American Indians and Alaska Natives also have disproportionately high death rates from unintentional injuries and suicide, according to recent statistics collected as part of Healthy People 2010.

While Asians and Pacific Islanders generally have good health, Vietnamese women have a five-fold increase in cervical cancer compared to Caucasian women. Also, Asians and Pacific Islanders living in the United States are at an increased risk of developing hepatitis and tuberculosis.[1]

Strategies to address health disparities for minorities include health promotion education, risk factor modification, culturally competent health care delivery, and continued research on factors contributing to racial and ethnic variances in disease and injury.[1]

Income and education often go hand in hand because they relate to access to health care information, activities, and programming. Those with the greatest health disparities, regardless of gender or ethnicity, have the highest poverty rates and the least education. Individuals with low incomes and low levels of education are at increased risk for heart disease, diabetes, obesity, elevated blood lead level, and low birth weight. While wealthier populations make gains in their health, those groups with lower socioeconomic status have increasing disparities in their health.[1]

Recent studies examining factors linked to mortality found that childhood conditions, including lower socioeconomic status, family living arrangements, mother's work status, rural residence, and parents' nativity, played key roles in causing earlier mortality.[11,12,13] These findings suggest that economic and educational policies that are targeted at children's well-being are health policies with implicit effects that reach far into the adult life course. As health care providers, physical therapists must acknowledge their roles in promoting health education, particularly to disadvantaged children.

Education is a key factor in health care. According to data collected for Healthy People 2010, the overall death rate for those with less than 12 years of education is more than twice that for people with 13 or more years of education. The infant mortality rate is almost double for infants of mothers with less than 12 years of education compared with those with an educational level of 13 or more years. Both these statistics suggest that health promotion and usable health education needs to be provided early and targeted to those with limited education in order to substantially impact lifestyle behaviors.[1]

People with disabilities have health disparities related to their levels of physical activity. In addition, individuals with chronic illness or injury generally have higher levels of obesity, possibly due to their having activity limitations or their needing assistance to access health care services and facilities.[14] Research has shown that people with disabilities generally report more anxiety, pain, sleeplessness, and days of depression, leading to diminished quality of life.[14] Our role as health care providers includes advocating for health care access and facilities enabling those with disabilities to engage in meaningful physical activity and to maintain both a physically and mentally healthy lifestyle.

Unfortunately, individuals living in rural areas have even greater risks for injuries, heart disease, cancer, and diabetes.[14] To further complicate this problem, fewer preventive care services and emergency care facilities are available to those living in isolated rural areas. New technology that can reach out to rural communities needs to be employed to improve access to services and to enhance education for preventive care.

Homosexual and bisexual individuals also experience disparate health problems. Gay men have an increased incidence of sexually transmitted diseases, substance abuse, depression, and suicide, particularly male adolescents.[1] Lesbians reportedly have higher rates of smoking, are more overweight, are more likely to abuse alcohol, and experience more stress than heterosexual women. Furthermore, lesbians and bisexual women evidenced higher behavioral risks and lower rates of preventive care than heterosexual women.[15] Family and social acceptance of sexual orientation affect the individual's mental health and could help reduce this health disparity.

The role of health care providers encompasses the provision of preventive practices to ensure optimal health for all populations. The Healthy People 2010 initiative provides a framework for addressing these issues by identifying populations at risk for poor health and health disparities. These challenges must be addressed in each community to improve the health of our nation. A multidisciplinary approach that incorporates strategies to address barriers to each population at risk is needed to achieve health equity. Not only must health care providers provide education, resources, and access to health care, but they must also empower individuals to make their own informed decisions for embracing a healthy lifestyle.

Objectives to Improve Health

Healthy People 2010 contains 467 objectives to improve health, organized into 28 focus areas.[1] These 28 focus areas include the following: access to quality health services; arthritis; osteoporosis; chronic back conditions; cancer; chronic kidney disease; diabetes; disability and secondary conditions; educational and community-based programs; environmental health; family planning; food safety; health communication; heart disease and stroke; HIV; immunization and infectious diseases; injury and violence prevention; maternal, infant, and child health; medical product safety; mental health and mental disorders; nutrition and overweight; occupational safety and health; oral health; physical activity and fitness; public health infrastructure; respiratory diseases; sexually transmitted diseases; substance abuse; tobacco use; and vision and hearing.

Physical therapists are uniquely qualified to address specific focuses outlined by Healthy People 2010, particularly those related to physical activity and fitness. With the opportunities to directly provide therapy services through direct access, physical therapists provide a new avenue for accessibility to health care. During initial screening of patients or health screenings for populations at risk, physical therapists are capable of screening body systems for potential disease and risks for injury. Familiarity with pathologies and risks for disease enable physical therapists to screen for risk factors associated with pathology as well as signs and symptoms of arthritis, osteoporosis, chronic back conditions, cancer, chronic kidney disease, diabetes, heart disease, stroke, respiratory diseases, obesity, signs and symptoms of HIV, mental health problems, and sensory losses including hearing and visual impairments. The prevalence of these pathologies could be reduced with appropriate health and wellness screenings, referrals, and health education to reduce risk factors contributing to illness.

The role of physical therapists focuses on enhancing health, fitness, and wellness to reduce disability and secondary conditions associated with common pathologies; this role is broadened through providing health screenings for health risks, encouraging individuals to maintain updated immunizations, informing clients of potential work-related injuries and risks of physical inactivity, educating clients about healthy lifestyle behaviors exclusive of tobacco use, abuse of drugs and alcohol, good nutrition, and avoiding other potential health hazards.

The national goals for Healthy People 2010 provide guidelines for affecting the leading health indicators and promoting a healthier nation.[1] While the overarching goals are to increase the quality and years of healthy life and to eliminate health disparities among various populations, more measurable outcomes have been developed to focus on national health concerns and means to address these two primary goals. The national goals for Healthy People 2010 directly related to physical therapy practice include the following:

1. Increase the quality and years of healthy life
2. Increase incidence of people reporting "healthy days"
3. Increase incidence of people reporting "active days"
4. Reduce activity limitations, especially for older adults
5. Reduce days of pain for those with arthritis, osteoporosis, and chronic back pain
6. Increase the adoption and maintenance of daily physical activity
7. Increase leisure time physical activity
8. Increase proportion of people who regularly perform exercises for flexibility and muscle fitness
9. Reduce the incidence of and deaths from cancer
10. Increase the diagnosis of and reduce the incidence of type 2 diabetes
11. Decrease the incidence of depression
12. Decrease the incidence of heart diseases including stroke and high blood pressure
13. Decrease the incidence of high cholesterol levels among adults
14. Eliminate health disparities
15. Decrease personal stress levels and mental health problems
16. Reduce steroid use, especially among youth
17. Reduce accidents, destructive habits, and environmental pollution
18. Increase access of health information and services for all people
19. Increase the proportion of all people who eat well (meet dietary guidelines, eat no more than 30% fat calories, eat no more than 10% saturated fat, eat 5 servings of vegetables and fruit daily, eat 6 portions of grain, consume needed calcium and iron, and avoid excess sodium)
20. Increase the prevalence of healthy weight, and reduce prevalence of overweight

Health care providers need to be aware of all the goals contributing to national health. Physical therapists can play a key role in addressing all of these goals but not in isolation. Working in collaboration with other health care providers ensures a more comprehensive and collaborative approach to good health. The ultimate outcome of these collaborative efforts is tracked by the Centers for Disease Control and Prevention and those involved with Healthy People 2010. The efficacy of health promotion and injury prevention activities is monitored by federal agencies involved in tracking health-related statistics, such as disparities in access to health care and individual differences that influence health, fitness, and wellness. Certain factors are identified as key variables for monitoring health and serve as "leading health indicators" of the nation's health status.[1]

Leading Health Indicators

Health indicators are factors that provide information about the health and well-being of a population.[1] The national health indicators are used to help public policy makers and health professionals measure the general health and wellness of the United States. These indicators are not used individually, but rather as an overview of key national health concerns that need attention. The top ten leading health indicators of our nation are addressed by at least one objective from Healthy People 2010 and are monitored regularly to determine the effectiveness of health and wellness programs established to improve national health. The 10 leading health indicators follow:

- Physical activity
- Overweight and obesity
- Tobacco use
- Substance abuse
- Responsible sexual behavior

- Mental health
- Injury and violence
- Environmental quality
- Immunization
- Access to health care

Physical activity is the health indicator that is most appropriately addressed by physical therapists. With backgrounds in anatomy, physiology, pathophysiology, exercise physiology, kinesiology, biomechanics, and related sciences, physical therapists can design optimal exercise programs for both healthy and ill clients. A recent Surgeon General's report on physical activity and health concluded that moderate physical activity can substantially reduce the risk of developing or dying from heart disease, diabetes, colon cancer, and high blood pressure.[14]

According to Healthy People 2010, *physical activity* is "bodily movement that is produced by the contraction of skeletal muscle and that substantially increases energy expenditure."[1] *Moderate physical activity* includes "activities that use large muscle groups,"[1] such as walking, swimming, housework, bicycling, and occupational activities. *Vigorous physical activity* refers to "rhythmic, repetitive physical activities that use large muscle groups at 70% or more of maximum heart rate for age."[1] An exercise heart rate of 70% of maximum heart rate for age is about 60% of maximal cardiorespiratory capacity and is sufficient for cardiorespiratory conditioning.[1] Maximum heart rate equals roughly 220 beats per minute minus age. Examples of vigorous physical activities include jogging/running, lap swimming, cycling, aerobic dancing, skating, rowing, jumping rope, cross-country skiing, hiking/backpacking, racquet sports, and competitive group sports (eg, soccer and basketball).

Physical activity plays an important role in primary and secondary prevention of conditions such as coronary heart disease (CHD), a leading cause of death and disability in the United States.[1] Risks posed by physical inactivity are almost as high as several well-known CHD risk factors, such as cigarette smoking, high blood pressure, and high blood cholesterol. According to measures by Healthy People 2010, physical inactivity is more prevalent than any one of these other risk factors.[1] The prevalence of overweight people and those with type 2 diabetes has increased over the past few decades.[1] Additionally, physical activity levels generally decline during adolescence. Recent research has shown that physical fitness and physical activity during adolescence can serve as predictors of cardiovascular disease risk in young adulthood. One study concluded that changes in the levels of physical activity and physical fitness between adolescence and young adulthood, especially in aerobic fitness, seemed to be the best predictor of cardiovascular risk factor levels in young adulthood.[16] These findings suggest that physical therapists play an essential role in both the identification of inactive youth and prescription of appropriate aerobic exercises to reduce risks of cardiovascular disease.

People with musculoskeletal problems affecting bones and joints also benefit from physical activity. Individuals with arthritis and osteoporosis significantly benefit from weight-bearing activities that increase bone mineral density, improve aerobic fitness, and increase muscle strength.[17] Bone health benefits from sustained exercise that is properly prescribed to minimize risks of side effects.

The majority of adults in the United States are not involved in vigorous physical activity. According to Healthy People 2010, "only about 23% of adults in the United States report regular, vigorous physical activity that involves large muscle groups in dynamic movement for 20 minutes or longer 3 or more days per week. Only 15% of adults report physical activity for 5 or more days per week for 30 minutes or longer, and another 40% do not participate in any regular physical activity."[1] Physical therapists must address the issues confronting those who remain inactive. Some barriers to activity include limited access to facilities for exercising or safe environments. For example, older adults may have concerns about safety when walking in their neighborhoods, wearing proper attire, and tolerating conditions warranting special attention, such as hot weather and icy conditions. The goal to increase physical activity and fitness is a cooperative effort between public efforts and professional organizations devoted to improving national health. Physical activity programs in recreation centers, worksites, health care settings, and schools can be developed and monitored by physical therapists who are best equipped to customize programs for the needs of special populations.

Disparities in Levels of Physical Activity

Various cultural and ethnic groups experience disparities in their leisure-time physical activity. According to a report of the Surgeon General, women tend to have less leisurely physical activity than men, a difference that is even greater in minority populations, such as African-Americans and Hispanics. This trend is also true for less affluent, less educated, and older populations, putting elderly adults with fixed incomes at increased risk for health problems. Across the nation, these differences in physical activity also vary. Adults living in the northern central and western states engage in more activity than northeasterners and southerners. Most importantly, physical therapists need to focus on individuals with disabilities and health conditions who are less likely to engage in physical activity than those who are able-bodied. When addressing these disparities in physical activity, health promotion efforts should be directed toward reducing these discrepancies and providing resources to address barriers to engagement in an active lifestyle.[14] In a study examining the levels of physical activity and obesity in low-income populations, especially women of African-American and Hispanic heritage, a low fat diet, and moderate/vigorous physical activity program were found to be beneficial. Interestingly, interventions were delivered through Internet and video, encouraging those most at risk to consume 30% or fewer calories from fat and to engage in moderate and vigorous physical activity.[10]

Health Education Resources

Health care providers must provide education that identifies risk factors for poor health in target populations and discuss effective strategies that can positively affect the well-being of both that individual and the community. While it is important to emphasize the importance of self-responsibility in managing lifestyle behaviors and optimizing wellness through healthy habits, employing a team approach to health education and social support can expand access to needed resources for populations at the greatest risk for health disparities. The following topics target common health concerns for at-risk populations:

Parents of Young Children

- Healthy nutrition
- Fitness activities for young children
- Protecting young children from preventable injuries
- Effective discipline for young children
- Protection against childhood illness
- Protection in childhood sports activities
- Proper nutrition for physical activity
- Reducing childhood obesity
- Safety when swimming (including protection against skin cancer)

Children Ages 8 to 12 Years

- Good nutrition
- Fitness activities
- Safety issues for children
- Playing it safe (protection in sports activities)
- Proper nutrition for physical activity
- Getting in shape (managing childhood obesity)
- Safety at the swimming pool/protection against skin cancer
- Ergonomics for children (including wearing backpacks and playing at the computer)

Adolescents

- Good nutrition
- Fitness activities
- Principles of fitness training
- Safety issues for athletes
- Protection against infections
- Proper nutrition for physical activity
- Screening for fitness
- Red flags for depression
- Prevention and management of obesity
- Pregnancy—healthy behaviors for a healthy baby
- Pregnancy—ways to reduce back pain
- Child development for teenage mothers/pregnant teenagers
- Screening for poor posture (including scoliosis).
- Changing your life to engage in healthy lifestyle habits (starting exercise programs and/or quitting smoking or other behaviors putting health at risk)
- Screening for stress
- Stress management
- Ergonomics for the workplace (computer users)
- Ergonomics for the workplace (manual labor)

Young and Middle-Aged Adults

- Good nutrition
- Fitness activities
- Principles of fitness training
- Choosing the right shoes for fitness training
- Proper nutrition for physical activity
- Screening for fitness
- Ergonomics for the workplace (desk jobs/computer users)
- Ergonomics for the workplace (manual labor)
- Red flags for depression
- Prevention and management of obesity
- Pregnancy—ways to reduce back pain
- Child development for new mothers

- Screening for poor posture
- Healthy lifestyle habits (quitting smoking or other behaviors putting health at risk)
- Screening for diabetes
- Screening for heart disease
- Screening for fitness training
- Screening for stress
- Stress management
- Prevention of low back pain
- Medications—benefits and risks of commonly used over-the-counter drugs
- Prevention of skin cancer
- Prevention of osteoporosis

Older Adults

- Reducing the risks of falls
- Good nutrition
- Physical activities for health and wellness
- Principles of fitness training for older adults
- Choosing the right shoes for fitness training
- Proper nutrition for physical activity
- Red flags for depression
- How to maintain healthy bones
- Ergonomics for the computer uses
- Ergonomics for the home
- Screening for stress
- Stress management
- Medications—the more you take the more you need to know.

As advocates for good health and improved quality of life, physical therapists must carefully screen for potential health risks, clearly explain these risks in an understandable manner, and help individuals develop strategies to maintain healthy lifestyle behaviors that reduce the risk of disease and injuries. This book provides resources for identifying health risks, locating reliable health education resources, and developing strategies to promote general health and well-being. In addition, it discusses of physical therapists' roles as advocates for prevention practice and managers of preventive practice businesses.

The Healthy People 2010 website provides valuable information for health education and collaborative prevention practice.[1] Included on this website is a full description of the national health goals with data supporting leading health indicators. In addition, the site provides health education about how to "be a healthy person," listing health education materials; online health checkups; health information by age, gender, race or ethnic origin; and caregiver and family roles. Physical therapists seeking additional support can contact national organizations dedicated to specific health concerns. The Healthy People 2010 website lists health observances days, weeks, or months devoted to promoting particular health concerns as well as select toll-free numbers for organizations that provide health-related information, education, and support. The health education component of this website offers Healthfinder, reliable health information resources that have been carefully selected by the United States Department of Health and Human Services from over 1,700 government agencies and nonprofit organizations. This information includes access to quality health care, disease-specific information, physical activity and exercise information, and the public health infrastructure (including public health professionals, public health statistics, and plans for developing a national public health workforce). Finally, the Healthy People 2010 website offers a road map of how to implement health promotion through partnerships with federal agencies, the Healthy People Consortium, businesses, organizations, and communities. Collaborative efforts among physical therapists, other health care professionals, and community businesses and organizations can provide a more comprehensive and sustainable program to improve community health and wellness.

Summary

Physical therapists can play a key role in meeting the national health goals of Healthy People 2010. In particular, physical therapists are well prepared to identify risk factors for pathology and develop appropriate strategies for healthy interventions to promote good health. While recognizing the importance of self-responsibility in lifestyle behaviors, physical therapists can work collaboratively with others interested in health care to encourage universal access to health care, engagement in physical activity, and reduction in unhealthy habits.

References

1. Office of Disease Prevention and Health Promotion and the US Department of Health and Human Services. Healthy People 2001. Available at: http://www.healthypeople.gov. Accessed October 15, 2005.
2. Borrell LN, Diez Roux AV, Rose K, Catellier D, Clark BL. Neighbourhood characteristics and mortality in the Atherosclerosis Risk in Communities Study. *Intern J Epidemiol.* 2004;33(2):398–407.
3. Chan S, Lam TH. Preventing exposure to second-hand smoke. *Semin Oncol Nurs.* 2003;19(4):284–290.

4. Carter D. Healthy People 2010: A blueprint for the decade ahead. *Body Positive: A Magazine for People Living with HIV.* December 2000.
5. United States Department of Health and Human Services Public Health Service, Office of Public Health and Science, Office of Disease Prevention and Health Promotion. *Healthy People in Healthy Communities: A Guide for Community Leaders.* 1998.
6. Ottenritter NW. Service learning, social justice, and campus health. *J Am Coll Health.* 2004;52(4):189–191.
7. National Center for Health Statistics. Life expectancy. Centers for Disease Control and Prevention. Available at: http://www.cdc.gov/nchs/fastats/lifexpec.htm. Accessed October 15, 2005.
8. Moriarty D, Zack M, Kobau R. The Centers for Disease Control and Prevention's healthy days measures—population tracking of perceived physical and mental health over time. *Health Qual Life Outcomes.* 2003;1(1):37.
9. Klose M, Jacobi F. Can gender differences in the prevalence of mental disorders be explained by sociodemographic factors? *Arch Women's Mental Health.* 2004;7(2):133–148.
10. Ofili E. Ethnic disparities in cardiovascular health. *Ethnic Disparities.* 2001;11(4):838–840.
11. Lynch JW, Kaplan GA, Cohen RD, et al. Childhood and adult socionomic status predictors of mortality in Finland. *Lancet.* 1994;343(8876):524-527.
12. Beebee-Dimmer J, Lynch JW, Turrell G, Lustgarten S. Childhood and adult socioeconomic conditions and 31-year mortality risk in women. *Am J Edidemiol.* 2004;159: 481-490.
13. Galobardes B, Lynch JW, Smith GD. Childhood socioeconomic circumstances and cause-specific mortality in adulthood: systematic review. *Epidemiol Rev.* 2004;26:7-21.
14. United States Department of Health and Human Services. *Physical Activity and Health: A Report of the Surgeon General.* Sudbury, Md: Jones and Bartlett; 1998.
15. Mays VM, Yancey AK, Cochran SD, Weber M, Fielding JE. Heterogeneity of health disparities among African American, Hispanic, and Asian American women: unrecognized influences of sexual orientation. *Am J Public Health.* 2002;92(4):632–639.
16. Hasselstrom H, Hansen SE, Froberg K, Andersen LB. Physical fitness and physical activity during adolescence as predictors of cardiovascular disease risk in young adulthood. Danish youth and sports study. An eight-year follow-up study. *Intern J Sports Med.* 2002;23(Suppl 1): S27–S31.
17. Singh MA. Physical activity and bone health. *Aust Fam Phys.* 2004;33(3):125.

Chapter 3

Key Concepts of Fitness

Catherine Rush Thompson, PhD, MS, PT

"True enjoyment comes from activity of the mind and exercise of the body; the two are united."

~ALEXANDER VON HUMBOLDT

Being Fit

Fitness or the state of being fit is essential to mental and physical health. While mental fitness includes self-acceptance, open-mindedness, self-direction, and calculated risk-taking, physical fitness is reflected in an individual's metabolic fitness (physiological measures at rest) and performance-based fitness (measures of movement and physical skill). Overall, fitness involves commitment, motivation, and responsibility for one's physical and mental well-being. Both mental fitness and physical fitness are integral to maintaining a healthy mind and body.

Mental Health, Fitness, and Wellness

Mental health is far more than the absence of mental illness; it involves an individual's self-perception, a realistic perception of others, and having the ability to meet the demands of daily living. Mental health infers a mental condition characterized by good judgment. According to the *International Index and Dictionary of Rehabilitation and Social Integration*, mental fitness involves habits related to the maintenance, improvement, and recovery of mental health.[1] These habits include mental relaxation, reflection, meditation, intellectual stimulation, and creativity.

Mental fitness is a state of mind involving enjoyment of one's social and physical environment, belief in one's creativity and imagination, and using one's mental abilities to the fullest extent by taking risks, asking questions, accepting alternative points of view, and having an openness to continual growth and change.[1] Mental fitness combined with an optimistic life perspective offers the hope for achieving happiness and sustained health.

Maintaining mental fitness requires paying attention to one's lifestyle by balancing work and leisure, maintaining social contact with those who provide enjoyment, reviewing one's aims and goals in life, and planning to meet those goals. In addition, it is essential to be aware of the mind-body interaction and the need to get adequate diet, sleep, and exercise. Other key factors for maintaining mental fitness include relationships with trusted friends and family members for advice and support when problems arise as well as having an awareness of potential problems that arise from poor health and other risk factors in one's life. Finally, mental fitness relies on problem-solving abilities that incorporate the identification of problems, using personal and other resources judiciously, and taking the needed steps to resolve those problems. When serious problems arise and are handled ineffectively, an individual's mental health is jeopardized by the chronic stress these problems may cause.

Mental fitness allows a person to develop self-appreciation or the ability to assess both personal strengths and weaknesses. At the same time, mental fitness allows the individual to appreciate one's own and other peoples' unique and individual contributions. This appreciation helps to build strong affiliations with others that provide mutually supportive social networks.

Mental wellness, the more "holistic" concept of well-being, includes mental fitness and physical fitness as well as resilience or the ability to "bounce forward" from hardship. Some experts suggest that resilience or the ability to recover quickly from adversity is the overriding characteristic that predicts how well individuals handle both physical and mental challenges.[2] Mentally aware individuals are aware that all the answers to life's challenges are not self-evident and often require assistance from others and reflection on personal experiences. Mental wellness involves handling stressors through appropriate stress management techniques, such as relaxation and exercise. According to the *Mental Health Report of the United States Surgeon General,* protective factors for mental health include interpersonal forgiveness.[3]

While tools are being developed to assess mental fitness and wellness, no standardized tool is currently available. A simple visual analog scale for each of the characteristics of mental fitness (including self-acceptance, open-mindedness, self-direction, and calculated risk-taking) may provide some indication of an individual's personal perspective of mental fitness. The health professional's observations or inquiries of key traits (commitment, motivation, and responsibility for one's physical and mental well-being) could also be included in a subjective evaluation of an individual.

Stress assessments, such as the Holmes and Rahe Social Readjustment Rating Scale,[4] provide valuable information about an individual's life changes and potential stressors that could affect mental fitness. Often patients who are injured or ill, particularly those in the hospital setting, are under significant stress related to their illness, their social isolation, their financial burden of hospitalization, and other significant life changes. Appropriate referrals to resources for social, financial, or psychological support in times of need are important for managing stressors that affect mental fitness.

Physical therapists can play an important role in promoting mental health through exercise and physical activity. Numerous studies clearly support the benefits of exercise and physical activity, including improving mood state and self-esteem.[5,6,7] Acute aerobic exercise for 20 to 40 minutes can elevate mood and anxiety for several hours subsequent to activity. For healthy individuals, exercise is preventive, but for those with mild-to-moderate illness, well-controlled exercise can serve to promote both physical and mental health. The only cases where exercise has proven detrimental involve individuals who exercise excessively, as often observed in females with anorexia.[8] Therefore, the guidance of physical therapists can help prevent any problems arising from inappropriate levels of exercise. Later chapters discuss exercise prescription based on individualized needs.

Physical Fitness

While mental fitness reflects an individual's ability to handle mental stress, *physical fitness* enables an individual to withstand physiological stressors and extreme demands on the body. Individuals with pre-existing levels of physical fitness are less vulnerable to illness and recover from injury and disease more readily than individuals who are *hypokinetic* (physically inactive or sedentary).

Physical fitness is identified by two types of measures: those taken with the body at rest and performance-based measures. Metabolic fitness involves tests of bodily functions at rest, including vital signs and blood tests. Performance-based or motor fitness measures include health-related fitness measures of cardiorespiratory fitness, muscle strength, muscle endurance, flexibility, and posture as well as tests of motor skill, including balance, coordination, reaction time, power, speed, and agility.

Metabolic Fitness

Metabolic fitness reflects the health status of physiological systems at rest, such as blood lipid profiles, blood sugar, resting blood pressure, and insulin levels. While metabolic fitness shows positive responses to moderate physical activity and reduces the risk of chronic diseases, such as diabetes and heart disease, correlations between indicators of metabolic fitness and physical activity are often significant but consistently low.[9] Corresponding correlations with measures of aerobic fitness are also low with the exception of those between fitness and *high density lipoproteins (HDL),* which are more variable. Evidence for a relationship between physical activity and blood glucose and insulin is limited.

Physical inactivity is a major lifestyle risk factor, especially related to the metabolic fitness of muscle. Metabolic fitness of muscle tissue is proposed as

TABLE 3-1
TARGET LOW-DENSITY LIPOPROTEINS LEVELS

The following target LDLs depend upon the following risk factors:

- LDL less than 100 mg/dL (2.59 mmol/L) if you have heart disease or diabetes
- LDL less than 130 mg/dL (3.37 mmol/L) if you have two or more risk factors
- LDL less than 160 mg/dL (4.14 mmol/L) if you have 0 or 1 risk factor.

Courtesy of US Department of Health and Human Services. National cholesterol education program. National Institutes of Health Publication No. 01-3305. 2001

the ratio between mitochondrial capacity for substrate utilization and maximum oxygen uptake of the muscle.[10] Skeletal muscle is an extraordinarily plastic tissue, and metabolic fitness alters rapidly with changing levels of activity. When muscles are fit, they use more fat at rest and during exercise. The capacity for glucose metabolism is also enhanced in trained muscle. Research has shown that a certain regularity of physical activity is required to maintain high metabolic fitness.[10] Metabolic fitness is directly related to how much the muscle is used, with even low levels of physical activity having a beneficial effect on an individual's overall health.

LIPID PROFILE

The *lipid profile,* a common measure of metabolic fitness, involves a series of blood tests including total cholesterol, *HDL-cholesterol* (the "good cholesterol" that can increase with exercise), *LDL-cholesterol* (low density lipoproteins-cholesterol: the damaging cholesterol), and *triglycerides* (another type of fatty material found in the blood). Sometimes the lab report will provide ratio or risk scores based on lipid profile results, age, gender, and other risk factors. These lab values are often used to determine risk for coronary heart disease or stroke. Treatment is based on overall risk of coronary heart disease. Target LDL levels are listed in the Table 3-1.

While their role in heart disease is not entirely clear, it appears that as triglyceride levels raise, levels of HDLs fall. The complex interaction of these three types of lipids is altered when a person has *hypercholesterolemia* (high blood cholesterol). Certain genetic causes of abnormal cholesterol and triglycerides, known as *hereditary hyperlipidemias,* are often very difficult to treat. High cholesterol or triglycerides can also be associated with other diseases a person may have, such as diabetes. In most cases, however, elevated cholesterol levels are associated with an overly fatty diet coupled with an inactive lifestyle. It is also more common in those who are obese. While individual lipid values are important to note, the two most important values are the HDL/cholesterol and triglyceride/HDL ratios.[11,12] Dividing the total cholesterol by the HDL value and multiplying by 100 gives the HDL/cholesterol ratio. The HDL ratio should be above 25 and preferably in the 30s. An HDL ratio above 40 diminishes the risk of heart disease considerably. If, however, the HDL ratio is below 15, a heart attack is likely.[11] The triglyceride ratio should be below 2.0. Individuals with abnormal lipid levels need a referral to their physician for appropriate medical management.

Glucose Tests

The *oral glucose tolerance test* (OGTT or GTT, a test sampling venous blood and used to measure glucose use over time) helps to identify individuals with diabetes or at risk for diabetes. Another glucose test is the fasting plasma glucose test, requiring fasting prior to the blood sampling. The American Diabetes Association (ADA) recommends fasting plasma glucose (FPG) as the screening test of choice "because FPG is easier and faster to perform, more convenient and acceptable to patients, and less expensive."[13] In healthy persons glucose levels rarely rise above 140 mg/dL (7.8 mmol/L) following meals. However, in persons with increasing impairment of glucose tolerance, glucose levels rise following meals. According to Biswas et al, individuals with low fasting glucose (below 126 mg/dL or 7 mmol/L) are considered diabetic.[13] Glucose levels, however, may vary dramatically over time. Up to 40% of individuals with 2-hour plasma glucose values greater than 200 mg/dL experience a significant decline in their fasting glucose levels, dropping to less than 126 mg/dL between meals, the same range as diabetic individuals. For this reason, Fasting Plasma Glucose is an effective means of screening those individuals with glucose levels that uncommonly fluctuate greatly between meals and fall below healthy ranges for normal function.[13] The health care provider should be aware of test differences and their implications for diabetes risk screening.

Blood Insulin

The *blood insulin* or *insulin test* measures blood samples for the amount of circulating insulin, a hormone released from the beta cells of the pancreas and responsible for regulating blood glucose usage by surrounding tissue. This blood test provides information about how effectively the body can utilize glucose as well as synthesize and store triglycerides and proteins. High blood glucose following a meal stimulates the release of insulin, while low blood glucose inhibits insulin release. Normal values are 5 to 20 microunits per milliliter (μU/mL) while fasting. Lower than normal values suggest diabetes mellitus, type 1 or 2, and elevated above normal levels suggest possible diabetes mellitus type 2, obesity (secondary to the insulin resistance syndrome), or other insulin-related disease processes.[13] Obesity decreases the sensitivity of various tissues to insulin, which normally results in the pancreas overcompensating and making excess insulin. A person with potential diabetes or other insulin-related pathologies needs an appropriate medical referral.

Pulse Rate

The pulse rate is the number of throbbing sensations felt over a peripheral artery when the heart beats. This rate normally ranges from 60 to 100 pulses per minute and indirectly assesses the heart's activity as well as the status of blood flow through peripheral arteries. Assessment includes counting the number of pulsations, noting the quality of pulsations, and determining the rhythm of heartbeats. When counting the pulse rate, the examiner places a fingertip over an artery and senses the pulse through gentle pressure over the artery. Regular rhythms or pulse sensations may be counted for 30 seconds and multiplied by 2 for a 1-minute pulse rate. The quality of the pulse is reflected in pulse strength. Numerous factors influence pulse rate, including age, activity preceding measurements, increased temperature, medications, gender, stress, pain, emotions, blood volume, and body build. While age, gender, and body build tend to remain constant for an individual, other factors should be controlled as much as possible to improve reliability of the test. It is important that the tested individual be in a resting position, supine or sitting, for at least 5 minutes for resting pulse rates. Pulse examinations may have interobserver variation. Individuals who lack both *pedal pulses* (pulses measured at the top of the foot above the ankle) have a high risk of peripheral artery disease and should be referred for a thorough cardiovascular examination. Also, a *bruit* (high pitch sound during auscultation of vessels) suggests possible vascular problems, such as an aneurysm, arterio-venous fistula, or stenosis, and indicates the need for referral.

Blood Pressure

Blood pressure involves indirectly measuring the effectiveness of the heartbeat, the adequacy of blood volume, and the presence of any obstruction to vascular flow using a sphygmomanometer and a stethoscope. Pressure measurements include systolic, diastolic, and pulse pressure. Sites for placement of the stethoscope include the brachial artery, the popliteal artery, and the radial artery. "Normal" blood pressure is 120/80 with the top number representing the systolic pressure and the lower number representing the diastolic pressure. *Systolic blood pressure* is the rhythmic contraction of the heart, especially of the ventricles, driving blood through the aorta and pulmonary artery after each *dilation* (relaxation) or *diastole.* Blood pressure varies with age, gender, and body size. It is important to listen for Korotkoff sounds I through V. Korotkoff sounds are five sounds that are heard as the pressure in the syphgmomanometer cuff is released during the measurement of arterial pressure. Korotkoff I is a sharp thud; Korotkoff II is a loud blowing sound; Korotkoff III is a soft thud; Korotkoff IV is a soft blowing sound; and Korotkoff V is silence or the diastole.[14]

Blood pressure can also be obtained by palpation or by *doppler* (an ultrasound method of examining blood vessels). Abnormal blood pressure readings include *hypertension* (high blood pressure) and *hypotension* (low blood pressure). *Orthostatic hypotension* is commonly seen in patients with low blood pressure. Orthostasis means upright posture, and hypotension means low blood pressure.[14] Thus, orthostatic hypotension consists of symptoms of dizziness, faintness, or lightheadedness which appear only on standing and are caused by low blood pressure. Orthostatic hypotension may be caused by anemia, *hypovolemia* (low blood volume), medications, dialysis, neurological problems, or cardiac problems.[14] Altered blood pressure may require a referral for further examination.

HEALTH-RELATED FITNESS

Health-related fitness, also known as *physiological fitness,* is generally associated with a reduced risk of disease. Components of physiological or health-related fitness include cardiorespiratory fitness, muscular strength, muscular endurance, flexibility, and posture. While many view body composition as a component of physical fitness, it may also be considered a component of metabolic fitness as a nonperformance measure of fitness.

Cardiorespiratory Fitness

Cardiorespiratory fitness is the individual's aerobic capacity to perform large-muscle, whole-body (*gross motor*) physical activity of moderate to high intensity over extended periods. This type of physical fitness is particularly important for the prevention of heart disease and metabolic syndrome, a condition that predisposes individuals to heart disease, stroke, and diabetes. Cardiorespiratory fitness is assessed by a variety of measures examining oxygen utilization and endurance while performing functional movement such as walking and running. The best measure of cardiorespiratory fitness is *$V0_2$ max,* representing the volume (V) of oxygen (O_2) used when a person reaches his or her maximum (max) ability to supply oxygen to muscle tissue during exercise. This value may be compared to a resting value of oxygen usage, known as VO_2 resting. One MET (metabolic equivalent) is another unit of measure representing resting oxygen uptake. One MET equals approximately 3.5 milligrams (mg) of oxygen consumed per minute per kilogram (kg) of body weight. Since MET levels may vary between males and females, it is important to find current MET tables for reference. *Respiratory reserve* (VO_2 R) is the difference between the maximum oxygen uptake and resting oxygen uptake (VO_2 max - VO_2 resting). A percentage of this value is often used to determine appropriate intensities for physical activity. When testing an individual during exercise, the examiner can gauge the individual's perception of the physical effort needed to perform the activity by using *ratings of perceived exertion* (RPE). The subjective assessment of exercise intensity or RPE is based on how the participant feels during various levels of physical exertion over time. While RPE is considered a reliable tool, clinicians need to consider that clients, particularly those with brain injury, may interpret the words on the scale differently and should be cautious of other observations when evaluating exercise tolerance.[15]

The Rockport 1-mile walk test, the YMCA 3-minute step test, and distance walks/runs can be used to determine functional cardiovascular fitness or endurance. Other measures of cardiovascular endurance include maximal exercise performance (on a treadmill or cycle ergometer) while mechanically measuring the individual's oxygen consumption at moderate to high intensities of exercise.

Another factor used to assess cardiovascular fitness is the speed at which the heart rate returns to pre-exercise levels after performing extended exercise. In determining cardiovascular fitness, it is important to measure an individual's resting and maximum heart rate to know safe ranges of exercise. Maximum heart rate equals 220 minus the individual's age (in years) and is reported as HR_{max} (in beats per minute [bpm]). Resting heart rate is the individual's lowest heart rate, measured at rest. When determining a safe range of exercise, it is recommended that the health care provider use the threshold of training heart rate. The threshold of training heart rate is the maximum heart rate (HR_{max}) times 55% (*threshold of training* = HR_{max} x 55%).

Muscular Strength

Muscular strength is the ability of muscles to produce force at high intensities over short periods. Muscle strength is essential for the performance of daily activities of living and key to preventive care. *Sarcopenia,* or age-related loss of muscle mass, can be prevented with regular exercise. According to the Centers for Disease Control and Prevention,[16] sarcopenia, secondary to progressively decreasing physical activity, is one of the top five health risks for older adults. Sarcopenia is likely a multifactorial condition that impairs physical function and predisposes an individual to disability.[17] This disabling condition may be reduced with lifestyle interventions that include increased muscle strengthening.

Muscular Endurance

Muscular endurance is the ability to perform gross motor activity of moderate-to-high intensity over a long period. Quality of life is affected by reduced strength and endurance that limit a person's ability to remain physically active. When combined together (versus alone), muscle endurance training and strength training have a greater impact on walking distance, endurance exercise time, and the quality of life of patients with chronic obstructive pulmonary disease. It is estimated that 16 million people in the United States have chronic obstructive pulmonary disease, including emphysema, chronic bronchitis, and chronic asthma.[18] All of these individuals could benefit from exercise that improves both their strength and muscular endurance for activities of daily living.

Computer-controlled equipment can measure the muscular force used in generating an *isometric contraction* (involving no movement of body parts) and *isokinetic contractions* (involving controlled movement). These types of equipment are costly, may require specialized expertise, and are not always available in community or clinical settings. While these highly reliable types of quantitative assessments of muscle strength are desirable, there are a number of other options available to the clinician:

- *Manual muscle testing* (MMT) is used to evaluate the strength of individual muscles and muscle groups based on palpating muscle contractions or having the individual perform specific movements (either gravity-eliminated or with resistance provided by gravity or manual resistance).
- *Hand-held dynamometry* can be a reliable assessment technique when used by an experienced clinician. The hand-held dynamometer consists of a simple adjustable gripping device that is capable of measuring muscular force and is sensitive to detection of neuromuscular weakness.

The grip strength is a useful measure for overall arm strength and can be a helpful screening tool for fitness.

- The *one-repetition maximum strength test* (1-RM) is a popular method of measuring muscle strength. This test provides a measure of the maximal force (generally using free weights) an individual can lift with one repetition.
- The *YMCA bench press test* is used to evaluate strength and muscular endurance using a relatively light load. This test has separate loads for males and females (males are required to lift an 80-pound barbell and females are required to lift a 35-pound barbell).
- The *push-up test* involves performing standard push-ups while positioned with hands and feet touching the floor, the body and legs well aligned, and the arms extended and at right angles to the body. This test is primarily used for assessing upper body strength, including triceps and latissimus dorsi muscles.

Muscular endurance may be tested by examining the ability of muscles to repeatedly contract over time. All of the muscle strength assessments with repeated muscular contractions include a muscle endurance component and can be used to determine muscular endurance.

Flexibility

Flexibility is the ability to move muscles and joints (including soft tissue) through their full range of motion. Without flexibility, joints cannot move to their fullest extent for movement, despite having full muscle strength to complete the movement. Limited spinal flexibility can lead to functional limitations that impair independent living, such as functional reaching and maintaining balance. Since older adults are at an increased risk for falls, maintaining joint flexibility across the life span is important for maintaining functional independence and one's quality of life. Spinal flexibility is a contributor to *functional reach,* a measure of functional limitation and an established measure of balance control. The *sit and reach test* is commonly used to measure the overall flexibility of the body, but primarily tests the flexibility of the posterior legs, the back, the shoulders, the arms, the head, and the neck.[30] *Range of motion* measurements also provide information about the individual's ability to either actively or passively move the joint in all planes of motion. It is essential that the clinician be familiar with anatomy and well trained in the use of a goniometer, patient positioning, and the "end-feels" of the joint to assess range of motion accurately. Many factors influence joint range of motion, including disease processes or injuries affecting joint tissue, bone or surrounding tissues, inactivity or immobility, age (older adults tend to be less flexible), hormonal status (pregnant women tend to be more lax), and gender (men tend to be less flexible). Joint play is the normal looseness within a joint that allows movement to occur. The joint play movements are very small but precise in range. Movements of joint play are independent of the action of voluntary muscles, yet the summation of normal joint play movements allows pain-free and fluid motion. If muscles are imbalanced, impaired, or inactive, they may cause limitations in joint play movements unless the joint is passively moved to maintain joint motion. For example, individuals with tightness in their finger joints may have tightening of muscles or tissue surrounding the joint.

Posture

Posture is the maintenance of correct alignment of body parts. While many think of posture as maintaining static or unmoving positions, postural adjustments responsible for maintenance of good posture during rest and during activity involve continuous muscle adjustments and awareness of where the body is in space. Poor postural habits commonly lead to body malalignment and chronic musculoskeletal problems, such as low back pain. According to the Centers for Disease Control and Prevention, 15% of adult physician visits are related to back pain. Interestingly, the incidence of low back pain is highest in two groups: (1) sedentary individuals with poor sitting posture and weakened muscles and (2) individuals who injure their backs doing manual labor.[16] In both instances, proper posture while sitting or lifting large objects plays a key role in reducing the risk of low back pain and disability. Photographs are particularly useful for documenting postural problems or asymmetries. The forward bending test is a classic screening for spinal malalignment. *Lordosis,* commonly referred to as "sway back" or an increased lateral curve in the lower spine, is commonly detected and often leads to low back pain later in life. Proper exercise can alleviate some of the contributors to chronic back pain.

Body Composition

Body composition is the final aspect of health-related fitness. Body composition is often represented as two components: lean body weight and fat weight. The National Institute of Health (NIH) uses the body mass index (BMI) to define normal weight, overweight, and obesity since it correlates strongly (in adults) with the total body fat content. According to the NIH, overweight is defined as a BMI of 27.3% or more for women and 27.8% or more for men, while obesity is generally defined as a BMI of 30% and above.[19] It is important to note that very muscular people may

TABLE 3-2

BODY FAT PERCENTAGES

	Females	Female Athletes	Males	Male Athletes
Lean	<17%	<12%	<12%	<7%
Acceptable	17% to 18%	12% to 25%	12% to 21%	7% to 12%
Fit	21% to 24%		14% to 17%	
Moderately Overweight	28% to 33%		21% to 26%	
Overweight	>33%	>25%	>26%	>15%

Adapted from:
HealthCheck Systems. Understanding your body fat percentage. Available at: http://www.healthchecksystems.com/bodyfat.htm. Accessed October 15, 2005.
Am I Fat: Tests and Guidelines. Body fat percentage. Available at: http://www.am-i-fat.com/body_fat_percentage.html. Accessed October 15, 2005.

TABLE 3-3

BODY MASS INDEX SCORING

BMI	Classification
<18.5	Underweight
18.5 to 24.9	Normal
25.0 to 29.0	Overweight
30.0 to 39.9	Obese
≥40	Extremely Obese

Note: Women typically have more body fat than men.

Adapted from Aronne LJ. Classification of obesity and assessment of obesity-related health risks. *Obesity Research Supplement.* 2002;2:105S–115S.

have a high BMI without undue health risks. Body composition often focuses on body fat since a high percentage of Americans are obese and at risk for significant health problems. Assessing body fat and monitoring changes in body fat with exercise can be helpful in identifying changes in body composition over time. The calculation of percent body fat equals the fat weight divided by the total body weight with the result of this fraction multiplied by 100 (% body fat = (fat weight / total body weight) x 100). Table 3-2 gives general guidelines for body fat percentage levels for normal versus athletic men and women.

Health and fitness professionals use a wide range of tests to determine body composition, depending upon their clinical setting and available equipment. Some measures are very sophisticated and costly, while others involve low-cost equipment and precise measurement techniques for increased reliability:

- *Skinfold thickness* measurements are one method used to estimate the amount of an individual's body fat. Skin and subcutaneous adipose tissues are measured at several different standard anatomical sites around the body. Skin fold measures are converted to percentage body fat (%BF) using various equations depending on the individual tested.
- *BMI* is a key index for relating a person's body weight to height. The BMI is a person's weight in kilograms divided by their height in meters (m) squared. Weight scales and a stadiometer are the tools needed to assess weight and height. The BMI equation follows: BMI = M / (H x H), where M = body mass in kilograms and H = height in meters. A higher BMI score usually indicates higher levels of body fat. This calculation is accurate for normal populations but is not valid for elderly populations, pregnant women, or muscular athletes. Table 3-3 lists how the scores are used to categorize an individual's BMI.

Table 3-4 shows converted values for the calculation of BMI based upon an individual's height and weight.

When combining BMI with waist measurements, the health professional can determine an individual's risk for disease, particularly cardiac pathology. Table 3-5 lists the BMI scores with associated risk for disease.

- *Waist to hip ratio* is simply measured using a tape measure around the waist and largest circumference of the hips. The ratio is a simple

TABLE 3-4
BODY MASS INDEX CALCULATIONS

BMI (kg/m^2)	19	20	21	22	23	24	25	26	27	28	29	30	35	40
Height (in)	**Weight (lbs)**													
58	91	96	100	105	110	115	119	124	129	134	138	143	167	191
59	94	99	104	109	114	119	124	128	133	138	143	148	173	198
60	97	102	107	112	118	123	128	133	138	143	148	153	179	204
61	100	106	111	116	122	127	132	137	143	148	153	158	185	211
62	104	109	115	120	126	131	136	142	147	153	158	164	191	218
63	107	113	118	124	130	135	141	146	152	158	163	169	197	225
64	110	116	122	128	134	140	145	151	157	163	169	174	204	232
65	114	120	126	132	138	144	150	156	162	168	174	180	210	240
66	118	124	130	136	142	148	155	161	167	173	179	186	216	247
67	121	127	134	140	146	153	159	166	172	178	185	191	223	255
68	125	131	138	144	151	158	164	171	177	184	190	197	230	262
69	128	135	142	149	155	162	169	176	182	189	196	203	236	270
70	132	139	146	153	160	167	174	181	188	195	202	207	243	278
71	136	143	150	157	165	172	179	186	193	200	208	215	250	286
72	140	147	154	162	169	177	184	191	199	206	213	221	258	294
73	144	151	159	166	174	182	189	197	204	212	219	227	265	302
74	148	155	163	171	179	186	194	202	210	218	225	233	272	311
75	152	160	168	176	184	192	200	208	216	224	232	240	279	319
76	156	164	172	180	189	197	205	213	221	230	238	246	287	328

Adapted from National Heart, Lung, and Blood Institute. Body mass index table. Available at: http://www.nhlbi.nih.gov/guidelines/obesity/bmi_tbl.htm. Accessed Novemeber 20, 2006.

TABLE 3-5
BODY MASS INDEX AND RISK OF ASSOCIATED DISEASE

BMI	Category	Waist <40 (in Men) or <35 (in Women)	Waist >40 (in Men) or >35 (in Women)
≤18.5	Underweight	N/A	N/A
18.5 to 24.9	Normal	N/A	N/A
25.0 to 29.9	Overweight	Increased risk	High risk
30.0 to 34.9	Obese	High risk	Very high risk
35.0 to 39.9	Obese	Very high risk	Very high risk
≥40	Extremely obese	Extremely high risk	Extremely high risk

Adapted from Aronne LJ. Classification of obesity and assessment of obesity-related health risks. *Obesity Research Supplement.* 2002;2:105S–115S.

TABLE 3-6

WAIST-TO-HIP RATIOS

Examples of how waist-to-hip ratios (WHR) are calculated:

Waist	Hip	Ratio	Ratio
36 inch	40 inch	36/40	0.90
36 inch	36 inch	36/36	1.00
40 inch	32 inch	40/32	1.25

	Acceptable	*Unacceptable*
Male	<0.90	≥0.90
Female	<0.80	≥0.80

Adapted from Dobbelsteyn CJ, Joffres MR, MacLean DR, Flowerdew G. A comparative evaluation of waist circumference, waist-to-hip ratio and body mass index as indicators of cardiovascular risk factors. *Int J Obes*. 2001;25(5):652–661.

calculation of the waist girth divided by the hip girth. Table 3-6 gives general guidelines for acceptable levels for waist-to-hip ratio (WHR).

- *Girth measurements and body breadth measurements* are additional measures of the body's size and shape. Girth measurements or circumferential measures of various body parts indicate growth, nutritional status, and fat patterning. Body breadth measurements, used to determine body type and frame size, are taken at the hips, shoulders, extremities, and other areas of concern. The clinician can use these measurements over time to monitor changes in the body shape and size.
- *Hydrostatic weighing* has been called the "gold standard" for measuring body composition. For this assessment, the individual, dressed in minimal clothing, is weighed for the dry weight; the fully submerged underwater weight is then determined. Body density is than calculated taking into account the body weight, the density of water, the residual lung volume, and corrections for air trapped in the gastrointestinal tract.
- *Bioelectric impedance* involves measurement of the body's impedance or conduction of electrical currents through the body. It is important to consider that body hydration, body temperature, and other variables affect the body's conductivity and should be held constant for all measurements for improved reliability. The device measures the amount of fat-free mass that allows current flow. Bioelectric impedance analysis is based on the principle that the resistance to an applied electric current is inversely related to the amount of fat-free mass within the body.[20]
- *Dual-energy x-ray absorptiometry* (DEXA) uses x-rays to differentiate the components of soft tissue (fat and lean) and bone. DEXA also has the ability to determine body composition in defined regions (ie, in the arms, legs, and trunk). DEXA measurements are based in part on the assumption that the hydration of fat-free mass remains constant at 73%. Hydration, however, can vary from 67% to 85% and can be variable in certain disease states.[22] This assessment tool is highly expensive but offers accurate body composition analysis that can screen for additional problems, such as osteoporosis. Individuals may have total body scans for total body composition or regional body scans of areas at risk for osteoporosis. Total body scans may be helpful in diagnosing and monitoring the following conditions: obesity, growth hormone abnormalities and treatment effects, primary hyperparathyroidism, secondary hyperparathyroidism, anabolic steroids therapy, anorexia nervosa, Cushing's syndrome, muscular dystrophy, cachexic or wasting disorders (eg, AIDS, cancer), chronic kidney disease, and malabsorptive syndromes.[40]
- *Near infrared interactance* (NIR) method is based on light penetration (using a fiber optic probe) into various tissues with reflection off the bone. The NIR contains a digital analyzer that indirectly measures the tissue composition (fat and water) at various sites on the body. The NIR data is entered into a prediction equation with the person's height, weight, frame size, and level of activity to estimate the percent body fat. This assessment of body fat, while simple, fast, and noninvasive, is costly and not reliable for very lean or very obese individuals.
- *Magnetic resonance imaging* (MRI) is a diagnostic imaging tool that uses contrast materials to help provide a clear picture of body structure, using magnets and computers to create images or "pictures" of certain areas inside the body. Unlike x-rays, MRI does not involve ionizing radiation. The person lies within the magnet as a computer scans the body. High-quality images show the amount of fat and where it is distributed. The MRI takes about 30 minutes, but use is limited due to the high cost of equipment and analysis.
- *Computed tomography (CT)* scans the body, providing cross-sectional images of each scan. An x-ray tube sends a beam of photons toward a detector. As the beam rotates around a person, data is collected, stored, and applied to calculations that determine body composition. CT is

particularly useful in giving a ratio of intra-abdominal fat to extra-abdominal fat. While CT scans are noninvasive, they subject individuals to radiation and are extremely costly.

- *BOD POD (air displacement)* uses air displacement instead of using water to measure body volume. The BOD POD uses computerized sensors to measure how much air is displaced while a person sits within the capsule and then calculates to body density and estimated body fat.[22] This new equipment is very expensive and limited in availability but provides values highly correlated (r = .93) with the gold standard, hydrostatic weighing.[22]

While these measures provide a variety of indices for physical fitness, it is important to consider that physical fitness is influenced by genetics, environmental influences, and the individual's activity levels. Many factors offer insight regarding the individual's disease risk and health habits, including patterns of growth and development, a history of exercise and good nutrition, a medical and psychosocial history, as well as a history of significant others in that individual's environment. For example, genetic information can be used to trace potential health problems or to predict family characteristics, such as typical growth and developmental patterns.

Another aspect of physical fitness is skill-related or motor fitness. This type of fitness provides another array of tests offering insight regarding an individual's physical capabilities for performing complex motor tasks.

Skill-Related or Motor Fitness

Motor fitness is often associated with athletic competition but should be considered in the overall fitness of all individuals. Motor fitness is essential for effectively, efficiently, and safely performing activities of daily living and participating in the community. Components of motor fitness include balance, coordination, reaction time, power, speed, and agility.

Postural Balance

Postural balance, or equilibrium, can be described as the body's ability to maintain an intended position (*static balance*) or progress through various movements without losing postural control (*dynamic balance*). While standing balance or equilibrium normally develops in the first two years of life, various factors may affect an individual's ability to maintain balance. These factors include visual input, normal functioning of the vestibular system (responsible for sensing movement and head position in space), adequate muscle strength and joint range of motion to assume and maintain postures, and normal somatosenses or sensations regarding the body's position in space. This information is integrated in the central nervous system to coordinate all the inputs responsible for the maintenance of equilibrium at rest and while moving.

Some assessments of balance involve sophisticated equipment that can isolate the various factors contributing to balance problems, while other measures focus on functional skills for independent living. Athletes performing in high-level competition require tests designed to meet specific criteria that exceed normative values of the general population. Tests for highly skilled athletes are not included in this listing of postural balance tests. Various tests for postural balance include the following:

- The *dynamic posturography* measure of balance requires equipment that can isolate the various factors contributing to standing balance. The individual stands on a platform in an enclosed space that obscures vision. For safety purposes, the person wears a harness to prevent falls. During the test, the platform is moved to elicit equilibrium reactions or the visual field is altered to isolate possible deficits in balance. By isolating the various factors that contribute to the maintenance of standing balance, this test assesses movement coordination and the organization of visual, somatosensory, and vestibular information relevant to postural control.
- For the *one-legged stance test* (OLST), the individual is asked to stand on one leg while the examiner times the duration of stance on each leg (with eyes opened or closed).
- For the *sharpened Romberg test* (SR), the individual stands with both feet in tandem (feet touching heel-to-toe) while both arms are crossed at chest level as the examiner stands nearby for safety. This test is performed with eyes opened and eyes closed to isolate visual input that can mask problems with balance.

The following tests are standardized tests that have a wide range of functional tasks and balance criteria used to determine the balance capabilities of populations at risk, including older adults and individuals with motor problems.

- The *Berg balance scale*, a standardized scale, is a 14-item test that focuses on reaching, bending, transferring, standing, rising, and other functional tasks for a total of 56 points.
- The *clinical test of sensory interaction and balance* is a standardized assessment that measures static balance under three visual and two supported conditions.

- The *functional reach test* measures the difference in inches between a person's arm position at rest (with the shoulder flexed to 90 degrees) and the distance reached forward while maintaining a fixed base of support while standing.
- The *Tinetti balance test of the performance-oriented assessment of mobility problems* consists of 28 items related to balance while standing and moving.
- The *timed up and go test* is a balance test that measures the time needed to rise to standing from a chair, walk three meters, turn, walk back to the chair, and sit down.
- The *physical performance test* measures standing and moving balance, feeding, and writing; the majority of these items are timed.

Coordination

Coordination is harmonious movement, reflecting the coordination of muscle contractions and their timing for desired movement. Coordinated movement includes the smooth and controlled lay-up for a basketball goal performed by a skilled athlete and the graceful movement of a figure skater performing on ice. Likewise, coordinated movement can include placing blocks into a tower without error as well as performing jumping jacks with ease. Tests for coordination include the following:

- The *finger-to-nose test* is designed to observe the smoothness and timing of arm movement. The individual is asked to repetitively touch the nose using the index finger and then to touch the clinician's outstretched finger.
- For the *dysdiadokinesis test* or *rapidly alternating movements test,* the individual alternately taps the palm then the back of one hand on the thigh. The examiner observes this movement for smoothness and speed.
- The *lower-extremity coordination test,* the individual is tested for smoothness and speed of movement in the lower extremities or legs while trying to make precise movements with each leg, such as sliding the heel down the shin of the opposite leg.

Individuals with poor coordination may need a more thorough examination to determine if fatigue, neurological insult, or other factors contribute to poorly coordinated movement.

Reaction Time

Reaction time is the amount of time needed to produce movement in response to a stimulus. Reaction time is especially important for completing movements within a safe time frame for effective function. For example, reaction time is critical when driving a car, such as quickly pressing on the brakes at a red light. Computers, the more expensive option, can test reaction times to various visual stimuli with specialized programs and equipment providing the appropriate stimuli for the desired motor response. *The ruler test,* a quick and readily available test for reaction time, measures the response when a ruler is dropped over the individual's head. The aim is to catch the ruler before it drops past onto the floor.

Power

Power is the ability to generate force (measured in force units/time units [ie, watts]) or the ability to exert maximum muscular contraction instantly in an explosive burst of movements. Power is important for lifting objects and pushing objects, as observed in competitive football and weight lifting. The PWC170 test is used to predict the power output (watts) at a projected heart rate of 170 bpm. The individual is asked to perform two consecutive 6-minute bicycle ergometer rides with work loads selected to produce a heart rate between 120 and 140 bpm on the first session and between 150 and 170 bpm on the second session. For each session, the average heart rate (bpm) and power output (watts) are recorded.[23]

Speed

Speed is the rate of movement and is essential for performing daily activities in a timely manner. Speed is often a convenient measure used to determine the amount of time a person needs to ambulate from one point to another or perform work-related tasks, such as typing. Timed tests for skilled motor performance determine an individual's speed. Examples of timed tests include the *60-meter speed test,* assessing gross motor speed for normal or athletic populations; and the *Jebsen hand test,* a standardized assessment used to measure dexterity or the speed of fine motor movements. With seven subtests, this tool evaluates a broad range of hand functions used in daily activities using common items such as paper clips, cans, pencils, and other functional objects.

Agility

Agility is the ability to move in a quick and easy fashion or the ability to perform a series of explosive power movements in rapid succession in opposing directions. Agility is often demonstrated by maneuvering around objects, such a going through an obstacle course as quickly as possible without falling or losing control of movement. Agility may be measured by observing how an individual navigates around an environment or may include a battery of standardized tests that test movement in multiple directions. Tests of agility generally involve the ability to rapidly, easily change directions in one or more directions, and include the *hexagonal obstacle agility test,* the *Illinois agility run test,* and the *lateral changing of direction test.*

The *Bruninks-Oserestsky test of motor proficiency* is an example of useful test that can be used to screen for multiple areas of motor fitness. This measure is a norm-referenced, standardized test composed of eight subtests designed to evaluate the following skills: gross motor development, running speed and agility, balance, bilateral coordination, strength (arm, shoulder, abdominal, and leg), upper-limb coordination, fine motor development, response speed, visual-motor control, upper-limb speed, and dexterity. The examiner can select measures that best match the functional skills associated with the individual's occupation or leisure function for a customized screening test for any of these areas of motor fitness.

Conclusion

Health care professionals work with populations ranging in age from young neonates to older adults who can all benefit from physical activity to enhance all types of fitness. Chapter 4 provides information about physical activity and fitness training designed for the various populations. Screening for both physical fitness and mental fitness enables health care professionals to determine if individuals are both physically able and mentally able to meet the challenges of every day life.

References

1. Saltin B, Pilegaard H. [Metabolic fitness: physical activity and health]. *Ugeskr Laeger.* 2002;164(16):2156–2162. (ARTICLE IN DANISH)
2. Doll B, Lyon M. Risk and resilience: implications for the delivery of educational and mental health services in schools. *School Psychology Review.* 1998;27:348–363.
3. United States Public Health Services. Mental health: a report of the surgeon general. Available at: http://www.surgeongeneral.gov/library/mentalhealth/home.html#forward. Accessed October 15, 2005.
4. Holmes TH, Rahe RH. The social readjustment rating scale. *J Psychosom Res.* 1967;11:213–218.
5. Vance DE, Wadley VG, Ball KK, Roenker DL, Rizzo M. The effects of physical activity and sedentary behavior on cognitive health in older adults. *J Aging Phys Act.* 2005;13(3):294–313.
6. Elavsky S, McAuley E, Motl RW, et al. Physical activity enhances long-term quality of life in older adults: efficacy, esteem, and affective influences. *Ann Behav Med.* 2005;30(2):138–145.
7. Sacker A, Cable N. Do adolescent leisure-time physical activities foster health and well-being in adulthood? Evidence from two British birth cohorts. *Eur J Pub Health.* 2006;16(3):332–336.
8. Hughes CS, Hughes S. The female athlete syndrome. Anorexia nervosa—reflections on a personal journey. *Orthoped Nurs.* 2004;23(4):252–260.
9. National Institute on Aging. Determinants of aging and health across the life span: potential new insights from longitudinal studies. Report of the July 2003 meeting of the NIA Longitudinal Data on Aging Working Group.
10. Horvath P, Eagen C, Nadine MS, et al. The effects of varying dietary fat on performance and metabolism in trained male and female runners. *J Am Coll Nutr.* 2000;19(1):52–60.
11. Kinosian B, Glick H, Garland G. Cholesterol and coronary heart disease: predicting risks by levels and ratios. *Ann Intern Med.* 1994;121(9):641–647.
12. McLaughlin T, Abbasi F, Cheal K, Chu J, Lamendola C, Reaven G. Use of metabolic markers to identify overweight individuals who are insulin resistant. *Ann Intern Med.* 2003;139:802–809.
13. American Diabetes Association. Report of the expert committee on the diagnosis and classification of diabetes mellitus. *Diabetes Care.* 2003;26(Suppl 1):S5–S20.
14. Pickering TG, Hall JE, Appel LJ, et al. Recommendations for blood pressure measurement in humans and experimental animals: part 1: blood pressure measurement in humans: a statement for professionals from the subcommittee of professional and public education of the Americans Heart Association council on high blood pressure research. *Circulation.* 2005;111(5):697–716.
15. Dawes HN, Barker KL, Cockburn J, Roach N, Scott O, Wade D. Borg's rating of perceived exertion scales: do the verbal anchors mean the same for different clinical groups? *Arch Phys Med Rehabil.* 2005;86(5):912–916.
16. Newman AB, Lee JS, Visser M, et al. Weight change and the conservation of lean mass in old age: the health, aging and body composition study. *Am J Clin Nutr.* 2005;82(4):872–878.
17. Office of Disease Prevention and Health Promotion, United States Department of Health and Human Services. Healthy People 2001. Available at: http://www.healthypeople.gov. Accessed October 15, 2005.
18. National Center for Health Statistics. Centers for Disease Control and Prevention. Available at: http://www.cdc.gov. Accessed October 15, 2005.
19. Williamson DF. Descriptive epidemiology of body weight and weight change in US adults. *Ann Intern Med.* 1993;119(7[Pt 2]):646–649.
20. Ward L, Cornish BH, Patons NI, Thomas BJ. Multiple frequency bioelectrical impedance analysis: a cross-validation study of the inductor circuit and Cole models. *Physiol Meas.* 1999;20:333–347.
21. Buchholz A, Bartok C, Schoeller D. The validity of bioelectrical impedance models in clinical populations. *Nutr Clin Pract.* 2004;19(5):433–446.

22. McCrory MA, Gomez TD, Bernauer EM, Mole PA. Evaluation of a new air displacement plethysmograph for measuring human body composition. *Med Sci Sports Exerc.* 1995;27(12):1686–1691.

23. Gore C, Booth M, Bauman A, Neville O. Utility of pwc75% as an estimate of aerobic power in epidemiological and population-based studies. *Med Sci Sports Exerc.* 1999;31(2):348–351.

Chapter 4

Fitness Training

Catherine Rush Thompson, PhD, MS, PT

"On average, physically active people outlive those who are inactive. Regular physical activity also helps to maintain the functional independence of older adults and enhances the quality of life for people of all ages."

~HEALTHY PEOPLE 2010

Improving Physical Fitness

Exercise can be any physical exertion to improve mental and physical health, including prevention or correction of impairments. Exercise must be performed to a certain extent (number of repetitions or minutes) to reap any benefits. According to the Surgeon General's Report, moderate physical activity results in significant health benefits and improved quality of life. Even greater benefits can be achieved by increasing the duration and intensity of exercise. While a daily regimen of 30 minutes of moderate level activity, such as brisk walking, provides proven mental and physical health benefits, progressive increases in activity offer an inexpensive yet powerful preventive measure for health, fitness, and well-being.[1] These benefits include, but are not limited to, those found in Table 4-1.[1]

Types of Exercise

Aerobic Exercise

Clinicians use a variety of exercise terms describing body demands, forces involved, or the intention of exercise. Aerobic exercise is exercise requiring the continual use of oxygen or any activity that uses large muscle groups, can be maintained continuously, and is rhythmic in nature. Types of aerobic exercise include bicycling, cross-country skiing, in-line skating, fitness walking, jumping rope, running, stair climbing, and swimming. Low intensity aerobic exercise generally demands a small, yet continual, level of oxygen, so the body can sustain exercise for a longer period of time. The individual should be able to carry on a conversation while performing aerobic exercise. Aerobic fitness levels can improve with as little as 10 minutes duration of aerobic exercise, as long as exercise is performed often (2 to 3 times a day, 5 days a week).[1] To balance general fitness, health, body composition, and scheduling concerns, 30 minutes is optimal for many people. Benefits of aerobic exercise include improved cardiovascular fitness, muscular strength and endurance, improved body composition, and improved mental fitness. With sustained aerobic exercise, the cardiac muscle becomes more efficient pumping blood; the skeletal muscles build endurance and become more toned; the body increases lean body mass and reduces fatty tissue; and the individual can experience better sleep, less depression, and improved mood.

ANAEROBIC EXERCISE

Anaerobic exercise is performed in the absence of a continual oxygen source. Anaerobic activities are short in duration and high in intensity, involving short bursts of exertion followed by periods of rest. Examples of anaerobic exercise include activities with variable, yet demanding, physical activity, such as racquetball, downhill skiing, weight lifting, sprinting, softball, soccer, and football. The benefits of anaerobic exercise include increased calorie consumption, increased metabolism, shorter workouts, improved brain function, and increased lean muscle tissue.[2]

ISOMETRIC EXERCISE

Isometric exercise is active exercise performed against stable resistance without change in the muscle length. Strength can be increased if the isometric contraction is sustained for 6 to 8 seconds; however, any one isometric exercise will only increase muscle strength at one joint angle. Strengthening the other joint positions requires repetition of alternative exercises involving those joints. If an individual has cardiac disease or high blood pressure, isometric exercises can pose problems. Muscle contractions involving the upper body can increase intrathoracic pressure or pressure in the chest. Taking a deep breath and performing a contraction against a closed glottis causes a problematic effect on the body, the *Valsalva effect.* This increase in intrathoracic pressure is combined with the intrathoracic pressure caused by the weight of the specific lift. During the muscular contractions in this form of exercise, blood pressure can rise quite dramatically. Arterial hypertension produced during heavy weight lifting with the Valsalva effect is extreme. The resultant elevated blood pressure may be dramatically reduced when the exercise is performed with an open glottis, facilitated by proper breathing during heavy resistance isometric exercises.

ISOTONIC EXERCISE

Isotonic exercise involves muscle shortening to generate force. As each muscle moves through its range of motion, isotonic contractions tone muscles. Isotonic training provides a broad variety of movements, allowing the individual to exercise all major muscle groups. The disadvantages include uneven forces throughout the range of movement and unequal muscle tension for muscle groups.

ISOKINETIC EXERCISE

Isokinetic exercise is constant-velocity muscle actions that may be either *concentric* (muscle tension is generated as the muscle length decreases or shortens) or *eccentric* (muscle tension is generated as the muscle length increases or lengthens). Unlike isotonic exercise, isokinetic exercise provides muscular overload at a constant speed while the muscle mobilizes its force through the full range of motion. Isokinetic exercise machines include the Cybex and Biodex machines, both designed to vary the resistance to muscle contraction throughout the range of motion. See Table 4-2 for a comparison of isometric, isotonic, and isokinetic exercises.

TABLE 4-1

BENEFITS OF PHYSICAL ACTIVITY

- Lower overall mortality. Benefits are greatest among the most active persons but are also evident for individuals who reported only moderate activity.
- Lower risk of coronary heart disease. The cardiac risk of being inactive is comparable to the risk from smoking cigarettes.
- Lower risk of cancers, including colon cancer and breast cancer
- Lower risk of diabetes
- Lower risk of developing high blood pressure. Exercise also lowers blood pressure in individuals who have hypertension
- Lower risk of obesity
- Lower risk of developing depression
- Improved mood and relief of symptoms of depression
- Improved quality of life and improved functioning
- Improved function in persons with arthritis
- Lower risk of falls and injury
- Prevention of bone loss and fracture after the menopause
- Improved quality of sleep
- Improved memory
- Increased endurance
- Increased strength
- Reduced stress and tension
- Increased energy
- Slowed aging process
- Boosted confidence

SPORTS EXERCISE

Sports exercise is any type of exercise involving physical games and competition. Extensive scientific research shows that regular physical activity and playing sports are among the best forms of preventive medicine.[3] Participation in sports and fitness

TABLE 4-2

A COMPARISON OF ISOMETRIC, ISOTONIC, AND ISOKINETIC EXERCISES

	Advantages	Disadvantages
Isometric	Does not aggravate sensitive joint surfaces Easy to perform and remember Reproducible Easy to measure Convenient Cost effective	Not functional Any improvements are speed and angle specific Many contraindications Not efficient in terms of strength No endurance enhancements
Isotonic	Functional Easy to monitor Minimal equipment needed Convenient Best strength and endurance enhancements	Maximal loading only at specific angles Momentum key factor Synergists either limit progress or are undertrained Unsafe for joints Highest likelihood of injuries Gives delayed onset muscle soreness Many contraindications Difficult to monitor accurately
Isokinetic	Maximal loading throughout whole range of motion Objective, reproducible, and easily quantifiable Muscles easily isolated Safest form of exercise Few contraindications	Time consuming Requires a lot of training and skill to use Costly Not functional

Adapted from:
Smith MJ, Melton P. Isokinetic versus isotonic variable resistance training. *Am J Sports Med.* 1981;9(4):275-279.
Muller EA, Hettinger TW. The effects of isometric exercise against isotonic exercise on muscles. *Arbeitsphysiology.* 1954;15:452.

activities offers potential health benefits for individuals of all ages, such as combating obesity and osteoporosis, as well as enhancing cardiovascular fitness. Psychological benefits of sports include the development of a positive self-image and increased support for exercise adherence.[3] Negative consequences of musculoskeletal injuries sustained during sports participation, however, pose long-term health problems. Sports with the highest risks of injury per 1,000 hours of activity include skating, basketball, running or jogging, racquetball, and any competitive sport involving athletes who are nonprofessional.[4,5] Proper exercise equipment and prevention of injury through proper training can reduce injuries from high-risk sports.

THERAPEUTIC EXERCISE

Therapeutic exercise, sometimes referred to as corrective exercise, is designed to use bodily movements to restore normal function in diseased or injured tissues and to maintain well-being. The goals of therapeutic exercise include enabling or improving ambulation; releasing contracted muscles, tendons, and fasciae; mobilizing joints; improving circulation; enhancing respiratory capacity; improving coordination; reducing rigidity; increasing balance; promoting relaxation; increasing muscle strength; and improving exercise performance and functional capacity. Therapeutic exercise is prescribed to address individualized needs based on health status and fitness goals. Clinicians educate their clients regarding key concerns and goals for health and wellness, then subsequently design an exercise program, prevention strategies, and/or physical activities that meet the specific needs and personal goals of each individual.

ACTIVE EXERCISE

Active exercise is exercise performed independently. When an individual is unable to perform active exercise, assistance is provided. This assistance is referred to as *active-assisted exercise* (when the patient assists in the movement) or *passive exercise* (when the patient does not provide any assistance in the movement). Generally, active-assistive range of motion (AAROM) or passive range of motion (PROM) exercises are provided to those who are debilitated by injury or illness. These types of exercises are not recommended for individuals who have unstable tissue (such as a broken bone or dislocation) requiring stabilization.

Physical Activity

Physical activity generally refers to all forms of large muscle movements including sports, dance, games, work, and lifestyle activities. Physical activity is often measured by examining activities of daily living necessary for independent functioning. Popular physical activities among adults in the United States are walking, gardening (yard work), stretching exercise, resistance exercise, and jogging or running.

Therapeutic Activities for Special Populations

Aquatherapy

Aquatic therapy, or *aquatherapy*, refers to therapeutic intervention using the water as an environment for performing aerobic exercise or relaxation activities. Aquatic immersion provides various types of stimulation, including hydrostatic pressure, buoyancy, resistance, and heat (if the pool is properly thermoregulated). These various simultaneous inputs affect the cardiopulmonary, neurological, and musculoskeletal systems in individuals with and without impairments. According to the Halliwick Concept,[6] as learners adjust to the water environment, they develop control in rotation, improve balance, and execute movements more smoothly. Aquatic therapy, with its buoyant effect, is also used to support individuals with conditions impairing upright posture and/or weight bearing (eg, muscular dystrophy, spinal cord injuries, and rheumatoid arthritis).

Hippotherapy

According to the American Hippotherapy Association, hippotherapy (from the Greek word "hippos" meaning horse) refers to activities performed on a horse designed to improve sensorimotor processing. Neurological processing and movement of the client are stimulated by the variable, rhythmic, and repetitive movement of the horse's gait, facilitated through input similar to human pelvic patterns while walking.[7] Specific riding skills are not taught (as in therapeutic riding); however, hippotherapy can positively improve the balance, posture, mobility, and function of the client. Individuals who engage in hippotherapy include those with cerebral palsy, developmental delay, learning disabilities, multiple sclerosis, traumatic brain injury, and stroke. "A general psychotherapeutic and psychohygienic effect is created by joy, change, and a new impetus in rehabilitation as well as by the emotional contact with the 'comrade animal.'"[7]

Tai Chi

Tai chi is an ancient Chinese practice designed to exercise body, mind, and spirit. Over 100 Tai chi postures are included in exercises that gently work muscles while requiring the motor control to maintain balance while transitioning into a new posture. The slow, controlled movements are gentle, continuous, and circular. One study looking at middle-aged women found that a form of this exercise effectively induced improved physical fitness, psychological relaxation, and mental concentration, as measured by subjective reports and by physiological measures of respiratory rate, heart rate, electroencephalography, surface electromyography, and exercise tolerance.[8] Tai chi exercise is particularly effective in balance training and fall prevention for older adults.[9,10,11]

Yoga

Yoga has many connotations but is used in this text to describe a type of exercise involved in attaining bodily or mental control through a variety of postures. *"Yog,"* the root of yoga, means to bind or to connect, referring to the spiritual aspect of these exercises and suggesting a connection with the soul of God. Yoga exercises have been practiced for more than 5000 years and are designed to incorporate breathing and meditation to calm the mind. Hatha yoga is the physical path of yoga and uses physical poses and breathing techniques designed to develop a strong, healthy, and flexible body.[12]

Recent studies have shown that yoga training optimizes the sympathetic response to stressful stimuli and restores the autonomic regulatory reflex mechanisms in hypertensive patients.[13] Furthermore, yoga-based intervention may benefit individuals with chronic low back pain, reducing levels of depression and disability, as suggested by a pilot study featuring 22 participants (between the ages of 30 and 65) with chronic low back pain.[14] Finally, a study examining the use of yoga for adult patients with asthma demonstrated that those practicing yoga techniques reported a significant degree of relaxation, positive attitude, and better yoga exercise tolerance. There was also a tendency toward lesser usage of beta-adrenergic inhalers, but pulmonary function tests did not vary significantly between yoga and control groups.[15] Overall, practicing the breathing and postures of Hatha yoga offers beneficial effects for both healthy and chronically ill populations.

Considerations for Exercise and Physical Activity

Numerous factors must be taken into consideration when engaging in exercise or physical activity. These factors include weather conditions, proper attire, the optimal time of day, nutrition, illness, medications, and alcohol, among others.

WEATHER CONDITIONS

Bad weather can pose a significant health hazard to those seeking outdoor activity. Unless the body is conditioned to exercise in hot weather, it is not advisable to perform vigorous exercise when it is over 98°F, especially if the humidity is high.[16] In hot environments, water loss can cause dehydration, so plenty of water is needed for exercise. Electrolyte replacements, such as Gatorade or diluted fruit juice, can limit dehydration, but caffeinated beverages (such as coffee and cola drinks) are diuretics and will cause the body to lose more fluid. Age-associated changes in thermoregulation and an increased susceptibility to dehydration underscore the critical importance of adequate fluid intake by older adults.

PROPER ATTIRE

The individual should wear clothing that allows the body to "breathe," yet protects the body from excessive sunlight. Wearing light-colored clothing reflects sunlight; however, exercising early in the morning or late in the afternoon avoids exposure to harmful midday sunrays. Likewise, exercise should be limited when the temperature is below freezing accompanied by wind speed, contributing to the wind chill factor. During cold weather, the individual should wear layered clothing. Clothing should be ideally made of fabrics that fit close to the skin and pull moisture away from the body. A porous windbreaker warms the body while blocking wind, and a hat prevents significant heat loss.[17] Hands can be protected by mittens. Petroleum jelly can also be used to insulate the skin, keeping the exposed hands, nose, and ears warm.[17] To avoid unnecessary chill, the individual should avoid getting wet.

TIME OF DAY

For outdoor exercise, it is advisable to avoid times of peak sunlight to prevent increased risk for skin cancer (unless a suitable sunscreen is used). Whenever exercising, the individual should wait at least 2 to 3 hours after a meal before exercising to avoid cramps, nausea, or vomiting.[17] To fully recover from physical activity, a 30-minute break postexercise is suggested.

PROPER NUTRITION

Eating a balanced diet improves general health and reduces the risk of many diseases. The food pyramid illustrated at the website for the United States Department of Agriculture (see Appendix C) provides general guidelines for proper nutrition to maintain good health. This website offers specific nutritional guidelines based on an individual's age, gender, and level of physical activity.[18]

Hydration is a key factor to address during exercise because body sweat can dehydrate the body regardless of weather conditions. According to the American Dietetics Association, individuals should drink about 400 to 600 mL of water 2 to 3 hours before exercise, 150 to 350 mL during exercise (about every 15 to 20 minutes), and 450 to 675 mL after exercise for every 0.5 kg of weight lost during exercise.[19]

Small meals should be consumed about 4 hours prior to exercise to allow time for digestion. Examples of healthy meals prior to exercise include the following: (1) cereal, fruit, milk, and toast; (2) yogurt, muffin, and fruit; (3) pasta with tomato sauce; or (4) soup, a sandwich with lean meat, and milk. In general, individuals who are engaged in endurance activities need increased complex carbohydrates (whole grains, fruits, and vegetables) to maintain adequate energy sources for muscle contraction.[19] Athletes, in particular, demand a ready source of carbohydrates and fats for sustaining muscle contractions. Glycogen, available in the liver and skeletal muscles, also contributes energy sources for physical activity. During exercise, however, muscle glycogen reserves can be used up when activities last more than 90 minutes. Gradually decreasing the amount of training during the last 6 to 7 days before an important game, and simultaneously increasing the amount of dietary carbohydrates results in higher physical performance.[18] Also, a combination of carbohydrates and proteins is effective for accelerating recovery after exhausting exercise.

Older adults should monitor nutrient intake to ensure adequacy, especially of carbohydrates and proteins. Carbohydrates promote glucose storage and provide an energy source during exercise. Protein promotes strength-training-induced muscle hypertrophy or muscle building. Supplementation of certain vitamins and minerals (including the vitamins B2, B6, B12, D, E, and folate, as well as calcium and iron) is recommended. Nutrition is an essential tool that older adults should use to enhance exercise performance and health.[19]

ILLNESS

If the individual has a cold and no other medical conditions, low-intensity exercise is generally safe, unless symptoms include fever, sore muscles or joints, vomiting or diarrhea, or a productive cough. These symptoms should resolve before resuming physical exercise. Individuals with chronic illness or diseases need therapeutic exercise programs specifically designed to meet their needs. Any questions about an individual's health should be discussed with the patient's physician, and then proper precautions should be addressed in a customized exercise program. Chapters 12 through 16 address health issues and special considerations affecting exercise prescription for individuals with pathology.

MEDICATIONS

Exercise increases heart rate, and stimulants (eg, caffeine, cold medications, diet pills, allergy remedies, and herbal teas) may contain compounds that can further elevate heart rate. Any ingested medication, food, or beverage with significant stimulating effects should be carefully monitored before engaging in exercise.

Some medications have side effects that result in impaired coordination, poor judgment, drowsiness, and dehydration. Medications such as *antihistamines* can cause an individual to feel drowsy, resulting in increased reaction time (slower response), poor balance, and incoordination and should be avoided during certain exercises. These side effects pose a significant risk for individuals on treadmills, bicycles, or other similar sports equipment.

Certain types of medications may enhance performance, though often at some risk. The International Olympic Committee has banned the use of certain stimulants, pain relievers, steroids, diuretics, hormones, over-the-counter preparations (eg, Actifed, Sudafed, Dexatrim, Metabolife, Midol, Alka-Seltzer Plus, and Vicks Inhaler), and herbal teas with ephedrine.[20] Most of these drugs have acceptable alternatives. One class of drugs called *fluoroquinolones* has been linked to serious tendon injuries, often in the ankle, shoulder joint, or hand. When used in high doses, Cipro (a fluoroquinolone prescribed for infections) may have severe effects including tendon rupture.[21] Another class of drugs, *anti-inflammatory drugs* (available by prescription and over the counter), is commonly used to treat musculoskeletal pain and inflammation. These drugs are effective for relieving pain and inflammation but also can cause stomach bleeding and ulcers as well as permanent tissue damage with chronic use.[20] *Antianginal medications* used to control cardiovascular problems may also affect exercise tolerance. Beta-blockers, commonly used for high blood pressure and certain heart conditions, effectively lower the heart rate both at rest and during exercise.[20] Some eye drops used to treat glaucoma contain beta-blockers. Beta-blockers tend to keep the heart rate slower, so pulse rates do not reflect the level of exertion the body is experiencing. Measures other than pulse rate should be used to gauge exercise tolerance when working with individuals taking beta-blockers.

EXERCISE AND ALCOHOL

Alcohol should be avoided when an individual is engaged in aerobic exercise because of potential fluid loss and dehydration. Alcohol consumed during exercise decreases coordination and masks the warning signs of fatigue, resulting in subsequent injury.

Screening for Pre-Existing Medical Conditions

Anyone initiating a new exercise program should be screened for potential health problems. Screenings should include past and current medical information, medications (over the counter and prescription), family history of medical conditions, and lifestyle considerations: nutritional habits, exercise habits, stress, smoking, and alcohol consumption. Any contraindications to exercise indicate the need for a referral to the appropriate health professional. A helpful fitness-screening test is the Physical Activity Readiness Questionnaire (PAR-Q), which can be used to identify existing cardiovascular problems, orthopedic problems, and neurological problems.[22] Questions from the PAR-Q are listed in Table 4-3.

If the individual answers "yes" to one or more questions, this person should be seen by a physician before initiating a standard exercise program. If there are no positive responses, then this person is more likely to be safe starting an appropriate exercise program under supervision.

Preparation for Exercise

Warming up muscles prior to exercise can prevent *delayed-onset muscle soreness* (DOMS), the pain and discomfort felt in muscles following exercise.[23] Methods to decrease DOMS include the following: (1) beginning exercise gradually, (2) performing concentric (shortening) contractions before building in eccentric (lengthening) contractions; (3) performing a regular warm-up; and (4) performing moderate exercise whenever soreness is experienced.[23]

TABLE 4-3

PHYSICAL ACTIVITY READINESS QUESTIONNAIRE QUESTIONS

1. Has your doctor ever said you have heart trouble?
2. Do you frequently have pains in your heart and chest?
3. Do you often feel faint or have spells of severe dizziness?
4. Has a doctor ever said your blood pressure was too high?
5. Has your doctor ever told you that you have a bone or joint problem, such as arthritis, that has been aggravated by exercise or might be made worse with exercise?
6. Is there a good physical reason not mentioned here why you should not follow an activity program even if you wanted to?
7. Are you over age 65 and not accustomed to vigorous exercise?

Adapted from Thomas S, Reading J, Shephard RJ. Revision of the physical activity readiness questionnaire (PAR-Q). *Can J Spt Sci.* 1992;17(4):338–345.

STRETCHING TO WARM UP

Stretching warm-up exercises have the most benefit for activities involving bouncing and jumping, with a high intensity of *stretch-shortening cycles* (SSCs).[24] These types of activities, such as soccer and football, require a muscle-tendon unit that is compliant enough to store and release high amounts of elastic energy needed for powerful movements. With insufficient compliance, the muscle-tendon unit is easily injured. In activities with low intensity or limited SSCs, such as jogging, cycling, or swimming, there is less need for a compliant muscle-tendon unit. Stretching has little, if any, benefit as part of a warm-up exercise prior to participating in low intensity aerobic exercise.[24]

Various types of muscle stretching can be used to prepare for exercise. *Static stretch* involves placing the muscle at the end of its range and holding it for 15 to 30 seconds.[24] When performed correctly, static stretch effectively lengthens a tight muscle without injury. It can also be used to relieve muscle soreness and muscle spasms. *Proprioceptive neuromuscular facilitation* (PNF) is a technique that can optimize flexibility. With PNF, there is little danger of overstretching a muscle, and strength can be developed. Like static stretch, PNF may be used to relieve muscle soreness and cramps, but it uses a reflex rather than pressure to relax the muscle prior to elongating it. PNF uses a contract-relax technique that helps to relax the opposing muscle before contracting the desired muscle. With continuous repetitions, this technique is the most effective for lengthening muscle.[24] *Ballistic stretch* involves a rapid movement to quickly stretch a muscle to its full range. This technique prepares the muscle for sports involving vigorous movement, power, and speed. Once the ballistic stretch lengthens the muscle maximally, the individual holds the position for 15 to 30 seconds for optimal lengthening of the muscle.[24]

BALANCE OF ACTIVITY

The *Physical Activity Pyramid*[25,26] provides useful guidelines for balancing physical activity. The pyramid has four levels based upon the frequency of desired physical activity. The bottom, widest tier is described as *daily physical activity* or *incidental activity*. It is recommended that each individual perform 30 to 60 minutes of daily exercise, including stretching, walking, stair climbing, shopping, dancing, housework, gardening, and other light work. According to the pyramid, this is how most people should spend the majority of their time. The second tier, aerobic activity, should be performed 3 to 5 days per week at moderate-to-high intensities for an average of 30 minutes each day. Activity categories in this tier include brisk walking, running, jumping rope, swimming, bicycling, step aerobics, and other exercises of similar intensity. The third tier includes sports and active leisure activities, such as tennis, touch football, swimming, and weight training. This level of exercise should be performed 2 to 3 nonconsecutive days per week. For weight training, an individual should perform 1 to 3 sets of 8 to 12 repetitions of resistance exercise, using body weight, free weights, tubing, bands, or weight machines. The top tier of the Physical Activity Pyramid (Table 4-4) lists watching television, working at the computer, and playing board games, all sedentary activities that contribute little to physical fitness, but can contribute to mental fitness. In terms of physical activity, sedentary activities should be limited to allow time for more demanding types of exercise and activity.

WEIGHT TRAINING

Discretion should be used in selecting equipment used in weight training. There are advantages and disadvantages to various types of equipment selected for muscle strengthening and endurance. In comparing free weights and resistance machines, they vary in the requirements of the individual using the equipment, the benefits, the risks, and the costs. Free

TABLE 4-4

PHYSICAL ACTIVITY PYRAMID

Level of Activity	Frequency	Type of Exercise	Examples
I	Occasional	Sedentary activity	Television, computer, games.
II	2 to 3 times per week	Sports activities Leisure activities	Tennis, football, soccer Swimming, gardening, weight-lifting.
III	5 to 6 days per week	Planned aerobic activities	Thirty minutes total per day: walking 3 to 4 km, biking 12 to 16 km, stair climbing, skiing, cross-country running.
IV	Increased incidental activity	Continual movement throughout the day	Walking the dog, using the stairs rather than the elevator, not using the remote controls, getting up regularly from seated work or leisure activities.

Adapted from Rauramaa R, Leon AS. Physical activity and risk of cardiovascular disease in middle-aged individuals. *Sports Med.* 1996;22(2):65–69.

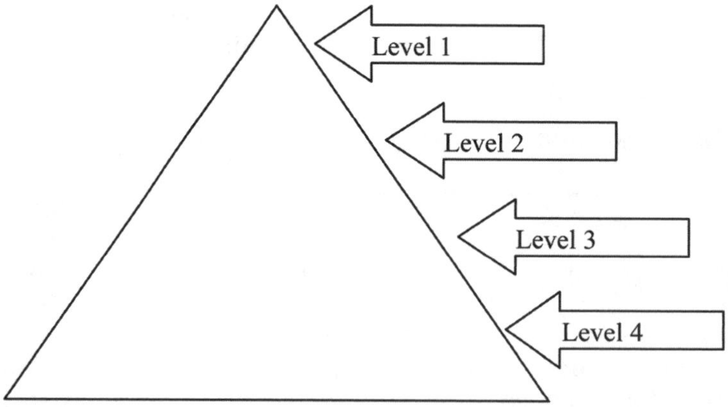

Level 1

Level 2

Level 3

Level 4

weights require adequate strength, balance, and coordination to handle and stabilize the weights without loss of postural control or dropping the weight. A spotter is indicated for safety purposes when using heavier weights. Free weights are more adaptive than resistance machines in terms of allowing free movement patterns and more activities closely resembling daily activities. As a low-cost alternative to weight machines, free weights tend to be durable, but also take more time for a complete workout than many weight machines. They can also create clutter if not stored properly. Resistance machines, the more costly alternative to free-weights, can isolate muscle activity and provide a safe environment for weight training. No spotter is needed, and changing weights on the machine is generally very simple. Movement is, however, generally restricted to certain ranges of motion and angles of movement. The equipment is often too expensive for an individual to own, so membership to a fitness club is an additional cost.

Exercise Prescription: The FITTE Formula

Exercises should be developed using the FITTE formula designed to progress an exercise program from appropriate levels of intensity and duration to more demanding exercises for improved fitness. The letters in the FITTE formula represents the following:

F = frequency of exercise (how often)
I = intensity of exercise (how hard)
T = time or duration of exercise (how long)
T = type of training (specificity of activity)
E = level of enjoyment

Ideally, the individual selects a favorite or highly enjoyable type of activity or sport (T = type, E = enjoyment) that can be performed at regular intervals (F = frequency) at a comfortable level of intensity (I = intensity, based on heart rate or 1 RM) for a desired duration (T = time). Using the FITTE formula

TABLE 4-5

BORG SCALE OF PERCEIVED EXERTION

Instructions for Borg Rating of Perceived Exertion (RPE) Scale:

The following scale is used to rate perception of physical exertion during physical activity. The perceived exertion should incorporate all feelings during exercise, including physical effort, fatigue, muscle pain, shortness of breath, and stress. Choose the number from the chart below that best reflects your level of physical exertion. Performing activities at level 13 helps to build endurance and working up to levels 15 to 17 result in greater muscle strength.

6	No exertion at all
7	Extremely light (7.5)
8	Very light
9	Very light exercise, like walking at a comfortable pace
9	Light
10	
11	
12	Somewhat hard
13	Somewhat hard to exercise, but it still feels okay
14	Hard (heavy)
15	
16	Very hard
17	Very strenuous, really pushing hard, feeling very heavy and very tired
18	Extremely hard
19	Maximal exertion, the most strenuous exercise they have ever experienced.

Adapted from Borg G. *Borg's Perceived Exertion and Pain Scales.* Champaign, Ill: Human Kinetics; 1998.

in conjunction with the Physical Activity Pyramid allows the clinician to design well-balanced and easy-to-follow exercise programs. The metabolic demands of each type of physical activity should also be taken into consideration when developing an exercise program. The Compendium of Physical Activities Tracking Guide lists MET values for over 600 different activities.[27]

General Exercise Principles

The body adapts to increasing levels of physical activity and "detrains" when exercise is not maintained over time. When prescribing an exercise program, lower levels of exertion are used to determine the body's tolerance to physical stress. Exercise tolerance must develop over time as the body builds the stamina and the strength to perform regular exercise with sufficient intensity and duration to increase cardiovascular endurance and strength.

Baseline levels of exercise may be 3 times per week at 5% to 60% intensity (maximum heart rate) for 30 minutes duration. At this level, the individual should be becoming familiar with the desired level of activity and determine the types of exercise that best suit personal needs and interests. While it is not advisable to begin an exercise program with vigorous exercise, the ultimate outcome should be moderate to vigorous activity most days of the week, according to the Surgeon General.[1]

The *overload principle* refers to the progressive increase in the amount of exercise needed to improve fitness levels. To experience overload, the individual must increase the frequency, intensity, or duration of exercise or modify the type of exercise to increase physiological demand (ie, to progress the exercise from lower frequencies, intensities, and durations to progressively higher demands in all three areas). Exercise prescription must be designed to optimally challenge the individual with sufficient frequency, intensity, and duration to promote improvements in muscular strength and endurance. For the intermediate athlete, exercise would be increased to 3 to 5 times per week at 60% to 75% maximum heart rate for 40 to 60 minutes. Higher levels of athletic performance would require increased training, such as increasing exercise to 5 to 6 times per week at 65% to 90% maximum heart rate for 60 to 120 minutes. Higher levels of performance would develop over time as the overload on muscles and the cardiovascular system would result in changes in both aerobic and anaerobic capacity, depending upon the type of exercise performed. The level of exercise an individual can tolerate can be judged using the Borg Scale of Perceived Exertion,[28] as discussed in Chapter 3 and illustrated in Table 4-5.

The *principle of specificity* refers to the training effects derived from different types of exercise. Low-resistance activities, such as long-distance walking, performed with increasing repetitions or for longer periods tend to increase endurance; on the other hand, progressively higher resistance activities, such as weight training, tend to build muscle strength. Another important aspect of prescribing exercise is the concept of periodization or prescribing exercise training to avoid over-training yet enhance performance accomplished through the manipulation of training frequency, intensity, duration, etc. Generally reserved for elite athletes, periodization involves alternating training loads to produce peak performance for a specific activity or training that involves progressive cycling of various aspects of a training program during a specific period. For example, periodization may be used in a resistance program to alternate high-resistance training with low-resistance training to improve different components of muscular fitness (eg, strength with higher resistance versus endurance with lower resistance). This system of training is typically divided up into cycles that may last as little as 7 days to as long as months according to the need to prepare for immediate competition versus the need to maintain fitness for subsequent seasons of competition. One benefit of periodization is reducing the boredom and monotony of performing the same exercise routine on a regular basis. The various types of health-related fitness (including cardiovascular endurance, muscle strength, muscular endurance, musculoskeletal flexibility, and body composition) and skill-related fitness (agility, speed, power, balance, and coordination) can be addressed using the principles of overload, specificity, and periodization.

Exercises That Can Cause Injury

Certain exercises that can predispose people to injury include the following:

- Hyperextending or overextending any joint
- Placing excessive stress on joints, such as performing double leg lifts
- Performing ballistic movements with the spine—either the low back or cervical spine
- Performing excessive hyperflexion of joints, potentially damaging ligaments, bursae, cartilage, and other joint structures
- Moving into positions that pinch nerves in the head, neck, trunk, and extremities

Before suggesting any specific exercises, all involved movements should be analyzed for stresses imposed on joints and soft tissue.

Hyperkinetic Conditions

Certain individuals are at risk of too much exercise. These individuals have a condition called *"activity nervosa"* characterized by too much activity and too little rest; this condition is often seen in conjunction with *anorexia nervosa* and *bulimia nervosa* (pathological eating disorders characterized by too little or too much eating, respectively).[29] Too much activity can result in joint injuries of the foot, ankle, or knee; stress fractures of the extremities; and/or muscle or connective tissue injuries such as shin splints, strained hamstring muscles, and calf pain. Individuals with psychological disorders, such as anorexia nervosa and body neurosis, also have an obsessive concern for an attractive body, often leading to excessive exercise accompanied by poor eating habits.

Special Considerations Before Prescribing an Exercise Program

Given the risks associated with exercise, it is advisable to get an informed consent from individuals who are receiving exercise advice or counseling. An informed consent provides sufficient information to enable individuals to make a well-informed decision about fitness testing and training. The informed consent form should provide clear explanations of the purpose, procedures, and risks associated with testing and exercise prescription as well as inclusion and exclusion criteria. Certain individuals may be precluded from exercise based on their medical histories, while other individuals may be at risk because of their age. Each individual should be screened for risk of harm from fitness training. The American College of Sports Medicine offers helpful information for screening and prescribing specific exercise programs for patients with chronic or debilitating disease in its book entitled, *Exercise Management of Persons with Chronic Diseases and Disabilities*.[30]

Individuals with high risk factors, as described by the American College of Sports Medicine, are those with unstable medical conditions that should result in exclusion from regular exercise, including cardiopulmonary disease and metabolic disease.[30] Other individuals who are excluded from exercise are those for whom the risk outweighs the benefits of exercise or those with pathologies exacerbated or worsened by exercise. Men 45 years and older and women 55 years or older are at moderate risk for exercise complications.[30] Also, younger individuals with two or more risk factors for coronary artery disease are at moderate risk for complications from exercise.[30] Physical therapists can modify exercise regimens to meet the needs of individuals at moderate risk for complications from exercise. Men younger than 45 and women younger than 55 (provided they have no more than one cardiovascular risk factor) are at little risk of cardiac problems associated with regular exercise provided it is properly prescribed for that individual.[30] Risks associated with exercise testing include risk of death (less than 0.01%), risk of myocardial infarction (0.04% or less), and risk of complications requiring hospitalization (0.02% or less).[30]

If fitness testing and training are conducted in a clinic or recreation center, emergency information should be clearly written with posted emergency plans. Also, the room layout should be designed for a safe exit, limiting the risk of accidents. Personnel should be certified in cardiopulmonary resuscitation in case of a medical emergency.

If equipment is used, it should be maintained, positioned for maximal visual supervision, and kept clean between uses.

Once the examiner has attained the desired performance on a fitness test, it is appropriate to discontinue testing, allowing the individual time to recover. Also, testing or exercise should be discontinued if the individual shows signs of distress, such as angina or chest pain, an excessive rise in blood pressure (BP) (systolic BP >260 mm Hg and diastolic BP >115 mm Hg), dizziness, lightheadedness, nausea, confusion, poor coordination, a pale complexion, cold and clammy hands, turning bluish in skin tone, severe fatigue, or changes in heart rhythm.[30] If there is a life-threatening situation, the emergency plan should be put into action. If the situation is not life threatening, the individual should be given time to cool down from the activity by slow steady movement, such as walking.

The range of mental and physical tests needed to assess an individual's fitness depends on the goals and types of fitness the person chooses to pursue. A physical therapist has the knowledge and skills to provide appropriate assessments and resources for both the mental and physical fitness of the people seeking their services. Referrals may be made to physicians or other health care providers, when appropriate. Fitness involves an individual's commitment, motivation, and responsibility for one's own well-being. One key physical therapy goal is to ensure that all individuals have the needed resources for maintaining fit minds and bodies.

Factors Influencing Maintenance of Physical Activity

Despite the proven benefits of physical activity, more than 50% of American adults do not get enough physical activity to provide health benefits, and 26% are not active at all in their leisure time.[1] Activity decreases with age, and sufficient activity is less common among women than men and among those with lower incomes and less education. Insufficient physical activity is not limited to adults. More than a third of young people in grades 9 to 12 do not regularly engage in vigorous physical activity.[1] Initiating an exercise program at any age requires significant contemplation and decision-making, while maintaining a program of physical activity requires some level of motivation. Initially, many believed that those who engaged in exercise on a regular basis did so because those individuals believed it would improve their health.

The Health Belief Model, developed in 1952 by Hochbaum, Kegels, and Rosenstock, was designed to test the hypothesis that health-related behaviors could be predicted based on an individual's beliefs about risks to their health and wellness.[31] This model has been used extensively in research exploring preventive health behavior. This theory has implications for providing health education about the benefits of exercise, the risks of not exercising, and the appropriate actions to take for age-appropriate exercise; however, little evidence supports this theory in terms of exercise adherence.

The Theory of Reasoned Action and Theory of Planned Behavior were developed by Ajzen and Fishbein in 1967[32] as an explanation of how attitudes or intentions are reflected in behavior. According to these theories, the most important determinant of a person's behavior is behavior intent. The individual's intention to perform a behavior, such as exercise, is a combination of attitude toward performing the behavior (ie, beliefs about the outcomes of the behavior and the value of these outcomes) and the subjective norm (ie, beliefs about what other people think the person should do, as well as the person's motivation to comply with the opinions of others). Two assumptions of this theory are (1) human beings are rational and make systematic use of information available to them and (2) people consider the implications of their actions before they decide to engage or not engage in certain behaviors. Given these two assumptions, the theory does not hold true for exercise behavior since the knowledge about the benefits of exercise is pervasive, yet not everyone engages in regular physical activity, as evidenced by the growing population of sedentary children and adults.

Social learning theory, also known as social cognitive theory, suggests that behavior change, such as exercising, is affected by environmental influences, personal factors, and attributes of the behavior itself.[31] A person must believe in his or her capability to perform the behavior (ie, the person must possess self-efficacy) and must perceive an incentive to do so (ie, the person's positive expectations from performing the behavior must outweigh the negative expectations). Additionally, a person must value the outcomes or consequences that he or she believes will occur because of performing a specific behavior or action. Several studies point to *self-efficacy* as the single most important characteristic that determines a person's behavior change, including exercise program participation. An individual's self-efficacy can be increased by providing clear instructions, adequate opportunities for skill development, training, and practice and by modeling the desired (and achievable) behavior in such a way that it evokes trust and respect from the individual.[33,34]

Factors that contribute to relapse include negative emotional or physiologic states, limited coping skills, social pressure, interpersonal conflict, limited social support, low motivation, high-risk situations, and stress. Principles of relapse prevention include identifying high-risk situations for relapse (eg, change in season, program location, instructor) and developing appropriate solutions (eg, finding a place to walk inside during bad weather, finding a stable location, or maintaining the same instructor).[33,34] Helping people distinguish between a "lapse" (eg, a few days of not participating in exercise) and a relapse (eg, an extended period of not exercising) is thought to improve adherence.

The Transtheoretical Model of Change provides a continuum of change through precontemplation, contemplation, preparation, action, and maintenance.[35] According to this theory, tailoring interventions to match a person's readiness or stage of change is essential. For example, for people who are not yet contemplating becoming more active, encouraging a step-by-step movement along the continuum of change may be more effective than encouraging them to move directly into action. Relapses are not uncommon, and maintaining a new action over a prolonged time may require motivators that are meaningful to the individual. The following questions can be used to guide others through the process of healthy exercise habits:

- *Precontemplation stage* – Goal: Individual will begin thinking about change.

  "What would have to happen for you to begin exercising?"

  "What warning signs would let you know that you need to begin exercising?"

  "Have you tried to exercise in the past?"

- *Contemplation stage* – Goal: Individual will examine benefits and barriers to change.

  "Why do you want to exercise at this time?"

  "What were the reasons for not exercising?"

  "What would keep you from exercising at this time?"

  "What are the barriers today that keep you from exercising?"

  "What might help you with that aspect?"

  "What people, programs, and behaviors have helped you exercise in the past?"

  "What would help you begin exercising at this time?"

- *Action stage* – Goal: Individual will develop self-efficacy in physical activity.

  "What questions do you have about exercise?"

  "Do you understand my explanations about exercise?"

  "Does my showing you how to do this exercise help you understand how it is done?"

  "Do you understand that repeated performance of this activity will help you learn it more easily? Practice is essential."

  "Do you feel comfortable performing exercise without any assistance?"

- *Maintenance stage* – Goal: Individual will integrate physical activity (exercise) into lifestyle.

  "Are you familiar with how to modify your physical activity for variation?"

  "Are you progressing or varying your exercises for interest?"

  "Would you like to do this activity with your friends and family?"

  "Does your community offer programs to support this activity?"

  "What motivates you to maintain your physical activity?"

A criticism of most theories and models of behavior change is that they emphasize individual behavior change processes and disregard psychosocial, cultural, and physical environmental influences on behavior. A health-promoting environment includes one that is sensitive to cultural issues, one that offers psychosocial support, as appropriate, and an environment that is conducive to a wide variety of activities, including outdoor recreational activities (bike paths, parks with walking paths, etc) and indoor facilities for times of inclement weather. Social support for physical activity or participation in an exercise program includes having a friend or family member provide company while walking, offer a ride to the activity, or provide emotional support during participation in the program. Sources of social support for physical activity include family members, friends, neighbors, coworkers, and exercise program leaders and participants. When developing exercise programs for each population, ecological perspectives should be considered because they influence health behaviors.

What motivates individuals to exercise? Some suggest that those who exercise regularly have either *intrinsic motivation* (ie, engaging in an activity for the

TABLE 4-6

BARRIERS TO EXERCISE ADHERENCE

Personal Barriers	Environmental Barriers
• Lack of time • Lack of motivation • Injury • Rapid fatigability • Misconceptions about exercise: "Animals sweat; men perspire; women do neither." • Physical discomfort (physical ailments including low-back injuries, knee joint degeneration, or restrictive and obstructive lung or heart disease, obesity, diabetes, peripheral neuropathies, other chronic illnesses) • Emotional discomfort (fear of injury, especially fear of falling in older adults) • Control in life • Attitude toward exercise • Assessment of the benefits of exercise • Self efficacy in performing exercises • Inertia: Difficulty changing lifestyle behaviors • Isolation	• Access: Some individuals do not have access to facilities to exercise. • Cost: Health clubs are too expensive for many people. • Climate: In northern climates, inclement weather and unsafe outdoor conditions due to ice and snow may cause many individuals, especially the elderly, to go without regular physical activity for 6 months or more. For those living in warmer regions, extremes of heat and humidity are obstacles to activity.

simple pleasure of it with no expectation of material rewards or external constraints) or *extrinsic motivation* (ie, engaging in the behavior as a means to an end and not at the sake of the activity itself).[36] However, relying exclusively on external influences can undermine intrinsic motivation, making it more difficult to maintain physical activity once the external influences are removed.[36] According to Dishman, who summarized the findings of numerous studies in his book *Advances in Exercise Adherence,* there are a number of diverse nonhealth-related participation motives for exercise.[37] According to Dishman, individuals are motivated to exercise by the desire to look good, lose weight, feel healthy, and improve fitness levels. Others have reported that individuals engage in regular exercise for fun because they enjoy the sensations that accompany the experience or the joy of being with other people. Motivators for exercise can be simply determined by asking the individual why he or she exercises. In addition to reinforcing motivators, as appropriate, the physical therapist should try to reduce the number of perceived barriers for maintaining adherence. Personal and environmental barriers that could interfere with exercise adherence are shown in Table 4-6.[8]

When prescribing exercises, physical therapists should be aware of potential barriers to exercise adherence and consider addressing any barriers that might interfere with their clients' success in both initiating and maintaining regular physical activity.

Community Support for Physical Activity

The most effective health behavior interventions occur on multiple levels: intrapersonal factors, interpersonal and group factors, institutional factors, community factors, and public policy. Interventions that simultaneously influence these multiple levels and multiple settings may be expected to lead to greater and longer-lasting changes and maintenance of existing health-promoting habits. Examples of how communities can meet the growing need for physical activity include the following:

- Provide safe, accessible, and attractive trails for walking and bicycling and sidewalks with curb cuts. This will make physical activity more enjoyable for everyone, including people with disabilities.
- Involve the widest possible variety of people, including people with disabilities, at all stages of planning and implementing community physical activity programs.

- Provide community-based physical activity programs that include aerobics, strength building, and flexibility. These programs should meet the needs of specific populations. These include racial and ethnic minority groups, women, older adults, people with disabilities, and low-income groups.
- Open schools for community recreation, form neighborhood watch groups to enhance safety, and encourage malls and other indoor or protected locations to provide safe places for walking in any weather.
- Ensure that facilities accommodate and encourage participation by people of all racial, ethnic, and income groups; women; older adults; and people with disabilities.
- Encourage health care providers to encourage people to add more physical activity into their lives.

Encourage employers to provide supportive worksite environments and policies that allow employees to incorporate moderate physical activity into their lives.

This is a promising area for the design of future intervention research to promote physical activity.

Summary

Physical therapists are uniquely qualified to provide a wide variety of exercises that meet the health-related fitness needs of individuals of all ages. While recognizing the basic principles of fitness training, physical therapists must be realistic about issues of exercise adherence and barriers to maintaining lifestyle habits that incorporate regular physical activity. Subsequent chapters provide information about exercise designed for specific populations, including children, adults, pregnant women, individuals performing manual labor, older adults, and individuals with impairments affecting their musculoskeletal, neuromuscular, and cardiopulmonary systems. Using key concepts of fitness training with a holistic health care approach can optimize preventive care.

References

1. United States Department of Health and Human Services. *Physical Activity and Health: A Report of the Surgeon General.* Sudbury, Md: Jones and Bartlett; 1998.
2. Cotman C, Engesser-Cesar C. Exercise enhances and protects brain function. *Exerc Sport Sci Rev.* 2002;30(2):75–79.
3. Tofler IR, Butterbaugh GJ. Developmental overview of child and youth sports for the twenty-first century. *Clin Sports Med.* 2005;24(4):783–804.
4. Koh JO, Cassidy JD, Watkinson EJ. Incidence of concussion in contact sports: a systematic review of the evidence. *Brain Injury.* 2003;17(10):901–917.
5. Kraus JF, Conroy C. Mortality and morbidity from injuries in sports and recreation. *Annu Rev Public Health.* 1984;5:163–192.
6. Lambeck, Johan Halliwick Method, course outlines 1996–2000.
7. Pesce T. Hippotherapy: horses provide sensory stimulation to enhance human muscle stability. Available at: http://bizntech.rutgers.edu/assayist/summer_2002/media/pesce.pdf. Accessed October 15, 2005.
8. Liu Y, Mimura K, Wang L, Ikuda K. Physiological benefits of 24-style Taijiquan exercise in middle-aged women. *J Physiol Anthropol Appl Human Sci.* 2003;22(5):219–225.
9. Fong SM, Ng GY. The effects on sensorimotor performance and balance with tai chi training. *Arch Phys Med Rehabil.* 2006;87(1):82–87.
10. Zhang JG, Ishikawa-Takata K, Yamazaki H, Morita T, Ohta T. The effects of Tai Chi Chuan on physiological function and fear of falling in the less robust elderly: an intervention study for preventing falls. *Arch Gerontol Geriatr.* 2006;42(2):107–116.
11. Choi JH, Moon JS, Song R. Effects of Sun-style Tai Chi exercise on physical fitness and fall prevention in fall-prone older adults. *J Adv Nurs.* 2005;51(2):150–157.
12. Herbal Healing. Introducing yoga. Available at: http://www.herbalhealing.co.uk/yoga_intro.htm. Accessed on February 6, 2006.
13. Parshad O. Role of yoga in stress management. *West Indian Med J.* 2004;53(3):191–194.
14. Sherman KJ, Cherkin DC, Erro J, Miglioretti DL, Deyo RA. Comparing yoga, exercise, and a self-care book for chronic low back pain: a randomized, controlled trial. *Ann Intern Med.* 2005;143(12):849–856.
15. Vedanthan PK, Kesavalu LN, Murthy KC, et al. Clinical study of yoga techniques in university students with asthma: a controlled study. *Allergy Asthma Proc.* 1998;19(1):3–9.
16. Tucker R, Rauch L, Harley YX, Noakes TD. Impaired exercise performance in the heat is associated with an anticipatory reduction in skeletal muscle recruitment. *Pflugers Arch.* 2004;448(4):422–430.
17. Gavhed D, Mäkinen T, Holmér I, Rintamäki H. Face cooling by cold wind in walking subjects. *Intern J Biometeorol.* 2003;47(3):148–155.
18. Position of the American Dietetic Association, Dietitians of Canada, and the American College of Sports Medicine. Nutrition and athletic performance. *J Am Dietetic Assoc.* 2000;100:1543–1556.
19. Silver M. Use of ergogenic aids by athletes. *J Am Acad Orthop Surg.* 2001;9(1):61–70.

20. Khaliq Y, Zhanel GG. Musculoskeletal injury associated with fluoroquinolone antibiotics. *Clin Plas Surg.* 2005;32(4):495–502.
21. Thomas S, Reading J, Shephard RJ. Revision of the physical activity readiness questionnaire (PAR-Q). *Can J Sport Sci.* 1992;17(4):338–345.
22. Thomas S, Reading J, Shephard RJ. Revision of the Physical Activity Readiness Questionnaire (PAR-Q). *Can J Sport Sci.* 1992;17(4):338-345.
23. Witvrouw E, Mahieu N, Danneels L, McNair P. Stretching and injury prevention: an obscure relationship. *Sports Med.* 2004;34(7):443–449.
24. Etnyre BR, Abraham LD. Gains in range of ankle dorsiflexion using three popular stretching techniques. *Am J Phys Med.* 1996;65(4):189–196.
25. United States Department of Agriculture. Physical activity pyramid. Available at: http://www.mypyramid.gov/pyramid/physical_activity.html. Accessed October 15, 2005.
26. Jump Start Eat Smart: A guide to healthy eating and healthy living. My physical activity pyramid. Available at: http://www.goerie.com/nie_jumpstart/my_physical_activity_pyramid.html. Accessed October 15, 2005.
27. The Compendium of Physical Activity Tracking Guide. Available at: http://prevention.sph.sc.edu/tools/docs/documents_compendium.pdf. Accessed October 15, 2005.
28. Dawes HN, Barker KL, Cockburn J, Roach N, Scott O, Wade D. Borg's rating of perceived exertion scales: do the verbal anchors mean the same for different clinical groups? *Arch Phys Med Rehabil.* 2005;86(5):912–916.
29. Solenberger SE. Exercise and eating disorders: a 3-year inpatient hospital record analysis. *Eating Behaviors.* 2001;2(2):151–168.
30. American College of Sports Medicine. *Exercise Management of Persons with Chronic Diseases and Disabilities.* Champaign, Ill: Human Kinetics; 1997.
31. American Society on Aging, Centers for Disease Control and Prevention. Planning and evaluating health promotion programs: the role of theory in a logic model. Available at: http://www.asaging.org/cdc/module7/phase5/phase5_10.cfm. Accessed October 15, 2005.
32. Bledsoe LK. Smoking cessation: an application of theory of planned behavior to understanding progress through stages of change. *Addict Behav.* 2006;31(7):1271–1276.
33. Bandura A. Self-efficacy: toward a unifying theory of behavioral change. Psychol Rev. 1977;84(2):191–215
34. Marcus BH, Selby VC, Niaura RS, Rossi JS. Self-efficacy and the stages of exercise behavior change. *Res Q Exerc Sport.* 1992;63(1):60–66.
35. Prochaska JO, Velicer WF. The transtheoretical model of health behavior change. *Am J Health Promot.* 1997;12(1):38–48.
36. King A, Friedman F, Marcus B, et al. Harnessing motivational forces in the promotion of physical activity: the community health advice by telephone (CHAT) project. *Health Edu Res.* 2002;17(5):627–636.
37. Dishman RK. *Advances in Exercise Adherence.* Champaign, Ill: Human Kinetics; 1994.
38. Fletcher G, Trejo JF. Why and how to prescribe exercise: overcoming the barriers. *Cleve Clin J Med.* 2005;72(8):645–649,653–654,656.

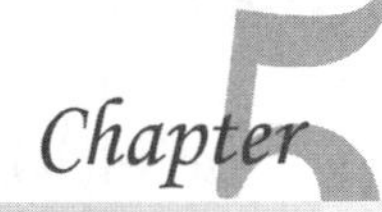

Screening for Health, Fitness, and Wellness

Catherine Rush Thompson, PhD, MS, PT

"Healing is a matter of time, but it is sometimes also a matter of opportunity."

~HIPPOCRATES

Screening Versus Examination

Screening is essentially checking for pathology when there are no symptoms of disease. A screening often includes simple measures to identify risk factors for illness and is used to determine the need for further examination. According to the *Guide to Physical Therapist Practice,*[1] common screening activities include (1) screening for lifestyle factors (eg, amount of exercise, stress, weight) leading to increased risk for serious health problems, (2) screening posture for scoliosis, (3) identifying high risk factors for slipping, tripping, or falling of older adults, and (4) performing prework screenings to identify risk factors in the workplace and the health status of potential workers.

Examination in physical therapy practice includes taking the client's history, reviewing the body systems for potential pathology, and performing specific tests and measures guided by the initial screening, patient/client history, professional judgment, and relevant clinical findings. The initial examination of a client involves screening but also incorporates specific tests and measures leading to a physical therapy diagnosis and/or a referral to another practitioner.

Evaluation, according to the *Guide to Physical Therapist Practice,*[1] is "the process in which the physical therapist makes clinical judgments based on data gathered during the examination. This process also may identify possible problems that require consultation with or referral to another provider."[1] Thus, screening a patient is always the initial step in physical therapy management to determine if further examination is needed or if referral is more appropriate. Screening for health, fitness, and wellness provides physical therapists with opportunities to prevent illness and refer potential pathologies before they become complicated and difficult to manage. Primary prevention involves screening at-risk populations for conditions that are not evident and helping the client to develop and maintain healthy lifestyle habits to ward off disease. Once risks for physical or mental health problems are identified, physical therapists can perform more extensive examinations to determine physical therapy needs and refer their clients to the appropriate professionals for health issues outside the scope of physical therapy practice.

Interviewing the Client

NONVERBAL COMMUNICATION

Appropriate interpersonal skills are essential to developing rapport with an individual during the screening process. The interviewer must be a good listener and have the ability to focus energy, attention, and thoughts on what the individual is saying. Effective attending skills include displaying an appropriate level of energy, using nonverbal communication that invites an open conversation, using appropriate types of questions to initiate conversation, active listening, and projecting clinical competence. When interviewing a person, the physical therapist needs to project a positive demeanor because first impressions are highly influential. The appropriate level of energy requires focusing both physical and mental energy on the individual speaking. Using a patient- or client-centered focus is an effective interviewing skill.[2] Too much energy may be intimidating; too little energy may suggest disinterest. The physical therapist must be able to read the patient's nonverbal communication to gauge what level of energy is optimal for interaction. Words have a 7% impact on interpersonal communication, and the tone of voice used in asking questions has a 38% impact; however, body language has a 55% impact on message delivery.[2] The unconscious mind automatically understands the meaning of every gesture, posture, and voice inflection. Five skills, if used effectively, can improve the enjoyment and outcome of interpersonal communication: (1) eye contact, (2) body position, (3) proper distance between the interviewer and interviewee, (4) gestures, and (5) facial expression.[3] There are some variations in communication across cultures, so the physical therapist must develop some level of cultural competency before interviewing individuals with different ethnic backgrounds.

Eye Contact

Eye contact is the most common and powerful nonverbal behavior. Optimal eye contact involves looking directly at the interviewee when speaking or listening, conveying sincerity and respect for the other person. Direct eye contact, however, is not always culturally appropriate. People in other parts of the world, including Latin America, Africa, and Asia, may believe that direct eye contact is a sign of disrespect.[4] In Arab countries, however, prolonged direct eye contact is a gauge of trustworthiness.[4] Poor eye contact, excessive self-consciousness, negative self-evaluation, and self-preoccupation are common characteristics of shyness.[5] If the interviewer suspects that an individual is shy, sensitivity to shyness can be demonstrated by glancing briefly around the eyes instead of looking directly into the pupils. Since eye contact expresses intimacy, prolonged eye contact can provide the interviewee with a sense of "safety" sharing private concerns.[6] However, uninterrupted eye contact may be too personal. It is important that the interviewer gauge the duration of eye contact based on other components of the interviewee's body language. Avoiding eye contact has negative implications, suggesting guilt, fear, or dishonesty. To make the interviewee more relaxed and comfortable, the interviewer must be careful to avoid staring, squinting, or excessively blinking during the interview.[6] Generally, more eye contact is experienced when topics are comfortable for both the interviewee and interviewer. Steady eye contact without staring indicates interest in the individual and pupil dilation indicates keen interest. Eye shifts indicate the individual may be processing or recalling information; however, darting eyes suggest that the individual is excited, worried, or wearing eye contacts. Furrowing of the brow suggests that the individual is perplexed or trying to avoid a topic. Staring with the eyes fixed on an object or lowering the eyes down and away indicate preoccupation with another concern or discomfort discussing a topic. Finally, lack of eye contact projects many possible interpretations, including respect, avoidance of interaction, discomfort, embarrassment, or preoccupation with another concern.[6]

Body Position

Ideally, the interview should be conducted with both the interviewer and interviewee comfortably seated with the eyes at the same level and shoulders squarely facing each other. Certain body positions confer possible meanings that should be taken into account during the interview process. A more open body posture (arms relaxed at both sides) is more welcoming than a closed body posture (arms crossed over the chest).[7] While a stiff posture indicates tension, anxiety, or concern, steady movement, such as rocking or squirming, suggests the person may be concerned, worried, or anxious. Leaning forward indicates eagerness, attentiveness, and openness to communication, but a person who is slouched, stooped, or turned away from the interviewer may be sad, ambivalent, or unreceptive to the interchange.[7] Good posture reflects confidence and assurance that the individual is paying attention to the information shared. Like eye contact, body posture can offer significant information regarding the interviewee's comfort level and general attitude during the screening process.

Distance

Physical distance between the physical therapist and interviewee is another key factor for interpersonal communication. Some individuals feel comfortable with physical proximity (one arm's length), while others may be offended. For example, southern Europeans (Italy and Greece) generally believe that touch is acceptable; however, individuals in northern Europe (England, France, and the Netherlands) expect little, if any, contact.[4]

Gestures

Gesturing is used instinctively to emphasize important points. While the lack of body gestures signals anger or lack of openness, gestures such as playing with clothing, hair, or jewelry are distracting. Again, cultural differences need to be considered. For example, Japanese men will tip the head backward and audibly suck air in through the teeth to signal "no" or that "something is very difficult." A Japanese gesture saying "I do not know," or "I don't understand," or "No, I am undeserving" is waving the hand back and forth in front of one's own face (palm outward).[4] The Taiwanese gesture to indicate "no" is to lift one's hand to face level, palm facing outward, and move it back and forth, sometimes with a smile.

Facial Expression

Incongruities between facial expression and verbal expression are not uncommon and often confound interpersonal communication. If facial expressions conflict with verbal messages, the listener will believe the nonverbal communication over what is said by the speaker. Certain facial expressions, such as wrinkling the forehead or speaking with a pursed or tight-lipped mouth, can indicate tension.[3] If someone says that she is fine but has a tense expression, more questions should be asked to elicit additional information. Yawning is an obvious sign of boredom or tiredness. Rolling the eyes can be a dismissive expression that has a negative effect on communication. Any of these facial cues should be carefully noted. Again, cultural differences exist. While many facial expressions tend to be universal, their interpretation may vary from one culture to the next. Generally, anxiety, fear, surprise, or joy can be easily observed in any individual; however, this is not always the case.

VERBAL COMMUNICATION

Nonverbal communication plays a key role in the interview process, but verbal communication is critical for eliciting responses needed for a medical history and identification of health risks. It is helpful to initiate the interview using open, general questions, gently put, to elicit sincere behavior from interviewees, allowing the individual the freedom to respond with presupposed answers. Open-ended questions generally begin with words like "how" or "why" and cannot be answered by a simple "yes" or "no." For example, the interviewer might ask the individual "How might your family health history impact your health status?" Responses to these broader questions provide an opportunity for the interviewee to express concerns and suggest safe issues to discuss. Closed-ended questions may be used to solicit simple "yes" or "no" responses related to specific screening questions. More directed questions are used to focus responses, such as identifying specific dates for previous health conditions. When the information is sensitive, the interviewer can provide an example that allows the respondent an opportunity to answer without embarrassment. For example, the therapist could state, "Women your age commonly have problems with controlling their bladder. Is this a problem that concerns you?"

Awareness of the individual's cultural background is critical to understanding the other person's point of view and relevant issues; the LEARN model, which emphasizes listening and sharing similarities and differences, can be used to effectively used to overcome cultural communication barriers.[5] The acronym LEARN represents the following key components of the model:

- L = Listen with sympathy and understanding to the client's perception of the problem.
- E = Explain your perceptions of the problem.
- A = Acknowledge and discuss the differences and similarities.
- R = Recommend a course of action.
- N = Negotiate an agreement.

Using the LEARN model enables the interviewer to effectively communicate with various individuals.

The purpose of active listening is to understand what the other person is meaning. The meaning is conveyed in the content (who, what, when, where, how, and why) as well as the affect of the person (emotions and feelings accompanying the content). An effective listener can understand the meaning of what is said and communicate that the information is important. The listener must take into account the speaker's frame of reference, congruous or incongruous verbal and nonverbal communication, previous patterns or experiences with this individual, and key themes or patterns of what is said. For example, if the individual repeatedly complains of pain while forcibly smiling, this incongruity suggests further exploration of pain issues. If the meaning is understood, the listener should try to be empathetic to elicit additional information. Most people speak at the rate of 110 to 140 words per minute, yet think at seven times that rate.[6] Full attention must be given to what is said. Throughout the interview, the interviewer may restate or summarize the interviewee's comments to confirm the meaning of what has been said. Both verbal and nonverbal agreement with these summary statements can give a clear indication of comprehension of what has been said by the interviewee. During the summation of discussion, the individual may be invited to elaborate on information shared to clarify any misunderstandings.

Projecting professionalism and clinical competence increases the sense of assurance during the interview process. Characteristics of professionalism include effective communication, professional appearance, timeliness, respect, and displaying tactful and courteous behavior.[2,7] Evidence of academic degrees, professional degrees, clinical specialist certifications, and professional memberships gives the individual more confidence in the interviewer's clinical competence and professionalism. A private area for the interview and a well-organized space for the screening process further provide the interviewee with a positive impression.

Screening for Mental Health

Mental health is directly or indirectly influenced by multiple factors, including memory, interpersonal relationships at work and at home, coping and stress management, social support, financial support, education, vocation, leisure activities, and personal values. Since genetics play a key role in mental health problems, family history of mental health dysfunction should be noted. Clues that suggest possible mental health problems include a negative affect, depression, anxiety, fear, aggression, or rage. Depressed patients tend to have reduced restlessness (leg and hand movements), reduced communication (fewer words and less gesturing), decreased active listening, and reduced eagerness (yes-nodding and no-shaking).[8] In general, depressed individuals display slowness of thought and speech, impaired ability to concentrate, and decreased motor activity. According to the National Institute of Mental Health, an estimated 5.3% of adults, or 17 million people, suffer from depression, and approximately 4% of adolescents get seriously depressed.[9] Gender differences exist with 12% of women and 7% of men experiencing depression at any one time.[9] Depression is a significant psychosocial problem affecting individuals' health, fitness, and wellness and, ultimately, their quality of life. A two-question initial screening test for depression has been developed and validated based on the *Diagnostic and Statistical Manual of Mental Disorders*[10] established criteria for the diagnosis of depression. The two questions are as follows:

1. During the past month, have you often been bothered by feeling down, depressed, or hopeless?
2. During the past month, have you often been bothered by little interest or pleasure in doing things?

A positive response to either of the two following questions is extremely sensitive and identifies more than 90% of patients with major depression. However, it is only approximately 60% specific and requires confirmation using a detailed clinical interview or more specific diagnostic tools.[10] If the screener suspects that the individual is experiencing mental health problems, it is appropriate to do a stress assessment and consider a referral for psychological or social services, as appropriate. Clear documentation of observations is useful for future reference.

Motor behaviors suggesting other types of mental health dysfunction include restlessness or performing unusual, purposeless movements. Those describing nonexistent sounds most likely have mental problems and need a referral for further examination. Additionally, those with memory problems or problems performing tasks that require concentration may need a more thorough psychological examination.[10] Normal individuals are motivated to survive, so those who suggest or exhibit self-harm may have mental illness. Signs of poor mental health include an obsession with negative thoughts and negative consequences, loss of creative and imaginative thoughts and ideas, unclear decision making, or a foggy mental state. Other characteristics of mental health disorders include unrealistic thoughts and perceptions, inappropriate emotions, and unpredictable behavior (as compared to the social norm).

Stress Assessment

During the interview, it is important to note stressors commonly affecting health status. Stressors include recent life changes or losses (eg, loss of family or friends, relocation of home and/or business), changes in marital status, or significant financial concerns. Responses to life changes vary, as each individual's perception of a stressful situation differs. Some individuals may not show any symptoms of stress on the surface but may have emotional or physical changes that may not be easily detectable. Other individuals may demonstrate more obvious problems, such as unusual behaviors or mannerisms requiring further

TABLE 5-1

RED FLAGS FOR SUBSTANCE ABUSE PROBLEMS

- Frequent absences from school or work
- History of frequent trauma or accidental injuries
- Depression or anxiety
- Labile or variable hypertension
- Gastrointestinal symptoms, such as stomach ache, diarrhea, or weight changes
- Sexual dysfunction
- Sleep disorders
- Mild tremor
- Odor of alcohol on breath
- Enlarged, tender liver
- Nasal irritation (suggestive of cocaine insufflation)
- Eye irritation (suggestive of exposure to marijuana smoke)
- Labile or variable blood pressure, tachycardia or increased heart rate (suggestive of alcohol withdrawal)
- "Aftershave/mouthwash" syndrome (to mask the odor of alcohol)
- Odor of marijuana on clothing
- Signs of chronic obstructive pulmonary disease, hepatitis B or C, HIV infection

Adapted from Schulz JE, Parran T Jr. Principles of identification and intervention. In: Graham AW, Schultz TK, Wilford BB, eds. *Principles of Addiction Medicine.* 2nd ed. Chevy Chase, Md: American Society of Addiction Medicine; 1998:250–251.

psychological examination. Convenient psychological measures of stress include the *Holmes and Rahe social readjustment rating scale* (commonly used for adults) and Yeaworth's *the adolescent life change event scale,* a questionnaire listing personal, social, and family changes believed stressful to adolescents.[11,12] All of these assessments provide the clinician with valuable information about the interviewee's recent stressors and the likelihood of illness.

While minor psychological stress is ever present, unrelenting stress can be extremely dangerous. Adrenaline, noradrenaline, and cortisol released into the bloodstream increase heart rate, increase respiration, dilate the pupils, and flush the skin. The body is aroused, and rational thinking may be altered. This response is adaptive for primitive survival instincts but is not functional in inescapable stressful situations that can mount over time. While acute stress responses may temporarily disable rational responses, chronic stress can impair both psychological and physiological functioning. Physiological measures for acute stress may be a part of a more extensive examination, including electrocardiography (ECG) (measurement of heart electrical activity) and the galvanic skin response (GSR) (measurement of the skin resistance to the passage of electric current).[12] Both of these measures can be useful in detecting the less dramatic physiological changes occurring with stress. Over time, increased blood pressure at rest may result from chronic stress. Individuals with hypertension need an immediate referral for appropriate intervention. While stress measures are useful for identifying a variety of stress factors potentially contributing to illness, there are very few comprehensive measures designed to identify how well individuals address the multiple dimensions of wellness.

Screening for Substance Abuse

Physical therapists may note stress behaviors in their clients and suspect abuse or violence. Table 5-1 lists some of the red flags commonly seen when individuals are engaged in chronic substance abuse.[13]

If alcohol use disorder is suspected, specific questions are recommended. Several screening tools are available, but the CAGE questionnaire is the most efficient and widely used.[14] CAGE is a mnemonic for a questionnaire that asks about attempts to *C*ut down on drinking, *A*nnoyance with criticisms about drinking, *G*uilt about drinking, and using alcohol as an *E*ye opener.[14] The test takes approximately one minute to complete and, while it does not diagnose alcoholism or problem drinking, it should prompt further examination.

Another shorter screening test involves only two questions: "In the past year, have you ever drunk or used drugs more than you meant to?" and "Have you felt you wanted or needed to cut down on your drinking or drug use in the past year?" In one study, at least one positive response detected current substance-use disorders with nearly 80% sensitivity and specificity. As with all screening tests, performance varies with the prevalence of substance abuse in the particular population screened.[14]

Screening for Physical Abuse

Oftentimes, individuals come to a screening to get help but are embarrassed to admit that they are experiencing significant psychosocial problems. It is important to screen for possible violence since an individual may be experiencing significant stress in personal relationships. Since physical, sexual, and verbal abuse are prevalent in our society, a screening of intimate partner violence is essential. The following three questions can open up discussion about potentially life-threatening situations and address the issue of intimate partner violence[15]:

1. "Have you been hit, kicked, punched, or otherwise hurt by someone in the past year?"
2. "Do you feel safe in your current relationship?"
3. "Is there a partner from a previous relationship who is making you feel unsafe now?"

A positive screen is a "yes" answer to any of the three questions. This information should be shared with the individual's physician immediately. Chapter 11 on Health Protection discusses some of the issues associated with suicide, violence against intimate partners, sexual violence, child abuse, elder abuse, and alcoholism.

Screening for a Balanced Lifestyle

Clinicians who anticipate a long-term relationship with clients may choose to conduct a wellness screening for a more holistic approach to health care and prevention practice. A wellness screening includes a broad range of questions reviewing social wellness, physical wellness, emotional wellness, career/leisure wellness, intellectual wellness, environmental wellness, and spiritual wellness. This type of screening tool could prove especially helpful in educating the client about balancing the multiple dimensions in life. One general survey, developed at the University of Wisconsin–Seven Points, is brief, educational, and helpful in identifying potential risks or concerns affecting the individual's life (Table 5-2).[16]

This survey may be administered as part of an interview or may be filled out by the individual independently then shared in the screening. Scoring involves looking at the number of answers that are marked as "always," indicating consistency between statements and the respondent's agreement with that statement. On this survey, overall wellness is accomplished when the individual's self-perception matches the criteria for each wellness dimension with an "always" response. If the individual is seeking ways to achieve a more balanced life for wellness, the survey's statements provide some ideas for reflection and guidance to promote well-being. The clinician may make referrals, as needed, to spiritual, social, psychological, or other professionals to ensure adequate resources for the individual to achieve wellness.

Screening for Physical Wellness

Physical therapists are experts in physical health and wellness and have a variety of tools to examine the musculoskeletal, neuromuscular, cardiopulmonary, and integumentary systems. It is helpful to have a comprehensive physical checklist to address possible risk factors for pathology affecting all body systems. After a quick review, the physical therapist is alerted to potential risk factors and the need for a more complete examination to address areas of concern. Based on the client's history, age, and risk for pathology, the clinician can focus on the aspects most relevant to the client. For example, it is important to screen a young child for immunizations, a young adult for reproductive systems, and an older adult for factors that contribute to falls, such as poor vision and muscle weakness. The physical health screening checklist[17] identifies risk factors for specific body systems, taking into consideration the individual's family history and personal health habits. The checklist may be done as part of an interview or completed by the individual before a physical screening. If a person completing the checklist does not understand the questions, this situation offers the clinician an opportunity to educate the client regarding those aspects that are not clearly understood.

The *physical health screening checklist* (Table 5-3) notes the most common illnesses affecting Americans, including hypertension, stroke, metabolic syndrome, cancer, diabetes, allergies, arthritis, alcoholism, mental illness, seizure disorders, and kidney disease. Questions throughout the checklist provide additional opportunities to identify potential risk factors associated with specific body systems.

General Health

Observation of the individual's overall appearance provides various indicators of general health. If the person is obese, this person is at risk for a variety of health conditions and needs a referral for a more extensive examination. The checklist offers common signs and symptoms indicating the need for a medical referral if they are chronic and unexplained. These clinical manifestations include fatigue, fever, weakness, and malaise and are commonly associated with a variety of systemic diseases.

TABLE 5-2

ARE YOU BALANCING THE SEVEN DIMENSIONS OF WELLNESS?

INSTRUCTIONS: Please answer each statement honestly based upon your current status. This wellness assessment provides information about your awareness of and making conscious choices toward a balanced and healthy lifestyle. Check the response that best matches your current perception of how each statement relates to your life. Consider each aspect of wellness as a resource for improving your overall wellness and health.

SOCIAL WELLNESS

Social wellness is the process of creating and maintaining healthy relationships.

I communicate honestly and directly.	____never ____often or ____always
I resolve conflict in a healthy, timely manner.	____never ____often or ____always
I give and take equally in cooperative relationships.	____never ____often or ____always
I treat every person with respect.	____never ____often or ____always
I use my economic resources to support socially responsible choices.	____never ____often or ____always
I maintain a strong mutual, interdependent social support system.	____never ____often or ____always

Comments:

PHYSICAL WELLNESS

Physical wellness is the process of having a flexible, aerobically fit body.

I maintain a consistent exercise regime consisting of flexibility and muscular strengthening exercises and at least 30 minutes of aerobic exercise daily.	____never ____often or ____always
I balance the amount of food I eat with the amount of exercise.	____never ____often or ____always
My body fat is in a healthy range for my age and no more than 20% of my calories are coming from fat.	____never ____often or ____always
I manage stress and do some activity that elicits the "relaxation response" for at least 15 min/day.	____never ____often or ____always
I abstain from addictions including caffeine, nicotine, alcohol, and drugs both over the counter (OTC) and illicit.	____never ____often or ____always
I take proactive steps to avoid and prevent injury, illness, and disease (including STDs).	____never ____often or ____always

Comments:

EMOTIONAL WELLNESS

Emotional wellness is the process of creating and maintaining a positive, realistic self-concept and enthusiasm about life.

I recognize that I create my own feelings and am responsible for them.	____never ____often or ____always
I can express all ranges of feelings including hurt, sadness, fear, anger, and joy and manage related behaviors in a healthy way.	____never ____often or ____always
I accept and appreciate my worth as a human being.	____never ____often or ____always
I avoid blaming other people or situations for my feelings and behaviors.	____never ____often or ____always
I can realistically assess my limitations and cope effectively with stress and ego.	____never ____often or ____always

Comments:

CAREER/LEISURE WELLNESS

Career/leisure wellness is the process of making and maintaining choices that are meaningful and contribute to your personal growth as well as work.

I have chosen a job role that I enjoy and that matches my values and lifestyle.	____never ____often or ____always
I have developed marketable job skills and keep them current.	____never ____often or ____always
I balance work with play and other aspects of my life.	____never ____often or ____always
I earn enough money to meet my needs and save to provide economic stability for myself and/or family.	____never ____often or ____always
My work benefits individuals and or society.	____never ____often or ____always

Comments:

(continued)

TABLE 5-2 *(continued)*

ARE YOU BALANCING THE SEVEN DIMENSIONS OF WELLNESS?

INTELLECTUAL WELLNESS

Intellectual wellness is the process of using your mind to create a greater understanding of yourself and the universe.

I view learning as a lifelong process and question my views and change them in accordance with new information.	____never ____often or ____always
I listen to ideas different from my own and constantly re-examine my judgments on social, cultural, gender, race, ethical, and political issues.	____never ____often or ____always
I take risks, learn from my mistakes, and question authority.	____never ____often or ____always
I appreciate and explore the creative arts of theater, dance, music, and expressive art.	____never ____often or ____always
I seek opportunities that challenge my critical thinking skills.	____never ____often or ____always

Comments:

ENVIRONMENTAL WELLNESS

Environmental wellness is the process of making choices to create sustainable human and ecological communities, improving qualities in air, water, land, and space.

I am moving toward limiting my acquisitions to those that contribute to sustainability.	____never ____often or ____always
I eat low on the food chain and minimize eating products that require a disproportionately high cost to deliver.	____never ____often or ____always
I live in harmony with nature and the universe.	____never ____often or ____always
I take personal and social responsibility for creating sustainable communities with chemically free air, water, and soil.	____never ____often or ____always
I recognize my impact on the environment and take deliberate action to minimize my impact, including responsible population control.	____never ____often or ____always

Comments:

SPIRITUAL WELLNESS

Spiritual wellness is the process of "experiencing life" while seeking meaning and purpose in human existence. Spirituality allows one to have consistency between values and behaviors.

I have a deep appreciation for the depth of life, death, and understanding universal human connection or consciousness.	____never ____often or ____always
I recognize that there are many spiritual paths and that every spiritual tradition recognizes and teaches basic precepts or laws of wise and conscious human conduct.	____never ____often or ____always
I integrate my "spiritual practice" within everyday life of work, family, and relationships.	____never ____often or ____always
I appreciate the individual uniqueness, diversity, and need for connected-ness among all people.	____never ____often or ____always
I have a consistency between my beliefs, values, and behaviors.	____never ____often or ____always

Comments:

Adapted from School of Health Promotion and Human Development. Employee wellness. University of Wisconsin – Stevens Point. Available at: http://cps.uwsp.edu/hphd/wellquiz. Accessed on October 15, 2005.

TABLE 5-3
PHYSICAL HEALTH SCREENING

Family History

Do you have a family history of:
____Blood pressure
____Stroke
____Cancer
____Diabetes
____Allergies
____Arthritis
____Alcoholism
____Mental illness
____Seizure disorders
____Kidney disease
____Other

General Health

Weight:____
(normal range ___, overweight___, underweight___)
____Fatigue
____Weakness
____Malaise
____Fever
____Illness

Immunizations

Are immunizations current? Yes____ No_____
What is your travel history? ____________________

____

Birth History

Vaginal:_______
C-section:____________
Full-term? Yes____ No____
Any complications:____________________

Medications

List prescription and over-the-counter drugs: ________

____

Medical History

Serious accidents (date, injury, length of care): _____

____

Hospitalizations (date, injury, length of care): ______

____

Surgeries (date, injury, length of care): ____________

____

Serious illness (date, injury, length of care): ________

____

Skin

____Skin problems
____Sun exposure
____Any special needs for personal care: skin and hair

Vision

____Glasses
____Any problems with vision

Ears

____Earaches
____Infections
____Discharge from ear
____Ringing (tinnitis)
____Dizziness (vertigo)

Nose and Sinuses

____Discharge from the nose or sinuses
____Sinus pain
____Unusual and frequent colds
____Change in sense of smell

Mouth and Throat

____Pain
____Toothache
____Lesions or sores on the mouth or throat
____Changes in the mouth or throat
____Altered taste
____Jaw pain

Neck

____Neck pain
____Limitations in neck movement
____Lumps, swelling, tenderness, or other discomfort

Respiratory System

____History of asthma
____Chest pain
____Shortness of breath
____Cough
____Wheezing

Cardiovascular System

____Pain near heart—with or without exertion
____Dizziness when standing up
____Personal history of any heart problems
____Problems breathing when sleeping

Peripheral Vascular System

____Coldness
____Numbness
____Tingling
____Swelling of legs or hands
____Pain in legs
____Discolored hands or feet
____Varicose veins
____History of vascular problems

(continued)

TABLE 5-3 *(continued)*

PHYSICAL HEALTH SCREENING

Gastrointestinal System

____Changes in appetite
____Food intolerance
____Heartburn
____Abdominal pain
____Nausea and vomiting
____Flatulence (gas)
Frequency of bowel movement ______
____Recent changes in stool
____Constipation or diarrhea
____Rectal bleeding
____Rectal conditions
____Use of antacids or laxatives
____High fiber in diet

Urinary System

Frequency of urination____
____Problems with urgency
____Pain with urination
____Unusual color
____Other problems
____For women: Kegel exercises post-pregnancy

Male Genital System

____Penis or testicular pain
____Sores or lesions
____Discharge
____Lumps
____Hernia

Female Genital System

Menstrual history (last period, duration; cycle): ______
____
Pregnancy history: ____________________________
____Vaginal itching
____Discharge
____Age of menopause
____Menopausal signs or symptoms
____Postmenopausal bleeding.

Sexual History

____In relationship involving intercourse
____Aspects of sex satisfactory
____Contraception is satisfactory
____Awareness of sexually transmitted diseases
____Awareness of family planning
____Familiar with sex education
____Presence of STDs (sexually transmitted diseases)

Musculoskeletal System

____History of arthritis; gout; joint pain, swelling, or stiffness, deformity
____Range of motion limitations
____Muscular pain
____Muscle cramps
____Muscle weakness
____Gait problems (problems with walking)
____Problems with coordination
____Back pain
____Joint stiffness
____Limitations in movement
____History of back problems or disc disease

Neurological System

____History of seizures, blackouts, strokes, fainting; headaches
____Motor problems—tics, tremors, paralysis, or coordination problems
____Sensory—numbness, tingling
____Memory: loss, disorientation
____Mood changes
____Depression
____History of mental health dysfunction

Hematologic System

____Bleeding problems
____Excessive bruising
____Lymph node swelling
____Exposure to toxins and radiation
____Blood transfusions and reactions______________

Endocrine System

____History of diabetes
____Thyroid disease
____Intolerance to heat and cold
____Change in skin pigmentation and texture
____Excessive sweating
____Abnormal relationship between appetite and weight (describe) ______________________
____Abnormal hair distribution
____Nervousness
____Tremors
____Need for hormone therapy

Adapted from Swartz M. *Textbook of Physical Diagnosis*. 5th ed. New York, NY: Saunders-Elsevier; 2005.

IMMUNIZATIONS

Individuals who follow the prescribed schedule of immunizations are commonly protected from a variety of common infectious illnesses. Those who travel, particularly outside of the country, may be unprotected from less common infective agents. For example, individuals who traveled to China during the severe acute respiratory syndrome (SARS) epidemic would be at risk for developing this pathology even after leaving the country because of the incubation period of the virus.[17] Individuals who have not been vaccinated should be advised of the risk of missing vaccinations.

BIRTH HISTORY

An individual's birth history is most relevant for those who are very young or who have developmental problems affecting their growth and development. The method of delivery (vaginal versus cesarean section), the length of gestation, and complications during the birth process can pose significant risks to normal development. The mother's health status throughout and following pregnancy is also important to note. Generally, a physician closely follows individuals with complications or problems during birth until health problems resolve.

MEDICATIONS

People commonly take diet supplements, prescribed medications, vitamins, minerals, over-the-counter drugs, or diet supplements or seek alternative therapies that could influence their health and wellness. While physicians closely monitor prescribed medications, individuals may alter the effects of their medications by adding over-the-counter drugs, vitamins, minerals, herbs, or other extracts from natural sources. Pathology can develop when inappropriate dosages are used or various drugs and agents are incompatibly mixed together. It is essential that the clinician request a comprehensive list of all agents the client is ingesting whether or not they are prescribed. All ingested agents should be shared with the individual's primary physician. In addition, the clinician should ask the client if all medications are taken as prescribed to ensure that correct dosage is administered. Expiration dates of current drugs should be noted, if possible. If the individual takes expired drugs or is not compliant with drug prescriptions, a referral should be made to the physician to ensure proper medical monitoring.

MEDICAL HISTORY

A comprehensive medical history that includes serious accidents, hospitalizations, surgeries, and serious illnesses can identify individuals who are at risk for further pathology. Identifying the date, the type of injury, and the length of care for serious accidents allows the physical therapist to appraise future risk. For example, individuals with a history of traumatic brain injury are at a higher risk for subsequent head injuries. A child with a history of frequent injuries may be either clumsy or a victim of abuse. Likewise, a history of hospitalizations, including the cause of hospitalization, the history of the disease or injury, surgeries performed, and the length of care alerts the clinician to possible risk factors or medical conditions that require continual attention. A referral should be made, as needed, to monitor conditions that have worsened since the patient's discharge.

SKIN

Skin problems can be identified through a visual screening process, noting the skin's color, texture (smooth or rough), thickness (visibility of vessels), and elasticity (presence of wrinkles). Special products used for skin or hair care may be responsible for problems such as contact dermatitis. Individuals with chronic skin conditions, such as psoriasis and dermatitis, may need to be reminded to maintain their medical management if they are experiencing ongoing problems. If problems arise in spite of current medical management, a referral to the physician is needed.

VISION

Obvious visual aids, such as glasses, are easy to identify; however, many individuals have had eye surgeries, such as LASIK, or wear contacts to improve their vision. The clinician should ask about any aids or surgeries to correct vision as well as ask about any problems with vision, including eye infections or soreness. While an optometrist may examine visual acuity problems, infections or other visual impairments should be more thoroughly examined by a physician.

EARS

Ear problems are common across the life span. Young children are susceptible to ear infections, such as *otitis media,* because of the horizontal alignment of their Eustachian tubes. Infants who drink from bottles while lying on their backs are at particular risk for ear infections. Other ear problems, such as earaches, discharges from the ear (thick drainage could indicate a ruptured eardrum or possible infection), *tinnitus* (ringing in the ear), *dizziness* (vertigo), or problems hearing may be reported and would warrant a medical referral.[17] Pain in the jaw just below the ear accompanied with an audible sound with opening and closing the mouth is commonly associated with *tempomandibular joint (TMJ) syndrome*. If the pain is severe, diagnostic imaging may be necessary to identify pathology.

Nose and Sinuses

A history of unusual or frequent colds, sinus pain, changes in smell, and any signs of discharge from the nose or sinuses suggest potential pathology. *Sinusitis* (inflammation of the sinus passages located behind the upper portion of the face) is one of the most common medical conditions affecting individuals. Up to 30% of the population experiences sinusitis at one point.[17] Morning headaches and pain or tenderness in the upper jaws, teeth, cheeks, ears, neck, eyes, and nose are common with sinusitis. In addition, the individual may have a stuffy nose, experience a loss of smell, and have swollen eyelids with pain between the eyes. Using decongestant nasal sprays too often, smoking, and swimming or diving can increase the risk of getting sinusitis, so it is helpful to ask follow-up questions about these risk factors.[17]

Mouth and Throat

Risk factors for pathology of the mouth and throat include pain (such as a toothache, jaw pain, sore throat, or lesions in the mouth or throat), altered taste, or other changes in the mouth or throat region. All ages are susceptible to infections, such as strep throat, so complaints of a persistent sore throat need immediate medical attention. Other signs or symptoms that need attention include a painless lump on the inside of the lip (possible squamous cell skin cancer); a painless hard coating on the inside of the mouth or on the tongue (a precancerous condition common in smokers); small, open sores on the lips, tongue, or sides or back of the mouth (cold sores or canker sores potentially caused by a virus); red and swollen gums or around a tooth (possible gingivitis or dental cavity); or sores around the mouth (possibly caused by a vitamin deficiency).[17]

Neck

Problems in the neck may present as neck pain or tenderness, limitations in movement, or swelling. Neck pain can indicate problems not only in neck tissue but also in distant parts of the body. For example, neck pain may be referred pain from cardiac disease. The clinician can quickly determine if there are problems in blood flow, characterized by louder sounds on auscultation of the carotid arteries located on either side of the neck. Tenderness around the throat, especially accompanied by swelling, suggests inflammation of the lymph nodes along the jaw line. While enlarged lymph nodes may simply indicate a normal body response to a cold, this condition may also be a sign of lymphoma or thyroid problems. If any of these problems exist, a physician referral should be made.

Respiratory and Cardiopulmonary Systems

Discrepancies in vital signs, such as respiratory rate, chest excursion, blood pressure, and pulse, for age- and gender-matched normal populations suggest a compromise in these body systems. Patients with cardiopulmonary impairments commonly present with problems of pain in the chest, neck, shoulder, upper back, and left arm, shortness of breath, and coughing or wheezing. If these are new complaints, a physician referral is warranted. Details of screening and prevention of cardiopulmonary problems are discussed in Chapter 13.

Gastrointestinal System

Abdominal discomfort may be a sign of gastrointestinal problems, cardiovascular problems, or other possible pathologies. Generally, individuals with gastrointestinal pathology have changes in appetite, food intolerance, possible heartburn (often confused with myocardial chest pain), nausea and vomiting, *flatulence* (gas), irregular bowel movements (constipation or diarrhea), or recent changes in stool and are at risk for gastrointestinal pathology.[17] There is greater concern if there are complaints of rectal bleeding because this indicates likely pathology, possibly cancer. It is helpful to know about the individual's use of any antacids, laxatives, or fiber (dietary or herbal supplements) that may affect bowel function. One common condition, *gastroesophageal reflux disorder* (GERD), caused by excessive reverse flow of gastric acid, presents with persistent heartburn and acid regurgitation as well as trouble swallowing, hoarseness in the morning, and chest pain.[17] There is an increased risk for GERD if individuals drink substances that weaken the sphincters controlling the flow of gastric juices, such as coffee and alcohol. Likewise, foods such as spicy, fatty, and tomato-based foods as well as chocolate, peppermint, garlic, onions, and citric fruit have been associated with GERD. Additionally, conditions related to enlarged abdomens, being overweight or pregnant, are contributors to GERD. This condition is chronic and can be controlled with lifestyle changes as well as proper medical management under the supervision of a physician.

URINARY SYSTEM

Screening the urinary system for pathology involves asking questions about the frequency of urination, problems with urgency, pain with urination, unusual color, or other problems. This topic is sensitive and may require open-ended questions that allow the individual to share any concerns. It is important to point out risk factors that warrant concern. A physician should address any problems with the urinary system that have not had prior medical attention to determine etiology and pathology.

MALE GENITAL SYSTEM

If talking to a male, it is best to follow up questions regarding continence with those related to the genital system. Prostate cancer, a "silent" but slow-growing disease, often develops with little early warning. Men with benign prostate hyperplasia, an enlarged yet noncancerous prostate, often have problems with increased frequency of urination, nighttime urination, pain with urination, and/or inability to urinate or trouble with ejaculation.[17] While these signs and symptoms may be benign, they could also be related to prostate cancer, so a medical referral is needed. Other concerns related to the male reproductive system include penis or testicular pain, sores or lesions, and any type of irregular discharge, lumps, or hernias. Since bladder cancer is the fifth leading cancer in the United States, any unusual signs or symptoms indicate a medical referral.

FEMALE GENITAL SYSTEM

When screening a woman, it is important to get a thorough menstrual history (last period, duration, and cycle) and a pregnancy history, as well as information about vaginal itching or discharges. If a woman has already reached menopause, note the age of onset as well as menopausal signs and symptoms. Menopause manifestations include hot flashes (a hot sensation generally starting at the waistline and extending to the head), night sweats, irritability, insomnia, and vaginal dryness.[17] It is also important to check if women are engaged in regular exercise for their pelvic floor muscles. Kegel exercises, designed to tone pelvic floor muscles, are particularly important postpregnancy to restrengthen muscles stretched by a vaginal birth and to prevent incontinence. While bleeding several years postmenopause is not unusual, this sign should be examined by a physician to ensure that any pathology is identified.[17] Additional issues related to women's genital system are described in Chapter 8 on Women's Health.

SEXUAL HISTORY

History of a relationship involving intercourse may put an individual at risk for sexually transmitted diseases (STDs). Sexual history questions should delicately explore personal issues, including sexual satisfaction, contraception, and education about STDs, sex education, and family planning.[17] These concerns may be referred to professionals who commonly deal with sexual issues, including physicians, nurses, psychologists, and medical specialists in men's and women's health. The presence of STDs warrants an immediate medical referral.

MUSCULOSKELETAL SYSTEM

Screening the musculoskeletal system can reveal conditions related to muscles, ligaments, tendons, and other joint structures as well as other conditions that present with similar patterns of pain or dysfunction. An individual reporting a family history of musculoskeletal problems, such as arthritis or muscle pathology, is at an increased risk for developing similar problems. The classic signs of arthritis include joint pain, swelling, and stiffness. With pathological progression, the joints may have limited motion and ultimate deformity. Any of these clinical manifestations indicate a medical referral. The clinician should also inquire about complaints of muscle pain, muscle cramps, muscle or joint stiffness, or inflexibility to determine possible causes of these problems related to varying levels of physical activity. A more thorough musculoskeletal examination is in order if these signs and symptoms limit the individual's work, leisure, or other activities. Individuals should also be asked specifically about back pain or a history of back pain. If there are complaints of any pain, it is important to ask about current exercises or activities that tend to ameliorate or exacerbate (increase) the pain, noting the frequency, intensity, duration, and types of activities, as appropriate. Bone pain, on the other hand, is suggestive of something related to bone disease and should be examined carefully to eliminate the possibility of cancer. During the screening, the clinician may note problems with motor control, such as abnormalities in gait or incoordination. Movement should be observed with shoes removed to avoid the confounding possibility that footwear might contribute to any presenting problems. If motor control problems exist, a more extensive examination should be performed to determine possible causes of any problems.

Neurological System

Individuals with a history of seizures, blackouts, strokes, fainting, or headaches are at risk for possible neurological impairments that are transient or recurrent.[17] These problems, if persistent, need to be examined more thoroughly by a neurologist. Likewise, motor problems such as tics, tremors, paralysis, uncoordinated movement, or sensory changes (eg, numbness or tingling) may suggest more serious neurological pathology and should be referred for a more complete examination. Cognitive dysfunction, such as memory loss or disorientation, could be indicative of a progressive neurological problem or side effects of current medications. If the individual complains of these problems, medications and other agents taken by the individual may be suspect. Finally, emotional problems such as depression, mood changes, or mental health problems that interfere with function should be discussed with a psychologist or the primary physician to ensure that needs are met through appropriate exercise, proper counseling, and/or medication.

Hematologic and Lymphatic System

Individuals may have recent hematologic lab tests that prove valuable in determining possible pathology. If these values are available, they can guide the clinician in making appropriate recommendations for exercise and medical referrals. Of particular concern are excessive bruising, bleeding, vascular swelling, or lymph node swelling. These problems suggest hematological or lymphatic pathology and should be medically managed. If an individual has received a blood transfusion, any adverse reactions to this transfusion should be noted. With the risk of HIV infections from transfusions, a screening test for this risk is also recommended. Chronic hematologic disorders may lead to observable changes to the skin (causing it to become more pale or yellow), may cause weakness (especially with physical exertion), and may contribute to dyspnea (shortness of breath). Individuals complaining of swelling, congestion, pain in their extremities unrelated to muscle or joint pain, or faintness may result from irregularities in the cardiovascular or lymphatic system. All these conditions warrant a medical referral. Some individuals with lowered white blood cell count are at risk for infection and may present with a sore throat, a cough, or signs of infection (elevated temperature, chilling, sweating, or malaise). Additionally, these individuals may complain of painful urination. These individuals need immediate medical attention if they present with these acute clinical manifestations.

Sickle cell anemia, a genetic (autosomal dominant) disorder, is relatively common, particularly in African-Americans.[17] This pathology manifests in multiple body systems with signs and symptoms including joint pain, fatigue, breathlessness, rapid heart rate, delayed growth and puberty, ulcers on the lower legs (seen in adolescents and adults), jaundice or yellowing of the skin, attacks of abdominal pain, or fever.[17] While sickle cell anemia is commonly diagnosed in childhood, complaints of *hematuria* (bloody urine), excessive urination, excessive thirst, chest pain, or poor eyesight/blindness suggest progression of the pathology.[17] A physician should more carefully examine any of these clinical manifestations.

Finally, individuals who have been exposed to toxins or radiation are at an increased risk for developing hematological pathology and should have lab tests to determine levels of toxicity.

Endocrine System

The endocrine system controls the pituitary, thyroid, parathyroid, adrenal glands; pancreas; and gonads. Dysfunction of these glands may be apparent in other portions of the screening but may also present with unique signs and symptoms. Growth and development of connective tissue is controlled by the endocrine system, so excessive or delayed growth is one indication of abnormalities. In addition, signs associated with stress (increased respiration, increased perspiration, heart palpitations, changes in water retention or dehydration, increased blood pressure, increased pulse rate, or elevated body temperature) suggest potential problems with the endocrine glands. Signs and symptoms associated with musculoskeletal problems, including muscle weakness, fatigue, muscle pain, or muscle atrophy, could be related to endocrine problems, since these clinical manifestations are also associated with conditions such as Cushing's syndrome and thyroid disease.[17]

Clinicians should carefully screen for diabetes when screening the endocrine system. Diabetes insipidus is a pathology related to pituitary pathology, among other causes, and results from the kidney's inability to conserve water, leading to excessive urination and thirst.[17] Individuals with these symptoms or with a history of diabetes or thyroid disease need medical monitoring to ensure proper medical management. Diabetes mellitus type 1 classically presents with excessive urination, excessive thirst, weight loss, and blurred vision.[17] Type 2 commonly presents with similar signs and symptoms, but may also include foot pain, infections, and abnormal lipid profiles.[17] It is crucial to make an appropriate medical referral if any type of diabetes is suspected.

Other problems associated with endocrine pathology include intolerance to heat and cold, changes in skin pigmentation and texture, or abnormalities in appetite or weight. Neurological signs that are suspect for endocrine disease include nervousness and tremors. Individuals with hyperthyroidism may also present with drowsiness, abnormal sensations or sensory loss, depression or personality changes, fatigue, or hyperactive reflexes. Likewise, hypothyroidism presents with personality changes and a risk for convulsions.[17] Individuals presenting with any clinical manifestations of possible endocrine pathology should be more thoroughly examined by a physician. In addition, women using hormone replacement therapy should be carefully monitored by a physician for effective and safe maintenance dosages.

Screening for Health Behaviors

Most pathological conditions are a combination of genetics and lifestyle behaviors. A thorough medical history provides some indication of genetic risk, but a comprehensive assessment of lifestyle behaviors offers equally important information. Areas to screen for lifestyle behaviors include activity and exercise (including activities of daily living and exercise behaviors), leisure activities, sleeping/resting behaviors, and nutrition. Nutrition screening includes both positive and negative health behaviors, such as healthy diet and smoking, caffeine, and alcohol use. The Lifestyle Behaviors Screening Tool is a quick and easy tool to determine general lifestyle behaviors (Table 5-4). Additional age-related screening tools will be provided in chapters featuring specific populations with unique growth and development issues.

Screening for Alcohol Use Disorder

It may be important to more thoroughly screen for an alcohol use disorder, so more specific questions are recommended. The questions recommended by the American Academy of Family Physicians follow: "When was the last time you had more than five drinks in one day?" for men and "When was the last time you had more than four drinks in one day?" The responses include: "Never," "In the last three months," or "More than three months ago." A positive screening response for either males or females is "in the last three months." The individual's physician should be informed of possible alcohol use disorder to ensure proper follow-up and management of this problem.

Assessment of Spiritual Beliefs

Current research supports the positive effects of spirituality for health and well-being. It is helpful to know if an individual relies on a particular spiritual belief system for improved health, fitness, and wellness. Knowledge of this belief system can alert the clinician to values contributing to or contradicting traditional medical beliefs. Cultural sensitivity is particularly important whenever assessing a person's level of spirituality. Simple questions might include, "How would you describe the role that spirituality plays in your health, fitness, and wellness?" It is inappropriate for the interviewer to guide an individual into a personal religious belief system, but it is appropriate to suggest that the individual's personal belief system can contribute to wellness. Those with spiritual concerns or those seeking spiritual guidance should be referred to a hospital chaplain or should be advised to explore their spirituality through local centers of worship. People with strong beliefs should be encouraged to engage in meaningful spiritual activities.

Screening for Holistic Health

A comprehensive screening for holistic health includes questions related to the mind, the body, and the spirit. The Holistic Health Score Sheet (Table 5-5) may be used to explore an individual's health more comprehensively, including the individual's physical and environmental health ("body"), the individual's mental and emotional health ("mind"), and the individual's social and spiritual health ("spirit").[18] Scores on this survey categorize the individual as striving, nourishing, maintaining, sustaining, or surviving as indicators of the individual's overall health.

Regular Medical Screening Tests and Immunizations

During the screening, it is helpful to advise individuals to participate in other medical screenings for annual check-ups or as recommended by their physicians. Individuals should be reminded to follow the recommendations of the Centers for Disease Control and Prevention, including regular immunizations, lab tests, screening tests for cancer, and follow recommendations for injury prevention. In addition, children and adults alike should be reminded to have regular dental examinations for preventive care.

TABLE 5-4

LIFESTYLE BEHAVIORS SCREENING TOOL

Describe each of the following:

Activity and Exercise

Daily Activities: Do you have problems with your activities of daily living? Yes ___No ____ If so, please describe:

Dressing: ______________________________
Bathing: ______________________________
Hygiene: ______________________________
Self-care: ______________________________

Leisure Activities: How would you describe the type, intensity, and duration of your physical activity (on a weekly basis)? If you do a variety of activities, please note these activities separately.

Type: ______________________________
Duration: ______________________________
Frequency: ______________________________
Intensity: ______________________________

Type: ______________________________
Duration: ______________________________
Frequency: ______________________________
Intensity: ______________________________

Sleep and Rest

How would you describe your sleep behavior?

Sleep patterns: ______________________________
Typical duration of sleep: ______________________________
Typical sleep posture: ______________________________
Does your partner interfere with your sleep? If so, how? ______________________________
Other comments:

Nutrition

How would you describe your eating behavior?

Overall diet: ______________________________
Alcohol intake: ______________________________
Caffeine (tea, coffee, cola drinks) intake: ______________________________
Smoking: ______________________________
Drugs (illicit): ______________________________
Use of vitamins: ______________________________
Food allergies or intolerance: ______________________________
Mealtime habits: ______________________________

TABLE 5-5

HOLISTIC HEALTH SCORE SHEET

Instructions:
Score each statement as follows:
0 = never
1 = very rarely
2 = sometimes
3 = often
4 = very often
Then score each section separately to determine areas of strengths and needs.

BODY: Physical and Environmental Health

1.	Do you regularly eat a healthy and well-balanced diet?	_____
2.	Each day, do you drink 0.5 oz of water for each pound of body weight? (eg, 120 lbs = 60 oz)?	_____
3.	Is your environment healthy (water, air, free of toxins)?	_____
4.	Do you engage in regular and healthy sensual and sexual practices?	_____
5.	Do you regularly do activities to relax muscles or relieve tension (eg, body massages, meditation)?	_____
6.	**Do you perform moderate exercise regularly (at least 3 times/week for 30 minutes)?**	_____
7.	Is your body free of chronic pains, injuries, or other problems?	_____
8.	Are you free of any drug or alcohol dependency?	_____
9.	Are you within 20% of your ideal body weight?	_____
10.	Do you have a healthy waist-to-hip ratio?	_____
11.	Do you have a healthy body mass index (BMI) score?	_____
12.	**Do you perform daily flexibility exercises?**	_____
13.	Do you perform daily strengthening exercises?	_____
14.	Do you perform daily cardiovascular endurance activities?	_____
15.	Do you perform daily deep breathing, meditation, or similarly relaxing activities?	_____
16.	Do you feel healthy?	_____
17.	Do you sleep between 7 and 9 hours per day?	_____
18.	Do you regularly awaken in the morning feeling well-rested?	_____
19.	Do you have daily, effortless bowel movements?	_____
20.	**Do you engage in healthy dental hygiene?**	_____

PHYSICAL AND ENVIRONMENTAL HEALTH SCORE _______

75 to 80 points = OPTIMAL
65 to 74 points = THRIVING
55 to 64 points = STRIVING
45 to 54 = NOURISHING
35 to 44 = MAINTAINING
25 to 34 = SUSTAINING
Less than 25 = SURVIVING

MIND: Mental and Emotional Health

1.	Do you have specific goals in your personal and professional life?	_____
2.	Do you have the ability to concentrate for extended periods of time?	_____
3.	Do you have a sense of humor?	_____
4.	Do you generally have an optimistic outlook on life?	_____
5.	Are you willing to take risks or make mistakes in order to succeed?	_____
6.	**Do your vocation(s)/avocation(s) provide sufficient challenges to match your talents?**	_____
7.	Are you free from a strong need for control or the need to be right?	_____
8.	Is your job enjoyable and fulfilling?	_____
9.	Do you give yourself more supportive messages than critical messages in the course of a day?	_____
10.	Do you sleep soundly?	_____
11.	**Are you able to adjust beliefs and attitudes as a result of learning from painful experiences?**	_____
12.	Are you able to fully experience your painful feelings (eg, fear, anger, and sadness)	_____

(continued)

TABLE 5-5 *(continued)*

HOLISTIC HEALTH SCORE SHEET

MIND: Mental and Emotional Health (continued)

13. Can you freely express your feelings? ______
14. Do you use visualization to enhance your goal achievement and/or performance? ______
15. Can you meet your financial needs and desires? ______
16. Do you easily adapt to change? ______
17. Do you have positive self-regard? ______
18. Do you maintain peace of mind and tranquility? ______
19. Do you make time for play? ______
20. Are you accepting of all your feelings? ______

MENTAL AND EMOTIONAL HEALTH SCORE ______

75 to 80 points = OPTIMAL
65 to 74 points = THRIVING
55 to 64 points = STRIVING
45 to 54 = NOURISHING
35 to 44 = MAINTAINING
25 to 34 = SUSTAINING
Less than 25 = SURVIVING

SPIRIT: Social and Spiritual Health

1. **Do you have faith in a God or any other spiritual entity?** ______
2. **Do you listen to your intuition ("gut feelings") and take risks?** ______
3. **Do you see the good in others?** ______
4. **Do you regularly engage in meditation, prayer, or reflection?** ______
5. **Are creative activities a regular part of your work or leisure?** ______
6. **Have you demonstrated the willingness to commit to a marriage/long-term relationship?** ______
7. **Do you have one or more close friends to whom you talk openly?** ______
8. **Do you feel close to your family?** ______
9. **Have your experiences of pain enabled you to grow spiritually?** ______
10. **Do you engage in regular social gatherings with family and/or friends?** ______
11. **Can you let go of self-interest in deciding the best course of action for a given situation?** ______
12. **Are playfulness and humor important to you in your daily life?** ______
13. **Do you have the ability to forgive yourself and others?** ______
14. **Do you experience intimacy, besides sex, in your committed relationship?** ______
15. **Do you routinely go out of your way or routinely give your time to help others?** ______
16. **Do you feel a sense of belonging to a group or community?** ______
17. **Are you grateful for the blessings in your life?** ______
18. **Do you take walks or have daily contact with nature?** ______
19. **Do you observe a day of rest away from work?** ______
20. **Do you experience unconditional love?** ______

SOCIAL AND SPIRITUAL HEALTH SCORE ______

75 to 80 points = OPTIMAL
65 to 74 points = THRIVING
55 to 64 points = STRIVING
45 to 54 = NOURISHING
35 to 44 = MAINTAINING
25 to 34 = SUSTAINING
Less than 25 = SURVIVING

Note: Individuals may improve their Holistic Health by balancing engagement in physical, environmental, mental, emotional, social, and spiritual activities, as suggested by questions in each section.

Adapted from:

Combined Health Care Professionals. Holistic health score sheet. Available at: http://www.chcp.com/tools/beginning.html. Accessed January 20, 2006.

Ivker RS, Zorensky EH. Thriving: A Man's Guide to Creating Optimal Health and Fitness. New York, NY: Random House; 1998.

Summary

Physical therapists play a key role in screening for primary, secondary, and tertiary prevention of pathology. Using simple screening tools in conjunction with effective communication skills can elicit key information leading to effective preventive care and management. Subsequent chapters will provide more details regarding age-appropriate screening tools and resources to help individuals manage their health and wellness.

References

1. American Physical Therapy Association. *Guide to Physical Therapist Practice.* 2nd ed. Alexandria, Va: APTA; 2003.
2. Heaven C, Maguire P, Green C. A patient-centered approach to defining and assessing interviewing competency. *Epidemiology of Psychiatric Sociology.* 2003;12(2): 86–91.
3. Thompson DW, Thompson NN. The art of interviewing your next CEO. *Trustee.* 2003;56(2):14–18.
4. O'Keefe M, Roberton D, Sawyer M, Baghurst P. Medical student interviewing: a randomized trial of patient-centeredness and clinical competence. *Family Practice.* 2003;20(2):213–219.
5. Berlin EA, Fowles WC Jr. A teaching framework for cross-cultural health care: application in family practice in cross-cultural medicine. *West J Med.* 1983;12(138):93-98.
6. Stern MA. Communication Tip: Maintaining Eye Contact. Available at: http://www.matthewarnoldstern.com/tips/tipps16.html. Accessed August 6, 2004.
7. Carducci B, Golant S. *Shyness: A Bold New Approach.* New York, NY: Harper Publishers; 2000.
8. Remland MS, Jones TS, Brinkman H. Interpersonal distance, body orientation, and touch: effects of culture, gender, and age. *J Soc Psychol.* 1995;135(3):281–297.
9. Goldin-Meadow S. The role of gesture in communication and thinking. *Trends in Cognitive Science.* 1999;3(11):419–429.
10. Thibault JM, Steiner RW. Efficient identification of adults with depression and dementia. *American Family Physician.* 2004;70(6):1101–1110.
11. Yeaworth RC, York J, Hussey MA, Ingle ME, Goodwin T. The development of an adolescent life change event scale. *Adolescence.* 1980;15(57):91–97.
12. Rahe RH, Meyer M, Smith M, Khaer G, Holmes TH. Social stress and illness onset. *J Psychomotor Research.* 1964;54:35–44
13. Schulz JE, Parran T Jr. Principles of identification and intervention. In: Graham AW, Schultz TK, Wilford BB, eds. *Principles of Addiction Medicine.* 2nd ed. Chevy Chase, Md: American Society of Addiction Medicine, 1998:250–251.
14. Mayfield D, McLeod G, Hall P. The CAGE questionnaire: validation of a new alcoholism screening instrument. *Amer J Psychiatr.* 1974;131(10):1121–1123.
15. Feldhaus KM, Koziol-McLain J, Amsbury HL, et al. Accuracy of 3 brief screening questions for detecting partner violence in the emergency department. *JAMA.* 1977;277:1357–1361.
16. Health Promotion and Human Development at University of Wisconsin at Seven Points. Are You Balancing the 7 Dimensions of Wellness? Available at: http://cps.uwsp.edu/hphd/wellquiz. Accessed February 6, 2006.
17. Swartz M. *Textbook of Physical Diagnosis: History and Examination.* 5th Ed. New York, NY: WB Saunders-Elsevier; 2005.
18. Ivker R, Zorensky E. The Holistic Health Score Sheet. Thriving: A man's guide to creating optimal health and fitness. Available at: http://www.chcp.com/tools/beginning.html. Accessed January 20, 2006.

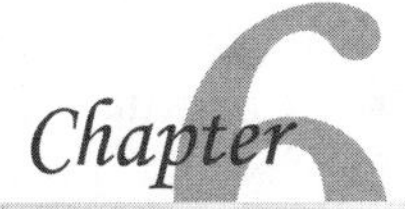

Health, Fitness, and Wellness Issues During Childhood and Adolescence

Catherine Rush Thompson, PhD, MS, PT

"It takes a village to raise a child."

~AFRICAN PROVERB

The Dynamic Process of Growth and Development

Neonates, infants, children, and adolescents face unique changes as they dynamically grow and develop into adults. Many people contribute to this dynamic process, involving families, communities, educators, and health care professionals. Health care professionals should be aware of physical and psychosocial transformations taking place early in life. These changes play a key role in promoting health for infants, children, and adults in various practice settings, ranging from pediatric intensive care units to community fitness centers and sports fields. Many of these settings afford children the opportunity to interact with healthy, fit siblings and peers as well as those at risk for health problems. Screening neonates, infants, children, and youth in these settings is an essential role of therapists practicing preventive care. A variety of screening tools are available that provide normative data for identifying children at risk or children with health impairments requiring appropriate interventions.

Genetics or "nature" plays a key role in a child's physical and psychological makeup; however, physical activity and other environmental influences can "nurture" a child, greatly influencing a child's healthy growth, proper development, increasing fitness, and emergent wellness. Combinations of genetic and environmental factors, including stressors the mother may be encountering, play key roles in these maturational processes. Certain aspects of growth are more strongly influenced by genetic factors, including dental development, the sequence of bone ossification, and sexual differentiation during puberty. Other aspects of growth and development are more strongly influenced by maternal lifestyle habits. Chapter 8 on women's health provides suggestions for promoting prenatal wellness through healthy lifestyle habits during pregnancy.

Early Childhood Screenings

Newborns are generally screened by obstetricians using the APGAR test, a screening tool describing the infant's *activity/muscle tone (A), pulse (P)* or heart rate, *grimace/infantile reflex response (G), appearance (A)* in terms of normal skin color, and *respiration (R) rate.*[1] These key indicators provide a quick screening of the newborn's body functions at 1 minute and 5 minutes after birth. Each of the 5 indicators is scored up to 2 points for optimal function. A score of 7 to 10 is considered normal, while 4 to 6 may require some immediate medical assistance. Infants with scores below 4 require immediate medical attention and are at increased risk for problems during infancy, including significant neurological dysfunctioning.[1] If a newborn is suspected of having problems prior to or during birth, the infant is generally referred to an early intervention program for further assessment. In some cases, these infants do not receive follow-up care and may need to be identified through additional screening opportunities. Health care professionals are commonly trained in performing the Denver II Developmental Screening Test (Denver II), a screening tool designed to detect problems in young children.[2] The Denver II, an updated version of the original Denver Developmental Screening Test, is a simple, sensitive, and convenient test developed to screen children from birth to age 6 years. This test battery includes screening of *personal-social skills* (getting along with others and taking care of self), *fine motor-adaptive skills* (eye-hand coordination and hand skills such as drawing and coloring), *language skills* (hearing, following directions, and speaking), and *gross motor skills* (total body movements such as sitting, walking, and jumping.) Any suspected delays in function should be reported to the child's physician for further examination. When performing any developmental screening test, it is helpful to make additional observations of structural and functional aspects of the child indicating potential problems. It is helpful to ask the parents, guardians, and/or teachers about the child's nutritional habits, developmental milestones, physical development, psychosocial interactions, communication skills, medical history of illness or injury, environmental hazards, and impairments such as hearing loss or visual deficits. Other considerations include observations for signs of child abuse and information about the safety and enrichment of the child's home environment. If there are any concerns, the family physician should be contacted for collaborative strategies to address the child's needs.

The child's height and weight should be measured and compared to normative data for age and gender to detect delayed or disproportionate growth of the body. According to the Center for Disease Control (CDC), being overweight is having a body mass above the 95th percentile for the child's age, while a body mass index (BMI) above the 85th percentile puts the child at risk of becoming overweight.[3] Some children who are very athletic may have a large muscle mass contributing to a high BMI, but the vast majority of children with high BMI scores are overweight and need help with weight management. A child with a BMI below the fifth percentile is considered underweight.[3] Again, if the child is developing normally, has a healthy diet, and is extremely active and energetic, this BMI may be normal. If the child has been ill with diarrhea and vomiting, has a poor appetite, or a low energy level, the child should be thoroughly examined to determine the cause of the problem.

Recent research indicates that there are racial differences in the timing of sexual maturation that can have significant impact on growth assessment in the use of the growth charts. Within age and gender groups, children who are sexually more mature tend to be taller and weigh more than less mature children.[4] Rapidly maturing children tend to have larger BMI values than those who are maturing slowly.[4]

Factors Influencing Growth and Development in Early Childhood

Genetics play a key role in a child's appearance and in some behavioral aspects of development yet it is not solely responsible for normal growth. More important are the environmental factors that facilitate, inhibit, and age tissue growth, such as gravitational forces, compression and traction forces, as well as other biomechanical forces that combine with healthy nutrition, adequate rest, and a healthy psychosocial environment. During the first 6 months of life, the body systems undergo dramatic changes to accommodate the dynamic physical changes of an infant. On average, babies grow 10 inches (25 centimeters [cm]) in height while tripling birth weight by their first birthday.[5] After age 1, a baby's growth in length slows considerably, and by 2 years, growth in height usually continues at a fairly steady rate of approximately 2.5 inches (6 cm) per year until adolescence. Children generally have a prepubescent growth spurt that begins at age 8 in girls and age 10 in boys. Throughout puberty, the growth spurt is accompanied by the development of secondary sex characteristics and the onset of menstruation for females. By age 18, most youths have reached physical maturity.[6] Additional factors that should be considered when screening a child for health fitness and wellness include considerations of the child's physical health, including proper nutrition, sleep, exercise, arousal and alertness, reflexes, and satiation of needs, such as eating, drinking, eliminating, and safety.

One area of great concern is the lack of physical activity by children. Nearly half of young people aged 12 to 21 years do not regularly engage in vigorous physical activity. This lack of activity leads to obesity and other significant complications, including increased risks for type 2 diabetes mellitus, problems with the musculoskeletal and cardiopulmonary systems, fertility problems, as well as psychosocial consequences in the form of a negative self-image, emotional and behavioral problems, and depression.[7] Many prevention programs are aimed at increasing physical activity, monitoring nutrition habits, and dealing with psychosocial issues.[8]

Common Health Problems of Infants and Young Children

Common childhood problems include acute health problems, chronic illness, and developmental or behavioral problems. Acute health problems may present as excessive crying, sleep disorders, fevers, ear infections, urinary tract infections, skin problems, and trauma. More chronic problems include allergies, asthma, chronic pain, problems with urination and constipation, and seizures. Developmental problems include developmental delays, attention-deficit/hyperactivity disorders, or other behavioral problems. In addition, structural problems related to the body systems can be observed when screening the child for normal growth and development.

Excessive Crying

Excessive crying in an infant under 3 months of age may indicate that the infant has colic, suggesting possible acute abdominal pain. If the crying persists beyond age 3 months, a referral should be made to the child's physician for examination to determine if the child has a pathology or dietary intolerance that needs addressing.[9]

Sleep Disorders

Sleep disorders, such as difficulty falling to sleep or problems staying awake, are generally noted when the child reaches school age, when 9 hours of sleep is recommended for elementary school children. A sizeable proportion of elementary school children sleep less than the recommended 9 hours.[10] While few pathologies are associated with pediatric sleep disorders, behavioral strategies may be recommended to help the parents deal with their child's sleeping problems. These sleep disorders are generally acute, but they can become chronic if they are not properly addressed. A referral to a child psychologist or the child's physician can provide the parents additional resources for resolving these problems.

Fevers

Fevers are common in children and should be addressed by the child's pediatrician. Fevers, however, do not always necessitate a doctor visit. According to Abraham Bergman, MD, criteria for an office visit include (1) any feverish child under the age of 3 months, (2) fever accompanied by significant localized pain (headache, chest, throat, or abdominal pain) or dysfunction (persistent vomiting, bloody diarrhea, limping, or altered state of consciousness), (3) fever lasting more than 4 days, duration unexplained by other illness, or (4) for the child who does not meet the above criteria but whose parents are very concerned.[11]

Otitis Media

Otitis media, an infection that leads to inflammation behind the eardrum, affects approximately 70% of children before their second birthday.[12] A child with otitis media may be irritable, cry or whine, have a reduced appetite, and have some difficulty sleeping. Fever is not always necessary for the diagnosis. While one child may complain that the ear hurts, an infant may simply rub or tug at the auricle or dig a finger into the auditory meatus as an indication of discomfort. In older children, chronic otitis media may lead to a hearing loss and complaints of ear stuffiness may be an indicator of the infection. Pain referred to the tempomandibular joint could also be an indicator of otitis media in the older child.[12] Children with these symptoms should be referred to the pediatrician for a definitive medical diagnosis.

Urinary Tract Infections

Urinary tract infections are common in children, often accompanied by fever in infants 0 to 23 months of age. Clinical manifestations of urinary tract infections include vomiting, diarrhea, irritability, and poor feeding. In addition, the urine may smell foul. Children with these signs and symptoms should see their doctor for a urinalysis to confirm the diagnosis.[13]

Skin Pathology

Skin problems may be noted during visual inspection of an infant or child. *Dermatitis* (inflammation of the skin) may be caused by irritants, such as diapers or infection; however, certain types are caused by a combination of genetic and environmental factors.[14] Often this skin condition presents with edematous patches and plaques on the face, the trunk, and extremities. Similarly, *impetigo* (characterized by small infectious vesicles on the skin's surface) presents with redness and skin irregularities.[14] *Hemangiomas* (tumors that may be superficial or deep) are similarly red but are generally singular and are often raised from the skin's surface. About 50% of these lesions resolve by age 9.[15] Warts are generally yellowish to brownish and are commonly seen on the hands. *Tinea capitis* (a scalp infection) appears as round or irregular patches of broken hairs on the scalp. Finally, *tinea corporis* (an infection on the body) presents as scaly, reddened patches with raised borders. Since many of these skin problems are infectious and all are treatable, immediate referral should be made to the physician for proper management.

TRAUMA—ACCIDENTAL AND INTENTIONAL

Trauma during childhood can result from a variety of accidents, including minor falls and burns, to near drowning and motor vehicle injuries. It is important to know if injuries are from accidents or intentionally inflicted. Some caregiver risk factors suggesting abuse are listed in Table 6-1.[15] If the clinician suspects any of these risk factors, contact must be made with the local child protection services.

TABLE 6-1

CAREGIVER RISK FACTORS FOR CHILD ABUSE

1. The explanation of the injury is not plausible.
2. The explanations are inconsistent or change.
3. The seriousness of the child's condition is understated.
4. There is a delay in obtaining treatment.
5. The caregiver cannot be located.
6. The male caregiver is not the child's father.
7. There is a history of domestic abuse.
8. There is a history of substance abuse.

Adapted from Bergman A. *Twenty Common Problems in Pediatrics.* St. Louis, Mo: McGraw-Hill; 2001:139.

The most common manifestation of abuse is bruises that are not on prominent surfaces over bones. Also, nonmobile infants rarely inflict wounds on themselves. Most suspect fractures are caused by twisting or pulling an extremity, causing damage to the *metaphysis* (the growing part of the long bone).[19] Perhaps the most difficult type of abuse to understand is *Munchausen by proxy syndrome* (MBPS), a situation in which the parent, usually the mother, fabricates information about the child's health and intentionally makes the child ill. This psychological disturbance of the parent can prove lethal. Victims of MBPS need immediate medical attention since these children are at an increased risk of death or dangerous injury.[16] Clinicians should collect information about witnesses to any traumatic event, any history of previous injuries, and past medical records. Suspected child abuse must be reported to the local authorities. A helpful website listing contact information is the Childhelp USA National Child Abuse Hotline (see Appendix C).

ALLERGIES

It is estimated that over 20% of children have seasonal allergies that present with nasal congestion, sneezing, and *rhinorrhea* (a discharge from the nasal mucous membrane).[17] Chronic congestion can lead to mouth breathing. Another common sign is constant rubbing of the nose in an upward direction. Finally, edematous or swollen eyes lead to suspicion that the child is having an allergic reaction to a seasonal *allergen* (agent causing the allergic reaction). These allergic reactions are commonly caused by the pollen from nonflowering, wind-pollinated plants.[17] Food allergies are more common in younger children and often decrease in prevalence once children reach the age of 4. In children, common allergy-provoking foods include cow's milk protein, hen's egg white, wheat, soybean or soybean products, codfish, peanuts, seafood, citrus fruit, and chocolate.[17] The oral allergy syndrome response is characterized by a red, itchy mouth and throat after eating the food. More generalized responses following the consumption of a large serving include rashes, flushing, abdominal pain, vomiting, diarrhea, and heart palpitations.[17] While an antihistamine is the most effective treatment for suspected allergic reactions, the physician should be contacted whenever allergic reactions are a concern. It is important that the parent record a description of the child's symptoms; the amount of time elapsed between ingestion and the initiation of symptoms; the type, quantity, and processing of food eaten (cooked, raw, processed with other foods); and the frequency of the allergic reaction. Since exercise may induce this allergic reaction, this should also be noted.[18]

ASTHMA

Asthma is a common pediatric condition limiting sports participation, causing sleep problems, leading to absences from school due to health care issues, and potentially reducing growth and development.[18] Asthma further affects the child's family in terms of recreational opportunities as well as economic costs of dealing with this chronic illness. Whenever asthma is suspected, an immediate medical referral should be made to confirm the diagnosis. Once the diagnosis is established, caretakers should eliminate asthma triggers, including airborne allergens; upper respiratory tract infections; smoke and other lung irritants; cold, dry air; and various types of medications (aspirin and other nonsteroidal anti-inflammatory drugs and beta-blockers) while encouraging "normal" breathing and normal physical activity. Swimming improves cardiorespiratory fitness in children with asthma and is asthmogenic (less likely to induce asthma than other forms of exercise).[19-22] Exercise training has health-related benefits and improves the quality of life of children with asthma.

CHRONIC PAIN

Chronic pain can be a potent stressor to children and family members. Certain pains are expected, such as teething pain accompanying tooth eruption in early childhood.[23] "Growing pains" are generally experienced in the legs of young children during growth spurts, often between the ages of 3 and 10 years.[23] The complaints of pain are generally in the evening, and both legs are affected, though pains rarely awaken the child during sleep and are often resolved by morning. Massaging the affected area can effectively reduce the pain. Recurrent abdominal pain affects up to 11% of children and may be caused by a variety of factors. While food allergies are often suspected, recurrent abdominal pain may be caused by irritable bowel syndrome, gastroesophageal reflux, or infection.[24] In some instances, abdominal pain is associated with psychological distress. Since pain is a subjective sensation, it is important to tell parents that the pain should not be over-emphasized. In addition, parents should encourage the child's normal engagement in daily activities if no organic cause is determined.

Headaches can be a concern if they are recurrent. While recurrent headaches could suggest intracranial disease, migraine headaches can occur in childhood and can be treated with over-the-counter medications. Fatigue, exercise, or long periods in the sun can trigger headaches as well as nuts, caffeine (including cola drinks), and spiced meats. Since there are many etiologies of headaches, it is important to have recurrent headaches examined by a physician. According to recent research, relaxation training and thermal biofeedback are promising treatments for pediatric headache, reducing both the severity and frequency of headaches.[25] Chest pain is less common and can generally be attributed to a musculoskeletal problem, such as overuse from coughing or novel physical activity. "Heartburn" or esophageal pain can also occur in children and may be related to digestive problems. If they persist, a medical referral is appropriate.

ENURESIS AND CONSTIPATION

About 15% to 20% of first graders have nocturnal *enuresis* (urinary incontinence)[26] and up to 2% have *encopresis* (involuntary defecation),[27] causing considerable concern to parents. Nearly 90% of these cases resolve over time; however, if these problems are not dealt with in a timely manner, they may cause subsequent maladaptive behaviors. A variety of medical and behavioral programs offer parents and their children considerable relief.[26,27]

SEIZURES

Seizures accompany high fevers in 2% to 5% of all young children. Approximately 50% of these infants under the age of 12 months have a second seizure, indicative of epilepsy.[28] Seizures may present in a variety of ways but often last less than 5 minutes and cease on their own. Any seizurelike activity, such as a loss of consciousness, involuntary movements, or total body convulsions, should be reported to the child's physician. The various seizure types are described at the emedicine website.[29]

DEVELOPMENTAL DELAYS

Therapists play in key role in diagnosing developmental delays in children. Approximately 12% of children between birth and 21 years of age receive special educational services for developmental disabilities, ranging from mental retardation to physical impairments.[30] Causes of developmental delay include emotional disturbance, specific learning disabilities, health impairments, visual impairments, traumatic brain injury, mental retardation, speech or language impairment, physical impairment, autism and other developmental disorders, hearing impairment, and developmental delay in two or more areas of physical development, cognitive development, communication development, social or emotional development, or adaptive development.[30] A thorough examination by the physical therapist is important to help establish the degree of impairment limiting function. Pervasive developmental disorders (PDDs) are becoming more prevalent in the United States.

PDDs are characterized by severe or pervasive impairment in social interaction skills, communication skills, or the presence of stereotyped behavior, interests, and activities generally presenting by age 3. According to the National Dissemination Center for Children with Disabilities, children with PDD "have difficulty in talking, playing with other children, and relating to others, including their family."[30] PDD disorders include autistic disorder, Rett's disorder, childhood disintegrative disorder, Asperger's disorder, and pervasive developmental disorder not otherwise specified. Children presenting with signs and symptoms indicating any of these disorders should have a complete examination by a psychologist to determine causality and diagnosis. The National Information Center for Children and Youth With Disabilities has a website devoted to educational materials for families

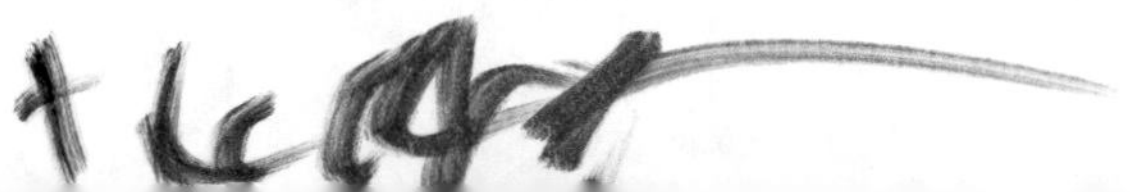

TABLE 6-2

CRITERIA FOR ATTENTION-DEFICIT/HYPERACTIVITY DISORDER

The diagnosis of ADHD is based upon the child presenting with six or more of the following criteria, which have persisted for at least 6 months to a degree that is maladaptive and inconsistent with the child's developmental level. In addition, these behaviors were present before age 7; were present in two or more settings; significantly impair the child's social, academic, or occupational functioning; and are not better accounted for by another mental disorder.

Inattention

- Often fails to give close attention to details, or makes careless mistakes in homework, work, or other activities.
- Often has difficulty sustaining attention in tasks or play activities.
- Often does not seem to listen when spoken to directly.
- Often does not follow through instructions, and fails to finish schoolwork, chores, or duties in the workplace (not due to oppositional behavior or failure to understand instructions).
- Often has difficulty organizing tasks and activities.
- Often avoids, dislikes, or is reluctant to engage in tasks that require sustained mental efforts.
- Often loses things necessary for tasks or activities (eg, toys, school assignments, pencils, books).
- Is often easily distracted by extraneous stimuli.
- Is often forgetful in daily activities.

Hyperactivity/Impulsivity

- Often fidgets with hands or feet or squirms in seat.
- Often leaves seat in classroom or in other situations in which remaining seated is expected.
- Often runs about or climbs excessively in situations in which it is inappropriate (in adolescents or adults, may be limited to subjective feelings of restlessness).
- Often has difficulty playing or engaging in leisure activities quietly.
- Is often "on the go" or often acts as if "driven by a motor."
- Often talks excessively.

Impulsivity

- Often blurts out answers before questions have been completed.
- Often has difficulty awaiting turn.
- Often interrupts or intrudes on others (eg, butts into conversations or games).

Adapted from Centers for Disease Control and Prevention. Symptoms of ADHD. Available at: http://www.cdc.gov/ncbddd/adhd/symptom.htm. Accessed October 15, 2005.

with developmental disabilities.[30] This website serves as an excellent resource for parents of children with suspected or diagnosed developmental disabilities. Children who have developmental delays may receive special education services within the first year of life through the Individuals with Disabilities Education Act (IDEA), Part C. Additional information about children with developmental disabilities is presented in Chapter 15.

ATTENTION-DEFICIT/HYPERACTIVITY DISORDER

According to the National Institute of Mental Health, up to 5% of all American children have attention-deficit/hyperactivity disorder. This disorder presents with features of inattention, hyperactivity or the inability to sit still, and impulsivity or uncontrolled interruptions of others.[31] Table 6-2 lists the criteria used to distinguish the various types of attention-deficit/hyperactivity disorder, commonly known as ADHD. Physical therapists can help families and educators identify and document these behaviors for diagnosis as well as provide structured learning environments in the home and at school. These children commonly are managed medically using a stimulant, such as Ritalin.[31]

OTHER BEHAVIORAL PROBLEMS

Other problems influencing a child's growth and development include a poor appetite, shyness or aggression, and spoiled behavior. These behaviors may be transitory but need to be recognized and discussed with parents. Pediatricians and psychologists are best trained to deal with these issues and can provide guidance, as needed.

OBESITY IN CHILDHOOD

BMI should decrease during the preschool years, then increase into adulthood.[4] Recently, however, the BMI has been increasing throughout childhood for individuals living in the United States. The percentage of children and adolescents who are defined as overweight has more than doubled since the early 1970s with about 15% of children and adolescents who are overweight.[4] Obese children and adolescents are more likely to become obese adults. All experts agree that weight management requires a combined approach of a sensible diet and regular exercise for weight loss. Before initiating a weight loss program for children with obesity, it is essential to contact the child's physician and a nutritionist to ensure a safe and enduring program for lifestyle changes that will safely manage the child's weight problem.[4] Most prevention programs include at least one of the following components: dietary changes, physical activity, behavior and social modifications, and family participation.[32] School-based prevention programs may also include elements related to the school environment and personnel. Primary prevention programs cannot usually restrict caloric intake, but may effectively reduce the energy intake by reducing the energy density of foods, increasing offering of fresh fruits and vegetables, using low-calorie versions of products, and reducing offering of energy-dense food items.[32] Physical activity interventions have recently focused more on reducing sedentary behavior, particularly television viewing. Physical therapists should work collaboratively with other professionals to ensure that physical activity is integrated into all prevention programs for childhood obesity.

ANOREXIA AND BULIMIA

Other weight problems, particularly during adolescence, include anorexia and bulimia. Individuals with anorexia suffer from a distorted self-image of being overweight when they may be grossly underweight. Chemical imbalances from anorexia can lead to heart arrhythmias and protein deficiencies. Likewise, individuals who engage in binge eating following by self-induced vomiting (referred to as bulimia) are equally at risk for poor health. If either of these two conditions is suspected, a physician or psychological referral should be made.

Factors Influencing Growth and Development in Children Ages 7 to 21

During preadolescent and adolescent years, lifestyle behaviors, including limited physical activity, poor nutrition, poor stress management, exposure to infective agents, sun exposure, substance abuse, delinquency, psychological disorders, sports-related injuries, sexually transmitted disease, and even homicide, pose significant health risks. Many of the leading causes of morbidity and mortality are interrelated, according to the Youth Risk Behavior Surveillance System (YRBSS)[33] that monitors priority health-risk behaviors contributing to unintentional injuries and violence, substance abuse, unintended pregnancy, sexually transmitted diseases, and obesity. Additional risks are related to riding with a driver who had been drinking alcohol. Nearly one-third of students do not participate in sufficient vigorous physical activity. Similarly, one-third of students in this age group watch television more than 3 hours per day on an average school day, providing evidence of sedentary behavior contributing to health risks. While excess body fat is a problem for certain students, taking laxatives and vomiting contributed to weight loss or was used as a strategy to prevent weight gain. Other health risks include significant underage alcohol use, cocaine use, desire to commit suicide, and cigarette use. For those engaged in physical activity, there is at increased risk of injuries if they are not wearing the appropriate protective gear. Chapter 11 offers preventive care for common sports injuries in this population.

Special Considerations for Screening Children and Youth

Screening preadolescents and adolescents may involve parents or may be performed in the absence of other adults. It is important to ask the youth about possible risk behaviors (sexual activity, substance abuse, psychological concerns, and physical inactivity) as well as growth pains that may accompany rapid growth spurts. Preadolescents and adolescents are particularly concerned about body image and self-concept. Questions should address potential eating disorders, depression, or suicidal thinking. Using indirect statements such as citing statistics related to risk behaviors might help the youth share more confidential information. Open questions could include the following: "How would you describe your extracurricular activities?" "How would you describe your general health?" "Have you had any loss of interest in favorite activities?" "What are your eating habits?" "What are your exercise habits?" and "Do you have a tendency to be worried or anxious?" The Activity Profile for Children and Youth is a short survey that can identify levels of physical activity, nutritional habits, and sedentary behaviors (Table 6-3).

A more comprehensive screening tool includes information about the teenager's medical history, school information, job/career information, family information, self information, health concerns, health behaviors, and family history. This survey could be modified, as needed, to focus on specific areas of concern. Screening tools for adolescents recommended by the American Academy of Pediatrics and the American Academy of Family Physicians are available on the web.[34] It is helpful to link high-risk behaviors related to physical health concerns, family dysfunction, sexual problems, substance abuse, emotional dysfunction, and school and social dysfunction. Early identification of potential problems provides an opportunity to help the youth make healthier lifestyle choices with support and knowledge. For positive findings in any areas of concern, clinicians should refer to the appropriate health care professional.

Fitness During Childhood

The average American child watches 28 hours of television a week, and studies have proven that parents rather than the children choose this activity for leisure-time activity.[35] Reasons given by parents for using the television as a planned activity include the following:

- Providing the parent freedom from entertaining the child
- Preventing the child from becoming bored
- Socializing in regards to popular television shows
- Watching television is not considered harmful

The drawbacks of watching so much television are self-evident. The child develops a sedentary lifestyle that can lead to obesity. Furthermore, watching television has been shown to slow the development of cognitive skills, especially imagination, and can lead to violent and aggressive behavior. Television should be limited to 1 to 2 hours per day and alternative games and activities, especially physical exercise, should be encouraged for healthy lifestyle behaviors.[35]

TABLE 6-3

ACTIVITY PROFILE FOR CHILDREN AND YOUTH

Child's name: ______________________
Grade: ________ School: ______________

Please answer these questions based upon behavior during a typical week:

1. How many hours each day do you watch television?
   - 0 minutes, I don't watch TV _____
   - 30 minutes to 1 hour (1 to 2 TV shows) _____
   - 1 to 2 hours per day (3 to 4 TV shows) _____
   - More than 2 hours per day _____
2. How much time do you spend exercising outdoors at school and at home?
   - 0 minutes _____
   - 30 minutes to 1 hour _____
   - 1 to 2 hours per day _____
   - More than 2 hours per day _____
3. How much time do you spend reading books, newspapers, or magazines at school and at home?
   - 0 minutes, I don't read at home _____
   - 30 minutes to 1 hour per day _____
   - 1 to 2 hours per day _____
   - More than 2 hours per day _____
4. How many servings of each food group do you eat on a typical day? Circle the answer.

Bread and cereal	1	2	3	4	5	6
Milk and cheese	1	2	3	4	5	6
Fruit and vegetables	1	2	3	4	5	6
Meat, chicken, fish, and beans	1	2	3	4	5	6

LIST YOUR FAVORITE PHYSICAL ACTIVITIES

____
____
____
____
____

Assessing Fitness in Children

Before recommending specific physical activities for children, a physical therapist should assess levels of fitness. The President's Challenge: Physical Activity and Fitness Program is a comprehensive program for children ages 6 to 17 incorporating activities designed to improve physical activity and physical fitness.[36] Tests used by this program to determine baseline levels of fitness include curl-ups or partial curl-ups, an endurance run for cardiorespiratory endurance, pull ups and push ups for upper body strength, a sit-and-reach test for flexibility, and BMI for body composition. Many educational settings employ the President's Challenge: Physical Activity and Fitness Program to address fitness needs of children and adults; nonetheless, children and youth are still prone to obesity and other health risks due to a predominantly sedentary lifestyle.

Exercise for Children and Youth

Physical activity produces overall physical, psychological, and social benefits for children and youth. Inactive children are likely to become inactive adults, so physical therapists need to encourage physical activity in children and youth as physiological buffers to illness. As with adults, physical activity can improve fitness in children and youth:

- Controlling weight
- Reducing blood pressure
- Raising HDL ("good") cholesterol
- Reducing the risk of diabetes and some kinds of cancer
- Improving in many areas of psychological well-being, including gaining more self-confidence and higher self-esteem

The American Heart Association (AHA) recommends that all children age 5 and older should participate in at least 30 minutes of enjoyable, moderate-intensity activities every day.[35] The AHA further recommends that children and youth perform at least 30 minutes of vigorous physical activities at least 3 to 4 days each week to achieve and maintain a good level of cardiorespiratory fitness.[35] Sufficient exercise for children with reduced endurance can be achieved by providing two 15-minute periods or three 10-minute periods in which they can engage in vigorous activities appropriate to their age, gender, and stage of physical and emotional development. The AHA has several key goals related to physical activity in its strategic plan for reducing disability and death from cardiovascular disease and stroke.[35] Physical activity goals related to children include the following:

- Communities will increase the number of youth who are complying with AHA—recommended guidelines for physical activity, as described previously.
- Communities will actively support accessible physical activity in accordance with AHA-recommended guidelines.
- Communities will mandate appropriate school-site physical activity programs in compliance with AHA—recommended guidelines.

The AHA strategic plan was developed by a panel of leading scientists and health educators:

- Increasing awareness of the physical, psychological, and social benefits of physical activity
- Increasing knowledge about the types and levels of physical activity that prevent cardiovascular disease and that promote overall health and fitness
- Increasing behavior-change skills that promote physical activity
- Increasing physical activity levels

This strategic plan targeted inactive youth as one of the primary populations for education and advocacy programs. Physical therapists need to play a significant role in the development and implementation of educational and physical activity programs that promote physical activity and behavior-change skills that reduce health risks posed by inactivity. The AHA suggests that programs be designed to help children and youth adopt the following behaviors[35]:

- Engage in regular, moderately intense physical activity for at least 30 minutes a day. Learn to enjoy physical activity.
- Engage in vigorous physical activity that helps develop and maintain cardiorespiratory fitness 3 or more days per week for at least 30 minutes per occasion.
- Learn and use self-management skills (eg, goal setting, monitoring, barrier minimization) to maintain active lifestyles.
- Know the amounts and types of physical activity associated with the benefits (ie, social, emotional, health, physical), and participate in a variety of these.
- Increase physical activity by reducing nonschool sedentary time spent watching TV, playing video games, etc.
- Develop skills and learn how to participate in developmentally appropriate physical activities.

In addition, recommendations for public policy were incorporated in the strategic plan to reinforce implementation of desired programs. These recommendations include the following:

- Helping establish standards for the quality and quantity of physical education classes and/or programs, such as requiring physical education classes for grades K through 12.

- Providing physical fitness and lifestyle management classes to children and youth.
- Integrating fitness testing into physical education programs that promote lifetime physical activity.

The AHA has ongoing efforts with several federal agencies and professional organizations to help implement its organizational strategic plan to meet goals for promoting physical activity. Other resources for promoting physical activity for children and youth include the following:

- Guidelines for School and Community Programs to Promote Lifelong Physical Activity among Young People. US Centers for Disease Control and Prevention. US Department of Health and Human Services. *Morbidity and Mortality Weekly Report*. Volume 46. March 7, 1997.
- *Promoting Physical Activity: A Guide for Community Action*. US Centers for Disease Control and Prevention. US Department of Health and Human Services. Human Kinetics Publisher, 1999.
- *Physical Best: Activity Guide (Elementary and Secondary Levels)*.
- Related AHA publications: *About Your Heart and Exercise* (for secondary students), *Just Move, Walking for a Healthy Heart, Walking: The Natural Way to Fun and Fitness, How Can Physical Activity Become a Way of Life* in the "Answers By Heart" kit (also in Spanish kit), and *Why Should I Exercise*.

Before any physical activity program is initiated, the child's physician should conduct a physical to ensure the child is not at increased risk for cardiopulmonary, neuromuscular, musculoskeletal, or other impairments from engaging in increased physical activity. Physical therapists are trained to modify exercise prescription based upon potential pathological conditions and can decrease the intensity, duration, or frequency of exercises to meet the individual needs of the child or youth. Chapter 15 discusses in greater detail developing health and fitness programs that best suit the needs of children with developmental disabilities. This chapter will focus on children without physical impairments restricting normal physical activity.

SUGGESTED SPORTS ACTIVITIES FOR CHILDREN AND YOUTH

Certain physical activities can be suggested for each age group based upon the normal physical and psychosocial development of children as they mature.[36] While individual differences might warrant exploring other options, it is important to offer a variety of activities that are age-appropriate.

Physical Activities for Children Ages 2 to 3

Young children are just learning to run, jump, and catch a ball, so competitive sports are inappropriate at this level. Physical activity offering variety and minimal structure will afford young children an opportunity to explore their bodies and their environment. Children tend to be more egocentric at this age and may not understand the concept of performing as part of a team. Activities that will most likely provide the appropriate physical activity include unstructured playtime with other children, running and walking in a yard or playground, swinging or sliding on a child-sized playground set, water play, toddler gymnastics classes, and tumbling. At this age, all physical activity should be closely supervised and provided on soft play surfaces.

Physical Activities for Children Ages 4 to 6

As children mature to elementary school age, they are capable of higher-level balance and coordination activities. They also are capable of sharing toys, such as a ball, and engaging in social activities with other children. Children ages 4 to 6 enjoy dancing, playing games like hopscotch or tag, jumping rope, playing catch with a lightweight ball, and riding a tricycle or a bike with training wheels.

Physical Activities for Children Ages 7 to 10

Children who are 7 and older are capable of understanding the concepts of team sports and are more cautious about safety issues. Sports activities popular with children in this age group include baseball, gymnastics, soccer, swimming, and tennis.

Physical Activities for Children Ages 10 and Older

As the child reaches adolescence and matures into an adult-sized physique, more demanding physical activity is allowable; however, precautions are needed to avoid overstressing developing musculoskeletal structures. Popular physical activities for children and youth who are 10 and older include biking, aerobic exercise and strength training, hiking, organized team sports, rowing, running, track and field events, and softball.

Precautions

Older children may be interested in prescribed exercise programs to increase health-related fitness and sports-related fitness. Special precautions should be applied to exercise prescriptions designed for children. Children and youth may experience a higher incidence of overuse injuries or damage to the epiphyseal growth plates of bones if exercise is too strenuous.[37]

Children must be careful when participating in activities that involve sudden, forceful external rotation of the ankle and foot. This kind of movement, especially in preadolescent children, can result in rotational injuries of the distal tibial growth plate.[37] Injury to the anterior cruciate ligament is one of the most common sports-related injuries of the knee, as are forearm fractures.[37] Children and youth should be advised to wear protective athletic gear and to avoid overuse injuries when participating in any types of sports activities. In addition, pre-participation physical examinations (PPEs) should include comprehensive screenings of all body systems to reveal potential risks related to the musculoskeletal and cardiopulmonary systems. Poorly healed injuries and joints unprepared for certain types of movement usually caused such disqualifications. Heart and vision problems were the next most common causes of disqualification.

Exercise Prescription for Children

When prescribing exercise for children and youth, it is important to recognize children do not have the same anaerobic capacity as adults. The ability to perform anaerobic or high intensity exercise for a short duration increases with age.[38] Likewise, blood lactate levels at maximal exercise also increase with age, possibly secondary to increases in energy stores, muscle mass, and improved neuromuscular coordination.[38] One study demonstrated a 10% to 15% increase in anaerobic power in 10- and 11-year-old boys engaged in a 9-week interval training program.[38] Training children requires knowledge of fitness training principles, including the overload principle, specificity, detraining, periodization, and individual differences.

Appropriate exercise prescription for children and youth requires minor modifications to standard exercise regimens to ensure that the growing child is not overstressed. Using the FITTE formula, the clinician should make the following modifications for strength training:

F = *Frequency:* ASCM suggests that strength training sessions should be limited to twice per week. Also, children and youth should be encouraged to participate in various forms of physical activity for fitness and enjoyment.[39]

I = *Intensity:* Since the musculoskeletal system is maturing, overstressing tissue should be avoided. Resistance exercises should not be done at maximal weights or to the point of muscular fatigue. To achieve training effects, the frequency rather than the intensity of weight training should be altered prior to puberty.[39]

T = *Time or duration:* Exercises should initially be performed slowly with an emphasis on proper technique and with adequate rest between exercises. The ACSM recommends performing 1 to 2 sets (with 8 to 12 repetitions per set) of 8 to 10 exercises emphasizing all major muscle groups.[39]

T = *Type:* Children and youth should perform a variety of exercises that work different major muscle groups during a workout.

E = *Enjoyment:* Children and youth should be encouraged to participate in physical activity for the sake of enjoyment rather than competition as much as possible.

The Mayo Clinic offers the following suggestions for youth strength training[40]:

- *Provide instruction.* Show the child proper breathing and exercise techniques to ensure safe execution of the desired movements.
- *Supervise.* Adult supervision is important to reinforce safety and good technique. Mentors serve as positive reinforcement for healthy lifestyle habits.
- *Warm up; cool down.* Have the child begin each workout with 5 to 10 minutes of a warm-up activity, such as walking, jogging in place, or jumping rope, to prepare the muscles for more dynamic activity. End each workout with a cool down, including some light stretching.
- *Think light weights, controlled repetitions.* One set of 12 to 20 repetitions at a lighter weight is all it takes. Resistance tubing can be just as effective as dumbbell weights, especially for younger children.
- *Rest between workouts.* Establish a rest period of at least a day between strength training workouts. Two or three sessions per week are adequate.
- *Track progress.* Teach the child how to fill out an exercise plan with a description of each exercise, how many repetitions need to be performed,

and what weights or resistance will be used during a workout. It will be helpful in monitoring progress.

- *Add weight gradually.* Only when the child masters proper form should weight be added.
- *Keep it fun.* Vary the routine often so that boredom and monotony are avoided.

Strength Training for Children and Youth

A growing number of children and adolescents are experiencing the benefits of strength training. Strength training can be a safe and effective activity for this age group, provided that the program is properly designed and competently supervised. It is important, however, to distinguish strength training from weight lifting and power lifting. *Strength training* refers to a systematic and progressive program of exercises designed to increase an individual's ability to exert or resist force. Professional organizations have published position stands on prepubescent strength training and offer the following guidelines and principles[40]:

- Strength training should be supervised and monitored closely by appropriately trained professionals who acknowledge that no matter how big, strong, or mature the individual appears, the individual is physiologically immature.
- The participant must be able to understand the key principles of strength training and acknowledge that physical fitness, and not power lifting and body building, are the goals of resistance training. Many 7- and 8-year-old boys and girls have benefited from strength training, and there is no reason why younger children could not participate in strength-related activities, such as push-ups and sit-ups, if they can safely perform the exercises and follow instructions.
- The primary focus should initially be directed toward learning proper techniques for all exercise movements (including warm-up and cool-down periods) and developing an interest in resistance training. Proper techniques, including proper breathing, should be taught before the gradual increase of resistance.
- Movements should be performed with control, avoiding any fast or jerky movements that could tear soft tissue and with an emphasis on full range of motion multi-joint exercises versus single-joint exercises. Strength training with maximal weights is not recommended because of the potential for possible injuries related to the long bones, growth plates, and back.

All fitness programs for children and adolescents should incorporate key fitness components, including flexibility, cardiovascular endurance, muscular strength and endurance, and improved body composition. Well-designed programs offer the added benefits of enhancing motor skills and improving sports performance. Strength training programs, in particular, can decrease the incidence of certain sports injuries by building strong muscles, resilient ligaments, and healthy bones. While muscle hypertrophy or enlarged muscle size is a common effect of strength training in most age groups, prepubescent children lack adequate levels of muscle-building hormones for observable changes in muscle bulk. Instead, changes in body composition, such as reduced body fat, are more frequently observed during childhood indicating that strength training may play an important role in reducing obesity during childhood and adolescence.

Flexibility Exercises for Young Athletes

While maintaining general fitness can be accomplished through a regular exercise program, most children and youth engage in sports activity to maintain fitness. To ensure that young athletes optimally benefit from sports activities, flexibility exercise can be helpful in preventing injury during competition. "Athletes must do each one of the exercises carefully, speed is not important. Once the exercise routine is learned, the entire program should take no longer than 10 minutes. It also is important to warm up before doing any of these exercises. Good examples of warm-up activities are slowly running in place and walking for a few minutes."[41]

Summary

The physical therapist plays a key role in the health, fitness, and wellness of children with impairments, functional limitations, and disabilities but must recognize how important it is to reach out to children and youth who are at risk for illness and potentially life-threatening injury. As part of the health care team, the physical therapist must communicate effectively with the obstetrician and gynecologist of pregnant women; the pediatrician or family physician regarding risk factors for children and youth; other professionals who support health, fitness, and wellness; and, most importantly, the family. Collaboration on all fronts offers the best opportunity for managing potential problems that threaten the health, fitness, and wellness of infants, children, and youth.

References

1. Psychosocial and Environmental Pregnancy Risks. Emedicine. Available at: http://www.emedicine.com/med/topics3237.html#selection~introduction. Accessed October 31, 2004.
2. Frankenburg WK, Dobbs JB. *Denver Developmental Screening Test II-Screening Manual.* Denver, Co: Denver Developmental Materials; 1990.
3. Brachlow A, Jordan AE, Tervo R. Developmental screenings in rural settings: a comparison of the child development review and the Denver II Developmental Screening Test. *J Rural Health.* 2001;17(3):156–159.
4. National Center for Chronic Disease Prevention and Health Promotion. Center for Disease Control. Available at: http://www.cdc.gov/nccdphp/dnpa/bmi/bmi-for-age.htm. Accessed November 10, 2004.
5. Tanner JM. Normal growth and techniques of growth assessment. *Clin Endocrinol Metab.* 1986;15(3):411–451.
6. Odegard RA, Vatten LJ, Nilsen ST, Salvesen KA, Austgulen R. Preeclampsia and fetal growth. *Obstet Gynecol.* 2000;96(6):950–955.
7. Renders CM, Seidell JC, van Mechelen W, Hirasing RA. Overweight and obesity in children and adolescents and preventative measures. *Tijdschr Geneeskd.* 2004;48(42):2066–2070.
8. Caballero B. Obesity prevention in children: opportunities and challenges. *Int J Obes Relat Metab Disord.* 2004;28(Suppl 3):S90–S95.
9. Rieser P. Patterns of growth. Human Growth Foundation. Available at: http://www.hgfound.org/patterns.html. Accessed November 11, 2004.
10. Spilsbury JC, Storfer-Isser A, Drotar D, et al. Sleep behavior in an urban US sample of school-aged children. *Arch Pediatr Adolesc Med.* 2004;158(10):988–994.
11. Bergman A. *Twenty Common Problems in Pediatrics.* St. Louis, Mo: McGraw-Hill; 1990.
12. Middle Ear, Acute Otitis Media, Surgical Treatment. Available at: http://www.emedicine.com/ent/topic211.htm. Accessed November 11, 2004.
13. Pediatrics, Urinary Tract Infections and Pyelonephritis. Available at: http://www.emedicine.com/emerg/topic769.htm. Accessed November 11, 2004.
14. Sidbury R. What's new in pediatric dermatology: update for the pediatrician. *Curr Opin Pediatr.* 2004;16(4):410–414.
15. Oral R, Blum KL, Johnson C. Fractures in young children: are physicians in the emergency department and orthopedic clinics adequately screening for possible abuse? *Pediatr Emerg Care.* 2003;19(3):148–153.
16. Munchausen syndrome by proxy. Available at: http://www.emedicine.com/ped/topic2742.htm. Accessed November 11, 2004.
17. Spergel JM, Beausoleil JL, Fiedler JM, et al. Correlation of initial food reactions to observed reactions on challenges. *Ann Allergy Asthma Immunol.* 2004;92(2):217–224.
18. Satta A. Exercise training in asthma. *J Sports Med Phys Fitness.* 2000;40(4):277–283.
19. Mellon M, Parasuraman B. Pediatric asthma: improving management to reduce cost of care. *J Manag Care Pharm.* 2004;10(2):130–141.
20. Asthma. Available at: http://www.emedicine.com/ped/topic152.htm. Accessed November 11, 2004.
21. Cabana MD, Slish KK, Lewis TC, et al. Parental management of asthma triggers within a child's environment. *J Allergy Clin Immunol.* 2004;114(2):352–357.
22. Rosimini C. Benefits of swim training for children and adolescents with asthma. *J Am Acad Nurse Pract.* 2003;15(6):247–252.
23. Evans AM, Scutter SD. Prevalence of "growing pains" in young children. *J Pediatr.* 2004;145(2):255–258.
24. Nygaard EA, Stordal K, Bentsen BS. Recurrent abdominal pain in children revisited: irritable bowel syndrome and psychosomatic aspects. A prospective study. *Scand J Gastroenterol.* 2004;39(10):938–940.
25. Powers SW, Mitchell MJ, Byars KC, et al. A pilot study of one-session biofeedback training in pediatric headache. *Neurology.* 2001;56:133.
26. Skoog SJ. How to evaluate and treat pediatric enuresis: behavioral modification, drug therapy are keys to controlling daytime, nighttime wetting. *Urology Times.* April 2004. Available at: http://www.urologytimes.com/urologytimes/article/articleDetail.jsp?id=92007&&pageID=2. Accessed November 17, 2004.
27. Von Gontard A, Hollmann E. Comorbidity of functional urinary incontinence and encopresis: somatic and behavioral associations. *J Urol.* 2004;171(6[Pt 2]):2644–2647.
28. Baumann R. Febrile Seizures from Emedicine. Departments of Neurology and Pediatrics, University of Kentucky. Available at: http://www.emedicine.com/neuro/topic134.htm. Accessed November 17, 2004.
29. Cavazos JE. Seizures and epilepsy: overview and classification. Departments of Medicine, Pharmacology, University of Texas Health Science Center at San Antonio, NM. Available at: http://www.emedicine.com/NEURO/topic415.htm. Accessed November 17, 2004.
30. The National Information Center for Children and Youth with Disabilities. Available at: http://www.nichcy.org/disabinf.asp. Accessed November 17, 2004.
31. National Institute of Health. Attention Deficit / Hyperactivity Disorder (ADHD). Available at: http://www.advantify.com/vani/adhd.htm. Accessed February 6, 2006.
32. Sawada Y. On the body composition of obese children and in particular, sexual, age, and regional differences of skinfold thickness. *J Human Ergol.* 1978;7(2):103–117.

33. YRBSS: youth risk behavior surveillance system. National Center for Chronic Disease Prevention and Health Promotion. Available at: http://www.cdc.gov/HealthyYouth/yrbs/index.htm. Accessed November 17, 2004.

34. American Academy of Pediatrics and the American Academy of Family Physicians. Lab Tests Online. Available at: http://www.labtestsonline.org/understanding/wellness/c_youngadult.html. Accessed February 6, 2006.

35. American Heart Association. Physical Activity: AHA scientific position. Available at: http://216.185.112.5/presenter.jhtml?identifier=4563. Accessed November 11, 2004.

36. President's Challenge: Physical Activity and Fitness Program. 2006. Available at: http://www.presidentschallenge.org. Accessed February 6, 2006.

37. Ippolito E, Postacchini F, Scola E. Skeletal growth in normal and pathological conditions. *Ital J Orthop Traumatol.* 1983;9(1):115–127.

38. Rotstein A, Dotan R, Bar-Or O, Tenenbaum G. Effect of training on anaerobic threshold, maximal aerobic power and anaerobic performance of preadolescent boys. *Int J Sports Med.* 1986;7(5):281–286.

39. Ashmore A. Strength training guidelines for children—CEU Corner. *American Fitness.* Sept–Oct 2003.

40. Mayo Clinic. Strength training: OK for kids when done correctly. 2006. Available at: http://www.mayoclinic.com/health/strength-training/HQ01010. Accessed February 6, 2006.

41. American College of Sports Medicine. Youth Strength Training. Available at: http://www.acsm.org/pdf/YSTRNGTH.pdf. Accessed February 2, 2006.

Health, Fitness, and Wellness During Adulthood

Catherine Rush Thompson, PhD, MS, PT

"Every human being is the author of his own health."

~ BUDDHIST QUOTE

Unique Challenges During Adulthood

The term "adult" suggests both physical maturation and a psychosocial transition from being dependent on others to becoming more self-reliant and responsible for personal behaviors. While the body is physically mature between ages 21 and 25, the adult's psychosocial dimensions continually develop. Key life skills developing throughout adulthood enable the individual to function independently in the home, in the community, and in the world, yet many of the psychosocial skills that enable the individual to function independently in varying contexts are taught early in life. Recognizing these foundational psychosocial skills, health care professionals need a broad perspective for managing the adult client. Independent function in the home, in the workplace, and in leisure activities is key to physical and mental health, yet interactions with others, including friends and family, play an essential role in wellness.

During adulthood, there are many common characteristics between males and females; however, priorities vary as men and women move from early to late adulthood. The primary life tasks that engage men and women are health, relationships with others (a spouse or partner, parents, and/or children), and financial security (property and income). Earlier in life, children dominate priorities, but income and property needed for financial stability and retirement become more important in later life. These priorities suggest key issues for preventive care: health, relationships, and income/property. Health care providers should promote the health of the individual while recognizing the importance of significant relationships and financial stability.

While children and youth deal with adapting to ever-changing physiques, psychologists suggest that individuals progressing through adulthood seek two basic needs: (1) *intimacy in human relationships* (affiliation, social acceptance, or love and belonging) and (2) *competence* (achievement, generativity, or productivity). Freud felt that the healthy adult has the ability to both love and work.[1] Erikson described the two crises of early adulthood in terms of intimacy versus isolation, followed by generativity versus stagnation.[3] 2Psychological health and happiness in adult years depend on how the individual envisions the future and what that individual does to bring about the desired vision. Generativity orients the individual toward the long-term goals in life and the future.

The key tasks of early adulthood include separating from parents, making choices in relationships, and achieving in the realms of education, career, community, and parenthood while accommodating social demands. As adults progress into adulthood, they become more conscious of their professional and personal goals, including issues associated with childbearing, career goals, social relationships, and mentoring others in life. Individuals with lower *socioeconomic status (SES)* often must leave school to begin work; they marry and often become parents at a younger age than other adults with more financial resources.[3] These additional responsibilities earlier in life can cause additional stresses that make people of low SES more vulnerable to stress and illness.[4] Minority populations with certain genetic backgrounds are put at an even greater risk for pathology when living in poverty.

Relationships with close friends or sexual partners may either serve as buffers against stress or as sources of stress for many individuals. Many intimate relationships in adulthood do not survive adulthood challenges, as evidenced by the divorce rate. The 2001 United States divorce rate for was 0.38% per capita per year according to the National Vital Statistic Report from the Center for Disease Control[4]:

> *Divorced adults, particularly divorced men, experience early health problems to a much greater extent than married individuals. Premature death rates for divorced men from such causes as cardiovascular disease, hypertension, and strokes double that of married men. The premature death rate from pneumonia is seven times larger for divorced men than for married men... The suicide rate for divorced white men was four times higher than for their married counterparts.*[4]

The importance of healthy adult relationships cannot be overrated.

Work during adulthood is often a key aspect of an individual's identity. For many people, work is central to their lives for more than economic reasons. Workers who have been laid off or disabled often feel lost, depressed, and empty. According to one study, the indirect cost of illness due to lost wages exceeds the cost of medical services by a large margin.[5] Social characteristics of persons with physical impairments are more important than the medical condition characteristics in predicting whether disability will lead to work loss.[6] Physical therapists can help adult clients reach their full potential by providing needed resources for physical, mental, and psychosocial health through education, fitness programs, and appropriate referrals to needed services, including psychologists and social workers.

The health, fitness, and wellness needs of adults vary between males and females. Both genders seek intimacy and generativity, but social roles as well as genetics lead to substantially different health risks.

Adult Health and Wellness Risks

Adults face health risks that affect all major body systems, including the integumentary, cardiovascular, neuromuscular, and musculoskeletal systems, commonly treated in physical therapy. In addition, risks for developing diabetes, cancer, chronic pain, substance abuse, gastrointestinal problems, migraine headaches, accidents, infections, and sleep disorders increase during adult years. Many of these conditions are covered in the chapters discussing musculoskeletal, neuromuscular, integumentary, and cardiopulmonary conditions. The physical therapist should be familiar with these risk factors to alert individuals to potential threats to health and to inform physicians of controllable factors potentially contributing to chronic illness.

SKIN CONDITIONS

Screening for skin conditions often occurs during a comprehensive examination but can be performed by asking questions related to common integumentary problems that arise in adulthood. While warts, acne, impetigo, and tinea pedis are more common in youth and adolescents, adults often present with chronic skin problems, such as dermatitis and psoriasis.

Dermatitis (eczema) is commonly seen as skin inflammation, generalized redness, edema or swelling, and possible oozing, crusting, and scaling, when long-standing.[7] *Contact dermatitis* is oftentimes produced by substances contacting the skin and causing toxic or allergic reactions. *Atopic dermatitis* has a genetic component that predisposes the individual to environmental agents or factors that precipitate skin inflammation. While elimination of precipitating factors alleviates contact dermatitis, it does not ameliorate atopic dermatitis.[7] *Psoriasis* is a common, chronic, recurrent skin disease that is characterized by dry, well-circumscribed, silvery, scaling papules and plaques of various sizes.[8] This skin condition often presents in a characteristic pattern on extensor surfaces of elbows and knees, scalp, back, anogenital region, and/or nails but may also appear on flexor surfaces, the tip of the penis, or the palms.[8] The physical therapist can ask about possible skin conditions or note skin rashes or irregularities during a physical examination. If an individual reports skin inflammation, itchiness, redness, soreness, or open wounds that fail to heal, medical attention is needed. All suspected skin conditions should be referred to a physician for a medical diagnosis and proper medical treatment.

To prevent skin problems, individuals need proper hydration. The skin is particularly vulnerable to changes in hydration and relies on fluid ingestion and humidity for a supple and soft appearance. According to the Merck Manual, 60% humidity in the environment is needed for keeping skin optimally hydrated.[11] At levels below 15% humidity, the corneum or outer surface of the skin tends to crack and shrink, making the skin vulnerable to infections and other skin irritations. Sweating allows evaporation of fluid from the body, so efforts to rehydrate the skin or prevent evaporation can benefit the skin in conjunction with drinking adequate amounts of fluid.[11] Dry and scaly skin can be treated by soaking the area with water for approximately 5 minutes and by reducing evaporation. Barriers to evaporation, such as oils and ointments, can help to reduce evaporation if used as recommended, generally once or twice daily. In areas with increased sweating, such as the armpit (axilla) and groin, barriers to evaporation are generally not recommended.[9]

When humidity increases to over 90%, the skin becomes overhydrated. With overhydration, such as when a foot is soaked for a long time, the cells of the skin are widely separated as tight junctions between cells are replaced by weaker connections. Ultimately, the skin loses it effectiveness as an environmental barrier. In these cases, air drying the affected area is recommended to reduce skin overhydration and risk of infection or injury.[9] When physical therapists are working in environments that are especially dry or humid, they can prevent skin problems by keeping the air optimally hydrated. In addition, offering their clients water frequently as well as having moisturizing lotions on hand can help alleviate skin problems associated with reduced hydration.

Skin Cancer

Skin cancer should always be considered as a threat to all adults, most particularly fair-skinned individuals. Skin cancers, which are usually curable, are the most common type of cancer; most arise in sun-exposed areas of skin.[10] *Malignant melanoma* is a fatal tumor affecting the skin, mucous membranes, eyes, and the central nervous system. The incidence of melanoma has more than tripled in the white population during the last 20 years, resulting in an estimated 7770 deaths in 2005 (4910 men, 2860 women).[11] More information about skin screening and protection is provided in Chapter 15.

Type 1 Diabetes Mellitus

Type 1 diabetes mellitus (type 1 DM) can occur at any age, but most commonly develops in childhood or adolescence and is diagnosed before age 30.[12] *Type 2 diabetes mellitus* (type 2 DM) is more commonly diagnosed in individuals over the age of 30 years, but it also occurs in children and adolescents. DM has diverse presentations, but both type 1 and type 2 DM generally present with *hyperglycemia* (high blood glucose). Symptoms of hyperglycemia include *polyuria* (frequent urination) followed by *polydipsia* (excessive thirst) and weight loss from dehydration. Other clinical manifestations of hyperglycemia include blurred vision, fatigue, and nausea as well as susceptibility to fungal and bacterial infections.[12] Type 2 DM is commonly associated with obesity, especially of the upper body (visceral/abdominal), and often presents after a period of weight gain. Most patients are treated with diet, exercise, and oral drugs, with some patients requiring insulin to control symptomatic hyperglycemia. Type 2 DM patients with visceral/abdominal obesity may have normal glucose levels after losing weight.[12]

According to the American Diabetes Association, a recent study by the Diabetes Prevention Program (DPP) demonstrated that people at risk for type 2 DM can improve their health through diet and increased levels of physical activity, potentially restoring blood glucose levels to a healthier range.[13] Diet and exercise may be even more effective than some medications designed to treat prediabetic patients. The DPP also demonstrated that 30 minutes a day of moderate physical activity in conjunction with as little as a 5% reduction in body weight produced a 58% reduction in diabetes.[13] The American Diabetes Association has extensive, up-to-date information about diabetes prevention, including diet and nutrition recommendations.

Cancer or Uncontrolled Cellular Proliferation

Cancer or uncontrolled cellular proliferation, by definition, is malignant but not necessarily fatal. Most cancers are curable if detected in their early stages, and patients can help recognize early signs of possible malignancies. All individuals should be encouraged to perform self-examinations, including for skin cancer and breast cancer (both males and females are vulnerable), and have appropriate diagnostic testing to screen for cancers that affect specific populations, such as cervical cancer in adult females and prostate cancer in adult males. According to the American Cancer Society (ACS) and the United States Preventative Services Task Force, beginning at age 50, both men and women should follow one of the following five testing schedules: (1) yearly *fecal occult blood test (FOBT)*, a test examining blood in the stool, (2) a flexible *sigmoidoscopy* (a tests that involves the doctor visualizing the lower bowel through a small, flexible, lighted tube inserted through the rectum and lower colon) every 5 years, (3) yearly *FOBT plus flexible sigmoidoscopy* every 5 years (preferred over either alone), (4) *double-contrast barium enema* every 5 years, or (5) a *colonoscopy* (an examination of the rectum and entire colon using a lighted instrument) every 10 years.[14]

Physical therapists should also be on the alert for common symptoms that are associated with cancer, including a change in usual bowel habits (constipation, diarrhea, or both); stools that are narrower than usual; blood in or on the stool; general stomach discomfort such as bloating, fullness, and/or cramps; frequent gas pains; a feeling of incomplete bowel emptying; weight loss with no known reason; and constant fatigue. Note the following cancer screening recommendations by the ACS in Table 7-1 as well as common symptoms noted in individuals with cancer, listed in Table 7-2.

OBESITY

Obesity is the fastest growing health problem in the United States with over 64% of adults either overweight or obese.[15] There are, however, great disparities in the prevalence in obesity. While 33% of all women and 28% of all men are obese, Mexican-American men have a higher prevalence of overweight and obesity (75%) than non-Hispanic, white men (67%) and non-Hispanic, black men (61%). Fifty percent of African American women and 40% of Hispanic women are obese compared with 30% of white women. In general, women and men from lower-income families experience a greater prevalence of obesity than those in higher-income families.[15]

Health risks associated with obesity include premature death, type 2 DM, hyperlipidemia, hypertension, coronary artery disease, stroke, certain types of cancer, gastroesophageal reflux disease, gallstones and gall bladder disease, gout, nonalcoholic fatty liver disease, pregnancy complications, menstrual irregularities, bladder control problems, osteoarthritis, obstructive sleep apnea, infertility, and psychological disorders such as depression, eating disorders, problems with body image, and low self-esteem.[16] The American Medical Association suggests that health professionals recognize the significant consequences of obesity with devastating medical, economic, and social consequences. According to a study of national costs attributed to both overweight (BMI 25.0 to 29.9) and obesity (BMI greater than 30), medical expenses accounted for 9.1% of total United States medical expenditures in 1998 and may have reached as high as $78.5 billion ($92.6 billion in 2002).[17] Measures to decrease obesity are listed in Table 7-3.

METABOLIC SYNDROME

As many as 22% of American adults may have a sinister sounding disorder called *syndrome X* or *metabolic syndrome*, a condition significantly increasing a person's risk of developing life threatening chronic diseases.[18] See Table 7-4 for risk factors commonly associated with metabolic syndrome.

When metabolic syndrome is diagnosed early in its development, it can be slowed and, in some cases, even reversed.[18] Changes in diet and exercise can help significantly reduce the risk of developing this pathology. If an individual presents with risk factors for metabolic syndrome, the physician should be contacted for appropriate medical management. With obesity as a primary risk factor, physical activity under the supervision of a physical therapist is advisable.

HEART DISEASE

Heart disease has many of the same risk factors as metabolic syndrome. Now affecting men and women as a leading cause of death in adulthood, this condition is discussed in greater detail in Chapter 13.

INSOMNIA

Insomnia is an individual's perception that sleep quality is inadequate or nonrestorative despite having the opportunity to sleep. Insomnia includes difficulty falling asleep, sleeping too lightly, being easily disrupted with multiple spontaneous awakenings, or early morning awakenings with an inability to fall back asleep.[19] Insomnia is considered a disorder when it disrupts or impairs daily functioning. If an individual reports any difficulty with sleeping, the physical therapist should note the duration of the symptom. Transient insomnia lasts less than 1 week; short-term insomnia lasts 1 to 6 months and is usually associated with persistent, stressful situations (such as death or illness of a loved one or environmental factors, such as loud environmental noises); and chronic insomnia lasts more than 6 months.[19] Insomnia can lead to depression and anxiety, abnormalities in metabolism, daytime sleepiness, and memory problems. Insomnia may be a problem of hyperarousal rather than mere sleep deprivation associated with stress. Individuals with insomnia should be referred to a physician for a more comprehensive examination and possible medical management.[19]

SEXUALLY TRANSMITTED DISEASES

Sexually transmitted diseases (STDs) have serious and sometimes fatal complications. Sexually active teens and young adults are at highest risk, but STDs can affect all age groups. Those who are at increased risk of infection[20] include the following:

TABLE 7-1

CANCER SCREENING RECOMMENDATIONS FOR AVERAGE-RISK ADULTS

	Test	Recommendations
Breast	Self-examination (BSE)	Monthly for women over age 20 with education that the risk of breast cancer increases with age *Education:* Increase vegetable intake, increase physical activity, limit alcohol intake, avoid becoming overweight, and take folic acid supplements.
	Clinical breast examination	Every 3 years (during regular physical examinations) from age 20 to 40 and annually thereafter *Education:* Same as for all breast cancer screening tests (see above)
	Mammography	Annually age 40 and older *Education:* Same as for all breast cancer screening tests (see above)
Cervix	Papanicolaou (PAP) test	Annually beginning within 3 years after first vaginal intercourse or no later than age 21. After age 30, women with three normal tests may be screened every 2 to 3 years. Women may choose to stop screening after age 70 if they have had three normal (and no abnormal) results within the last 10 years. *Education:* Increase vegetable and fruit intake, increase physical activity, and avoid becoming overweight.
Colon	Fecal occult blood (FOB) testing and rigid sigmoidoscopy	Annual FOB testing combined with rigid sigmoidoscopy can increase the identification of cancer more accurately than either test conducted alone. Barium enema and colonoscopy are also considered reasonable alternatives. *Education:* Increase vegetable and fruit intake, limit intake of red meat, increase physical activity, avoid becoming overweight, limit alcohol intake, take folic acid supplements, and take selenium supplements.
	Double-contrast barium enema	While this is not the screening test of choice, it may be used to detect larger growths. *Education:* Same as for all colon cancer screening tests (see above)
	Colonoscopy	Colonoscopy can be used to detect larger growths; however, it poses more risk than other screening measures, including the risk of perforation and bleeding. *Education:* Same as for all colon cancer screening tests (see above)
	Digital rectal exam (DRE)	DRE is not recommended because of its limited ability to detect colon cancer. Less than 10% of patients with colorectal cancer have growths than are within the reach of the examining finger. *Education:* Same as for all colon cancer screening tests (see above)
Prostate	Prostate specific antigen (PSA) blood test	DRE and PSA tests should be offered annually to men age 50 and older who have at least a 10-year life expectancy; those at high risk should begin their testing at age 45. High-risk groups include men of African descent and those whose relatives were diagnosed at a young age. *Education:* Increase vegetable and fruit intake, limit intake of red meat, take vitamin E supplements, take selenium supplements, and take selenium supplements.
Other	Cancer-related checkup	Every 3 years for men 20 to 40 and annually thereafter; should include counseling and perhaps oral cavity, thyroid, lymph node, or testicular examinations. Those with family histories of cancer or other related risk factors should consult their physicians about more frequent examinations. *Education:* Increase vegetable and fruit intake, limit intake of red meat, increase physical activity, avoid becoming overweight, and limit alcohol intake. *Note:* The use of dietary supplements and nutritional intake is dependent upon the individual's cancer risk for a particular type of cancer. Generally, consuming soy foods and taking supplements (beta-carotene, vitamine E, vitamin C, folic acid, and selenium) may provide some benefit.

Adapted from:

Pignone M, Rich M, Teutsch S, Berg A, Lohr K. Screening for colorectal cancer in adults at average risk: a summary of the evidence for the US Preventive Services Task Force. *Ann Int Med.* 2002;137:132–141.

Smith R, von Eschenbach A, Wender R, et al. American Cancer Society guidelines for the early detection of cancer: update of early detection guidelines for prostate, colorectal, and endometrial cancers. *CA Cancer J Clin.* 2001;51:38–75.

Smith R, Saslow D, Sawyer K, et al. American Cancer Society guidelines for breast cancer screening: update 2003. *CA Cancer J Clin.* 2003;53:141–169.

Byers T, Nestle M, McTiernan A, et al. American Cancer Society guidelines on nutrition and physical activity for cancer prevention: reducing the risk of cancer with healthy food choices and physical activity. *CA Cancer J Clin.* 2002;52:92–119.

TABLE 7-2

CANCER SYMPTOMS

- Persistent cough or blood-tinged saliva
- A cough that lasts more than a month or with blood in the mucus that is coughed up
- A change in bowel habits
- Blood in the stool
- Unexplained anemia (reduced red blood cells), commonly experienced as unexplained fatigue
- Breast lump or breast discharge
- Lumps in the testicles
- A change in urination
- Hematuria (blood in the urine)
- Hoarseness.
- Persistent lumps or swollen glands
- Obvious change in a wart or a mole
- Indigestion or difficulty swallowing
- Unusual vaginal bleeding or discharge
- Unexpected weight loss, night sweats, or fever
- Continued itching in the anus or genitals
- Nonhealing sores
- Headaches
- Back pain, pelvic pain, bloating, or indigestion

Adapted from eMedicineHealth. Cancer Symptoms. The American Cancer Society. Available at: http://www.emedicinehealth.com/articles/9786-2.asp. Accessed October 15, 2005.

TABLE 7-3

PREVENTIVE CARE FOR OBESITY

1. Advocate lifestyles to promote a healthy weight.
2. Alert individuals to the risks of inappropriate weight gain and the benefits of weight loss.
3. Take baseline measures of weight, height, BMI, waist circumference, and blood pressure to monitor the individual's progress.
4. Assess the current levels of physical activity, eating habits, and readiness to make long-term lifestyle changes.
5. Guide individuals toward weight management programs under the supervision of their physician.
6. Provide ongoing support and encouragement for individuals in weight treatment programs.
7. Recognize behavioral and environmental factors that may contribute to overweight and obesity.
8. Identify health professionals in the community who are critical to the treatment of adults who are obese, including registered dieticians, bariatric surgeons, and mental health professionals.
9. Provide relevant health education materials.
10. Become aware of and share community resources that can assist in the management of overweight and obesity problems.

- People who have had multiple sex partners, especially those who have exchanged sex for money or drugs
- Males who have sex with males
- Injection drug users and their sex partners
- Individuals with exposure to HIV/AIDS, gonorrhea, syphilis, chlamydia, genital herpes, and genital warts

According to the Centers for Disease Control and Prevention, an estimated 850,000 to 950,000 persons in the United States are living with human immunodeficiency virus (HIV), including 180,000 to 280,000 who do not know they are infected.[21] The number of new infections is an estimated 40,000 per year for the past decade, indicating that more preventive measures are needed to reduce HIV infections.[21]

Physical therapists can help educate the public about the continued risk of HIV infection and the need to practice safe sex with all partners. In addition, therapists can be aware of the signs and symptoms of HIV infection, as listed in Table 7-5.[22]

Health Risks for Adult Males

In the United States, the top five health risks for men are heart attacks, motor vehicle accidents, lung cancer, HIV, and alcohol abuse.[23] Stroke and violence are sixth and seventh. Heart disease is the greatest health threat to men in the United States today. According to the American Heart Association, men have a greater risk of heart disease and have heart attacks much earlier in life than women do. All men need to take this disease seriously and understand that this number-one killer can often be prevented. Physical and mental health problems can arise with the increasing family and work responsibilities that adult males face.

CANCER

According to the ACS,[23] the most common cause of cancer death for men is lung cancer, and 90% of these deaths are linked to cigarette smoking. Prostate cancer is the second leading cause of cancer death among men. More than half the men older than age 50 have an enlarged prostate caused by a noncancerous condition called *benign prostatic hyperplasia (BPH)*. About one-third of all cancer deaths are related to nutrition or other controllable lifestyle factors.

TABLE 7-4

RISK FACTORS FOR METABOLIC SYNDROME

- Abdominal or "central" obesity (waist size of greater than 40 inches in men, greater than 35 inches in women)
- High levels in the fasting blood of triglycerides (fats) greater than 150 mg/dL
- Low levels of HDL (good) cholesterol (men less than 40 mg/dL and women less than 50 mg/dL)
- High blood pressure (greater than 130/85)
- High levels of glucose (as measured by a "fasting" glucose test) greater than 110mg/dL
- Insulin resistance

Adapted from American Heart Association. Metabolic syndrome. Accessed January 28, 2006. Available at: http://www.americanheart.org/presenter.jhtml?identifier=534.

TABLE 7-5

CLINICAL SIGNS AND SYMPTOMS OF HIV INFECTION

- Chronic dry, scratchy cough, shortness of breath, tightness or pressure in the chest
- Rapid weight loss
- Profuse night sweats
- Continuous unexplained fatigue
- Diarrhea longer than a week (found in both early and late stages of HIV)
- Swollen lymph glands (lymphatic nodes in the neck, armpits and groin)
- Sores, white spots, or blemishes in the mouth, gums, and on the tongue
- Burning sensation and an altered sense of taste.
- Pneumonia
- Shingles
- Excessive bruising and bleeding
- Herpes simplex affecting the rectal, genital, and esophageal regions of the body
- Loss of appetite
- Red, pink, brown, or purplish blotches on and/or under the skin
- Pain or difficulty swallowing
- Constant headaches
- Confusion or forgetfulness
- Unexplainable change in vision
- Chronic yeast infections (women)
- Pelvic inflammatory disease (women)
- Cervical abnormalities (women)
- Skin conditions such as rash, hives, lump, lesion, sore, spots, or abnormal growths
- Chronic monolike illness
- Receding gums
- Constant fevers

Adapted from Daveyboy. HIV/AIDS symptoms and signs. Available at: http://www.hivaidssearch.com/facts/hiv_aids_common_symptoms.htm. Accessed Octobr 15, 2005.

CHRONIC OBSTRUCTIVE PULMONARY DISEASE

Chronic obstructive pulmonary disease (COPD) is an overall term for a group of chronic lung conditions including emphysema and chronic bronchitis. The main cause of COPD is smoking, and it is strongly associated with lung cancer, the number-one cause of cancer death in men.[23] A smoker is 10 times more likely to die of COPD than a nonsmoker.

STROKE

Stroke, also commonly called a cerebrovascular accident, is one of the leading causes of disability in males living in the United States.[23] High blood pressure, smoking, lack of exercise, and a diet high in fat and cholesterol are risk factors that are controllable and that should be considered in preventive care.

ACCIDENTS AND UNINTENTIONAL INJURIES

Accidents and unintentional injuries killed nearly 64,000 men in 2000, the leading cause being motor vehicle crashes. About twice as many men (28,352) as women (13,642) died in traffic accidents.[23]

DIABETES

In 2000, nearly 70,000 people died of diabetes and almost 32,000 of them were men.[23] Diabetes is a chronic disease that has no cure but may be preventable. Advanced diabetes can cause blindness, kidney disease, and severe nerve damage.

PNEUMONIA AND INFLUENZA

When associated with other chronic health conditions, pneumonia and influenza can be life threatening. People with COPD, asthma, heart disease, diabetes, and conditions that suppress the immune system are at high risk. Because both pneumonia and influenza affect the lungs, smoking increases the danger of pneumonia and influenza.

KIDNEY DISEASE

According to the National Kidney Foundation, 20 million Americans, or 1 in 9 American adults, have chronic kidney disease and another 20 million more are at increased risk.[24] Since high blood pressure and chronic kidney disease are closely related,[25] early detection of kidney disease through appropriate urine and blood pressure analysis as well as promoting healthy lifestyle behaviors can help prevent the progression of kidney disease into kidney failure.

LIVER DISEASE

Chronic liver disease and cirrhosis kill over 17,000 men in the United States annually. Alcoholic liver disease and chronic hepatitis C are the leading causes of cirrhosis.[25] *Cirrhosis* is the scarring that results when liver tissue is destroyed by infection, poison, or disease. While cirrhosis is serious and irreversible, liver diseases can be prevented. Preventive measures include avoiding excessive alcohol, practicing safe sex, avoiding street drugs, getting hepatitis B vaccinations, using precautions when using hazardous chemicals, and maintaining a healthy weight.[25]

SCREENING TESTS AND IMMUNIZATIONS

Physical therapists should be mindful of disease risks of the general population and aware of increased risk factors for males. While the physical therapist can ask questions related to lifestyle behaviors contributing to illness (eg, sedentary behavior, poor diet, smoking, use of alcohol or other substances), specific medical tests can screen for pathophysiological changes that clearly identify pathology. The Table 7-6 offers screening guidelines, tests, and immunizations for adult males that should be encouraged by all health care professionals.[26]

Prostate Cancer Screening Test

The prostate-specific antigen (PSA) test is a blood test that measures the amount of a protein secreted by the prostate gland and is used to screen for possible prostate cancer. According to the ACS, both the PSA blood test and digital rectal examination (DRE) should be offered annually, beginning at age 50, to men who have at least a 10-year life expectancy.[27] Men at high risk (African-American men and men with a strong family history of one or more first-degree relatives—father or brothers—diagnosed at an early age) should begin testing at age 45. Men at even higher risk, due to multiple first-degree relatives affected at an early age, could begin testing at age 40. Depending on the results of this initial test, no further testing might be needed until age 45.[27] Symptoms of prostate cancer are listed in Table 7-7.

While risk factors associated with age, gender, and genetics cannot be controlled, a healthy diet with reduced fats, moderate intake of fish with fatty acids (salmon, herring, and mackerel), and high in vegetables can result in lower rates of prostate cancer.[28]

Testicular Examination

A testicular self-examination can be performed to note any masses in the testicles or any change in size, shape, or consistency of the testes. Testicular cancer is the most common malignancy in American men between the ages of 15 and 34.[28] A testicular self-examination can be helpful in detecting a tumor. Guidelines for conducting a testicular self-examination can be found on the web.[28] Table 7-8 provides a helpful list of common symptoms associated with testicular cancer.

Dental Checkup

Bruxinism, or clenching the jaw and the grinding teeth, is a behavior that is commonly seen as a reaction to stress or because of tempomandibular joint (TMJ) dysfunction. Regular dental exams should be encouraged to monitor the teeth, gums, lips, and soft tissue as well as the alignment of the jaws for a proper bite. A more thorough physical therapy examination should be performed when oral motor dysfunction or TMJ impairment is suspected.

Screening Guidelines for Both Men and Women

In addition to performing a standard screening of adult clients, physical therapists need to remind adults of regular medical screening tests that are important for early detection of other common pathologies. Physical therapists should be familiar with the following common medical tests used to screen individuals for pathological changes in their body systems:

- *Blood cholesterol level test:* The level of blood cholesterol is a significant risk factor for heart disease, particularly coronary artery disease. A lipid panel should be routinely performed that measures total cholesterol, low-density lipoprotein (LDL) cholesterol (the "bad" cholesterol), high-density lipoprotein (HDL) cholesterol (the "good" cholesterol) and triglycerides.
- *Electrocardiogram (ECG):* An ECG can detect abnormalities such as heart damage after a heart

TABLE 7-6

SCREENING TESTS AND IMMUNIZATIONS FOR MEN

Screening Tests	Ages 18 to 39	Ages 40 to 49	Ages 50 to 64	Ages 65+
General Health				
Full check-up (including lifestyle behaviors, nutritional habits, weight, and height)	Annual checkup	Annual checkup	Annual checkup	Annual checkup
Heart Health				
Blood pressure test	Starting at age 21, then once every 1 to 2 years if normal	Every 1 to 2 years	Every 1 to 2 years	Every 1 to 2 years
Cholesterol test	Starting at age 35, then every 5 years	Every 5 years	Every 5 years	Every 5 years
Diabetes				
Blood sugar test	Discuss with your health care provider	Starting at age 45, then every 3 years	Every 3 years	Every 3 years
Oral Health				
Dental exam	1 to 2 times every year	1 to 2 times every year	1 to 2 times every year	1 to 2 times every year
Prostate Health				
Digital rectal exam (DRE)		Annual checkup	Annual checkup	Annual checkup
Prostate-specific antigen (PSA) (blood test)		Annual checkup	Annual checkup	Annual checkup
Reproductive Health				
Testicular exam	Monthly self-exam and part of a general check-up	Monthly self-exam and part of a general check-up	Monthly self-exam and part of a general check-up	Monthly self-exam and part of a general check-up
Sexually transmitted disease (STD) tests	If sexually active or have a history of infection	If sexually active or have a history of infection	If sexually active or have a history of infection	If sexually active or have a history of infection
Colorectal Health				
Fecal occult blood test			Yearly	Yearly
Flexible sigmoidoscopy (with fecal occult blood test is preferred)			Every 5 years	Every 5 years
Double contrast barium enema (DCBE)			Every 5 to 10 years (if not having colonoscopy or sigmoidoscopy)	Every 5 to 10 years (if not having colonoscopy or sigmoidoscopy)
Colonoscopy			Every 10 years	Every 10 years
Rectal exam			Every 5 to 10 years with each screening (sigmoidoscopy, colonoscopy, or DCBE)	Every 5 to 10 years with each screening (sigmoidoscopy, colonoscopy, or DCBE)

(continued)

TABLE 7-6 *(continued)*

SCREENING TESTS AND IMMUNIZATIONS FOR MEN

Screening Tests	Ages 18 to 39	Ages 40 to 49	Ages 50 to 64	Ages 65+
Eye and Ear Health				
Vision exam with eye care provider	Once initially between age 20 and 39	Every 2 to 4 years	Every 2 to 4 years	Every 1 to 2 years
Hearing test	Starting at age 18, then every 10 years	Every 10 years	Annual screening	Annual screening
Skin Health				
Mole exam	Monthly mole self-exam and during annual checkups	Monthly mole self-exam and during annual checkups	Monthly mole self-exam and during annual checkups	Monthly mole self-exam and during annual checkups
Mental Health				
Mental health screening	Annual screening	Annual screening	Annual screening	Annual screening
Immunizations				
Influenza vaccine	Discuss with your health care provider	Discuss with your health care provider	Yearly	Yearly
Pneumococcal vaccine				1 time only
Tetanus-diphtheria booster vaccine	Every 10 years	Every 10 years	Every 10 years	Every 10 years

Adapted from Screening tests and immunizations for men. Available at: http://www.4woman.gov/screeningcharts/mens.htm. Accessed August 15, 2006.

TABLE 7-7

SYMPTOMS OF PROSTATE CANCER

- A need to urinate frequently, especially at night
- Difficulty starting urination or holding back urine
- Inability to urinate
- Weak or interrupted flow of urine
- Painful or burning urination
- Painful ejaculation
- Blood in urine or semen
- Frequent pain or stiffness in the lower back, hips, or upper thighs

Adapted from MayoClinic.com. Prostate cancer prevention: What you can do. Mayo Foundation. Available at: http://www.mayoclinic.com/health/prostate-cancer-prevention/MC00027. Accessed January 28, 2006.

TABLE 7-8

SYMPTOMS OF TESTICULAR CANCER

- A lump in either testicle
- An enlargement of a testicle
- A feeling of heaviness in the scrotum
- A dull ache in the lower abdomen or the groin
- A sudden collection of fluid in the scrotum
- Pain or discomfort in a testicle or in the scrotum
- Enlargement or tenderness of the breasts

Adapted from MayoClinic.com. Testicular cancer. Mayo Foundation. Available at: http://www.mayoclinic.com/health/testicular-cancer/DS00046. Accessed January 28, 2006.

attack, an irregular heart rhythm, or an enlarged heart.

- *Chest x-ray:* A chest x-ray shows the size and shape of the heart and provides information regarding the lungs' condition.
- *Blood chemistry test:* An adult's blood chemistry reveals the functional status of the liver, kidney, and pancreas, measuring sodium, potassium, calcium, phosphorus, and blood sugar, as well as liver enzymes, bilirubin, and creatinine. Adults who have used certain medications are at increased risk for liver, muscle, and kidney damage. The American Diabetes Association recommends that adults 45 or older should have their fasting blood sugar level tested every 3 years.[30]
- *Complete blood count (CBC) with differential:* The complete blood count is used to identify cardiovascular and hematological problems. The CBC measures *hemoglobin* (an indication of the blood's oxygen-carrying capacity), *hematocrit* (the percentage of red blood cells in total blood volume), *leukocytes* (the number and types of white blood cells in the blood), and the number of *platelets* (an indicator of blood coagulability). A CBC can help detect the presence of many conditions, including anemia, infections, and leukemia.
- *Thyroid-stimulating hormone (TSH) test:* This blood test identifies levels of thyroid stimulating hormone (TSH), a pituitary-gland hormone used to produce the hormone thyroxine. This test is used to detect too little thyroxine (an indication of low thyroid activity, or *hypothyroidism*) or too much thyroxine (an indication of increased thyroid activity, or *hyperthyroidism*).[30]
- *Transferrin saturation test:* This blood test measures the amount of iron bound to transferrin—an iron-carrying protein in the bloodstream—and is used to detect *hemochromatosis*—a condition of iron-overload in the blood.[31] Hemochromatosis, a treatable hereditary disease, can lead to diabetes, arthritis, heart disease, or liver disease. Since this condition is often under-recognized, the physical therapist should encourage individuals to have their blood tested regularly during medical visits.
- *Urinalysis:* A urinalysis is helpful for detecting levels of glucose excreted from the body, the presence of red blood cells (signaling internal problems, including possible tumors in the gastrointestinal tract), white blood cells indicating infection, and elevated bilirubin suggesting liver disease.

Table 7-9 lists additional interventions that are typically performed on adults as part of prevention practice. Additional screening tests for women are discussed in Chapter 8.

Oral Health

Oral health is essential during adulthood. Healthy dentition is critical for eating a variety of textured foods and for the pronunciation of certain words. All clients should be counseled to stop the use of all forms of tobacco and to limit consumption of alcohol to reduce the risk of oral cancer as well as cardiovascular pathology. While clients generally have regular oral examinations by their dentists, physical therapists should be aware of the following potential indicators of disease[32]: (1) sore in the mouth that does not heal; (2) lump or thickening in the cheek; (3) a white or red patch on the gums, tongue, or lining of the mouth; (4) soreness or a feeling that something is caught in the throat; (5) difficulty chewing or swallowing; (6) difficulty moving the jaw or tongue; (7) numbness of the tongue or other area of the mouth; or (8) swelling of the jaw, causing dentures to fit poorly or become uncomfortable. Any of these signs or symptoms, commonly associated with cancer, should be immediately reported to the physician.

Fitness in Adulthood

Just as children and youth must complete a preparticipation examination, adults should be thoroughly screened prior to initiating a fitness program. Screening should provide the individual's personal medical information, information about any current medical information, medications (over-the-counter and prescription medications), a family history of medical conditions, as well as lifestyle behaviors (ie, nutritional habits, exercise habits, stress, smoking, alcohol consumption). Any contraindications indicate the need for a referral to an appropriate health professional.

Individuals with unstable medical conditions (cardiopulmonary or metabolic disease processes) or conditions exacerbated by exercise have what are considered high-risk factors according to the American College of Sports Medicine. Additionally, those with special testing or exercise needs require a more thorough examination before initiating any program of physical activity. In these cases, the risks of exercise or physical activity may outweigh the benefits.[33] Individuals at moderate risk for exercise include males who are 45 years or older, females who are 55 years and older, and individuals of either gender with two or more risk factors for coronary artery disease.[33] Those below these ages with no more than one

TABLE 7-9

PREVENTIVE INTERVENTIONS FOR PERSONS AT RISK

Condition	Preventive Measure	Risk Factors
Abdominal aortic aneurysm	Abdominal palpation, ultrasonography	Males older than 60 years who smoke Hypertension Vascular disease Family history of abdominal aortic aneurysm Signs and symptoms of pulsating of the abdomen
Bacteriuria	Dipstick testing for leukocyte esterase or nitrite	Older women People with diabetes Pregnant women Patients with infected kidney stones Kidney transplant patients
Carotid artery stenosis	Neck auscultation, carotid ultrasonography	High blood pressure Cigarette smoking Heart disease Diabetes Transient ischemic attacks
Dementia	Standardized mental status instruments	Older age Family history of dementia Stroke risk factors Endocrine disorders Metabolic disorders Nutritional disorders
Depression	Interview, standardized questionnaires	Gender (women > men) Women who are unhappily married, divorced, or separated Ages 20 to 50 with increasing incidence with older age Personal history of depression Family history of depression Postpartum Premenstrual dysphoric disorder Seasonal affective disorder Drug abuse Nutritional deficiencies Chronic stress Prolonged illness Death of friend or relative Sleeping problems Social isolation (especially in older adults)
Glaucoma	Funduscopy, tonometry, automated perimetry	African Americans older than 40 years Persons with severe myopia Diabetes Family history of glaucoma
Hearing impairment	Directed questioning, the whispered-voice test, or audiometry	Older age Exposure to noise above 85 decibels (DB)—blenders, hair dryers, lawn blower, leaf blower, garbage disposal, vacuum cleaner

(continued)

cardiovascular risk factor are considered low-risk individuals. Cardiovascular risk factors include hypertension (systolic greater than 135 mm Hg and diastolic greater than 90 mm Hg), a family history of myocardial infarction, coronary revascularization, sudden death before 55 years of age in a first-degree relative, hypercholesterolemia (total serum cholesterol greater than 200 mg/dl, HDL cholesterol less than 35 mg/dL, or LDL greater than 130 mg/dL), obesity (BMI of 30 kg/m2 or greater), a sedentary lifestyle (not

TABLE 7-9 *(continued)*

PREVENTIVE INTERVENTIONS FOR PERSONS AT RISK

Condition	Preventive Measure	Risk Factors
Hyperlipidemia	Measurement of serum cholesterol with or without lipoprotein	Gender (men > women) Men aged 35 to 65 years Women aged 45 to 65 years Type 1 diabetes and type 2 diabetes Hypothyroidism Cushing's syndrome Certain types of kidney failure Drug risk factors include use of birth control pills, hormones (eg, estrogen), corticosteroids, certain diuretics, and beta-blockers Dietary risk factors include dietary fat intake greater than 40% of total calories, saturated fat intake greater than 10% of total calories, cholesterol intake greater than 300 milligrams per day, habitual excessive alcohol use, and obesity. Cigarette smoking with hyperlipidemia increases the risk for heart disease.
Hypertension	Measurement of blood pressure	Family history of hypertension Men over the age of 45 Women over the age of 55 After age 75, more than three-quarters of all women have high blood pressure Family history of hypertension African descent Diabetes Sedentary lifestyle
Obesity	Measurement of weight or BMI	High blood pressure (hypertension) High LDL cholesterol ("bad" cholesterol) Low HDL cholesterol ("good" cholesterol) High triglycerides High blood glucose (sugar) Family history of premature heart disease Physical inactivity Cigarette smoking *Note: People with obesity-related diseases are at an increased risk for diabetes, hypertension, coronary artery disease, hyperlipidemia, or obstructive sleep apnea.*
Thyroid dysfunction	Serum thyroid-stimulating hormone	Women over age 50

Adapted from:
Lederle F. Ultrasound screening for abdominal aortic aneurysm. *Ann Int Med.* 2003;139:159.
US Library of Medicine and National Institutes of Health. Medline Plus. Available at: http://www.nlm.nih.gov/medlineplus/ency. Accessed November 30, 2006.

participating in regular exercise), current cigarette smoking, or impaired glucose fasting (fasting blood glucose of 110 mg/dL or greater).[33]

A more comprehensive fitness assessment includes information about the individual's knowledge of health-related fitness, the individual's current exercise program, and motivation for exercise. While the risks of death or myocardial infarction are relatively small (less than .04%),[34] this information should be shared with individuals undergoing submaximal exercise testing. Additional details about exercise for women are discussed in Chapter 8 on women's health.

Suggested Adult Physical Activities

Physical therapists should prescribe physical activity programs commensurate with those recommended by the Centers for Disease Control and Prevention and the American College of Sports Medicine (ie, 30 minutes or more of moderate-intensity physical activity such as brisk walking on most, and preferably all, days of the week).[35] A variety of adult-oriented activities are effective for burning calories and promoting general cardiopulmonary fitness. Table 7-10 lists the number of calories generally burned by an adult when performing each activity.[36]

A well-rounded exercise program should address all areas of health-related fitness, including muscular strength and endurance. A generic outline for a comprehensive exercise program, addressing all areas of health-related fitness, includes flexibility, strengthening, muscular endurance, cardiopulmonary endurance, and postural exercises.

TABLE 7-10

NUMBER OF CALORIES BURNED BY AN ADULT PER ACTIVITY

Activity	Calories Burned/Hour
Bicycling 6 mph	240
Bicycling 12 mph	410
Jogging 5.5 mph	740
Jogging 7 mph	920
Jumping rope	750
Running in place	650
Running 10 mph	1,280
Skiing (cross-country)	700
Swimming 25 yds/min	275
Swimming 50 yds/min	500
Tennis (singles)	400
Walking 2 mph	240
Walking 4 mph	440

Adapted from Exercise and Your Heart—A Guide to Physical Activity. National Heart, Lung, and Blood Institute. American Heart Association, DHHS, PHS, NIH. Publication No 93-1677.

Weekend Warriors

According to the 2005 Census Bureau, Americans spend more than 100 hours commuting to work each year, exceeding the normal vacation time many workers take per year.[37] This statistic gives credence to the reason some cite for not exercising: lack of time. Those who try to compress their exercise into their free time, often the weekend, are referred to as "weekend warriors." Do weekend warriors achieve the recommended amount of exercise?

A cohort study among 8,421 men (mean age, 66 years) in the Harvard Alumni Health Study,[38] without major chronic diseases, provided survey responses to questions about their levels of physical activity in 1988 and 1993. Men were classified as "sedentary" (expending <500 kcal/week), "insufficiently active" (500 to 999 kcal/week), "weekend warriors" (≥1,000 kcal/week from sports/recreation 1 to 2 times/week), or "regularly active" (all others expending ≥1,000 kcal/week). At baseline, 8,421 men were classified as follows: 17% as sedentary, 13% as insufficiently active, 7% as weekend warriors, and 62% as regularly active. The study showed many weekenders reaching their calorie expenditure by playing tennis, golf, or gardening. Among the weekend warriors, over 75% exercised two days per week rather than one. Between 1988 and 1997, 1,234 men died. The study found that among men without major risk factors, weekend warriors had a lower risk of dying compared with sedentary men (relative risk = 0.41; ie, less than half as likely to die) as compared to men with at least one major risk factor (relative risk = 1.02).[38] The researchers concluded that regular physical activity generating 1,000 kcal/week or more should be recommended for lowering mortality rates; however, among those with no major risk factors, even 1 to 2 episodes/week generating 1,000 kcal/week or more can postpone mortality. There was no such advantage for the high-risk weekend warriors.

Sedentary men (those with energy expenditures of less than 500 calories per week) had the highest risk of death, while those expending 1,000 calories or more had the lowest risk.[39] "Weekend warriors" (those who expended 500 to 1,000 calories per week but in only one or two sessions) generally did not differ in their health risks from others with the same energy expenditure spread over more sessions; however, the risk of death increased if the weekend warriors were overweight, smoked, had high blood pressure, or had high cholesterol.[39] Interestingly, the presence of risk factors did not inhibit exercise benefits in men who exercised regularly, but weekend warrior men who had any one of these risk factors had a risk of death similar to that of sedentary men.[38]

The Harvard Alumni Health Study provides evidence that the frequency of exercise is critical for effective prevention practice.[39] Men who engage in irregular exercise, particularly "weekend warriors" with unhealthy health habits, high blood pressure, and elevated cholesterol, should consult a healthcare provider for appropriate fitness training and exercise prescription.[38] While the Harvard Alumni Health Study only examined the risks of mortality for men, population at risk for increased mortality may also be more vulnerable to musculoskeletal injuries, such as sprains and strains.[38]

The Harvard study was conducted with only male participants, but it is likely that women who are "weekend warriors" may have similar risks of injury and needs for appropriate exercise prescription based on their risk factors for cardiopulmonary disease.

Summary

For adult clients it is important to recognize priorities that enable individuals to maintain a healthy lifestyle, manage stress, and sustain financial security while continuing healthy relationships at home and at work. Physical therapists can identify pathological risk factors, reduce stressors, address lifestyle habits that impair health, and recommend appropriate exercise programs to optimize limited time. A holistic approach to health care for adults includes an awareness of multiple responsibilities and needs affecting priorities and lifestyle habits. Chapter 8 offers additional suggestions to promote the health and wellbeing of women.

References

1. To love and to work. Adlerian thoughts on an anecdote about Freud. *Bulletin of the Meninger Clinic.* 1981;45(5):439–441.
2. Wikipedia contributors. Erikson's stages of psychosocial development. Wikipedia, The Free Encyclopedia. 2006. Available at: http://en.wikipedia.org/w/index.php?title=Erikson's_stages_of_psychosocial_developmen t&oldid=37220111. Accessed February 4, 2006.
3. McAdams DP, St. Aubin ED, Logan RL. Generativity among young, midlife, and older adults. *Psychol of Aging.* 1993;8(2),221–230.
4. Larson S, Larson D. Divorce: a hazard to your health? *Physician.* 1999;May/June:14.
5. Yelin E, Nevitt M, Epstein W. Toward an epidemiology of work disability. *Milbank Mem Fund Q Health Soc.* 1980;58(3):386–415.
6. Smith IM. Aging begins at 30: the burden of disease. University of Iowa Hospitals and Clinics Website. 2001. Available at: http://www.vh.org/adult/patient/internal-medicine/aba30/2001/diseaseburden.html. Accessed January 30, 2006.
7. Kantor J. Contact dermatitis. Medline. Available at: http://www.nlm.nih.gov/medlineplus/ency/article/000869.htm. Accessed January 28, 2006.
8. Kantor J. Psoriasis. Medline. Available at: http://www.nlm.nih.gov/medlineplus/ency/article/000434.htm. Accessed January 18, 2006.
9. Beers M. Psoriasis. *The Merck Manual of Medical Information.* 2nd home ed. Online version. Available at: http://www.merck.com/mrkshared/mmanual/section10/chapter117/117b.jsp. Accessed January 28, 2006.
10. Kopf A. Prevention and early detection of skin cancer/melanoma. *Cancer.* 1988;62(8 Suppl):1791–1795.
11. Parkin DM, Bray F, Ferlay J, Pisani P. Global cancer statistics, 2002. *CA Cancer J Clin.* 2005;55(2):74–108.
12. Votey S, Peters A. Diabetes mellitus, type 2—a review. Emedicine. 2005. Available at: http://www.emedicine.com/emerg/topic134.htm. Accessed January 28, 2006.
13. American Diabetes Association. Clinical practice recommendations. *Diabetes Care.* 1998;21(suppl 1):1–70.
14. Smith RA, Cokkinides V, Eyre HJ. American Cancer Society guidelines for the early detection of cancer, *2003. CA Cancer J Clin.* 2003;53(1):27–43.
15. Kumanyika S. Obesity, health disparities, and prevention paradigms: hard questions and hard choices. Preventing chronic disease. 2005. Available at: http://www.cdc.gov/pcd/issues/2005/oct/05_0025.htm. Accessed January 28, 2006.
16. National Institutes of Health, National Heart, Lung, and Blood Institute. Clinical guidelines on the identification, evaluation, and treatment of overweight and obesity in adults: the evidence report. *Obesity Research.* 1998;6(suppl 2):51–209
17. Finkelstein EA, Fiebelkorn IC, Wang G. National medical spending attributable to overweight and obesity: how much, and who's paying? *Health Affairs.* 2003;3:219–226.
18. American Heart Association. Metabolic syndrome. Available at: http://www.americanheart.org/presenter.jhtml?identifier=534. Accessed January 28, 2006.
19. Erman MK. Insomnia. In: Poceta JS, Mitler MM, eds. *Sleep Disorders: Diagnosis and Treatment.* Totowa, NJ: Humana Press; 1998:21–51.
20. Emedicine. Sexually transmitted diseases. Available at: http://www.emedicinehealth.com/articles/17489-1.asp. Accessed January 28, 2006.
21. Centers for Disease Control and Prevention. HIV/AIDS Surveillance Report, 2003. Atlanta, Ga: US Department of Health and Human Services, CDC. 2004;15:1–46. Available at: http://www.cdc.gov/hiv/stats/2003surveillancereport.pdf. Accessed March 16, 2005.
22. The HIV/AIDS Network. HIV/AIDS symptoms and signs. Available at: http://www.hivaidssearch.com/facts/hiv_aids_common_symptoms.htm. Accessed January 28, 2006.
23. MedicineNet.com. Men's top 5 health concerns. Available at: http://www.medicinenet.com/script/main/art.asp?articlekey=46826. Accessed January 28, 2006.
24. National Kidney Foundation. What is chronic kidney disease? Available at: http://www.kidney.org/kidneydisease. Accessed January 28, 2006.
25. MayoClinic.com. Men's top health threats: mostly preventable. Available at: http://www.mayoclinic.com/health/mens-health/MC00013. Accessed January 28, 2006.
26. US Department of Health and Human Services. Screening tests and immunizations guidelines for men. Available at: http://www.4woman.gov/screeningcharts/mens.htm. Accessed January 28, 2006.
27. MayoClinic.com. Prostate cancer prevention: what you can do. Mayo Foundation. Available at: http://www.mayoclinic.com/health/prostate-cancer-prevention/MC00027. Accessed January 28, 2006.

28. MayoClinic.com. Testicular cancer. Mayo Foundation. Available at: http://www.mayoclinic.com/health/testicular-cancer/DS00046. Accessed January 28, 2006.

29. American Diabetes Association. All about diabetes. Available at: http://www.diabetes.org/about-diabetes.jsp. Accessed January 28, 2006.

30. Beers M. Thyroid disorders. *The Merck Manual of Medical Information.* 2nd home edition. Online Version. Available at: http://www.merck.com/mrkshared/mmanual/section2/chapter8/8a.jsp 21 and 22. Accessed January 28, 2006.

31. Beers M. Iron overload. *The Merck Manual of Medical Information.* 2nd home edition. Online Version. Available at: http://www.merck.com/mrkshared/CVMHighLight?file=/mrkshared/mmanual/section11/chapter128/128a.jsp%3Fregion%3Dmerckcom&word=Hemochromatosis&domain=www.merck.com#hl_anchor. Accessed January 28, 2006.

32. Indiana State Department of Health. Oral health. Available at: http://www.in.gov/isdh/programs/oral/s-tobacco.html. Accessed January 28, 2006.

33. Thompson P, Buchner D, Piña I, et al. Scientific statement: exercise and physical activity in the prevention and treatment of atherosclerotic cardiovascular disease. *Circulation.* 2003;107:3109.

34. American Heart Association. Heart disease and stroke statistics—2004. Update American Heart Association. Available at: http://www.americanheart.org. Accessed January 30, 2006.

35. Pate RR, Pratt M, Blair SN, et al. Physical activity and public health: a recommendation from the Centers for Disease Control and Prevention and the American College of Sports Medicine. *JAMA*. 1995;273:402–407.

36. National Heart, Lung, and Blood Institute *Exercise and Your Heart—A Guide to Physical Activity.* American Heart Association, DHHS, PHS, NIH Publication No 93-1677.

37. US Census Bureau. US Department of Commerce. Americans spend more than 100 hours commuting to work each year. Available at: http://www.census.gov/Press-Release/www/releases/archives/american_community_survey_acs/004489.html. Accessed January 30, 2006.

38. Sesso HD, Paffenbarger RS Jr, Lee IM. Physical activity and coronary heart disease in men: the Harvard Alumni Health Study. *Circulation.* 2001;102:975–980.

Chapter 8

Women's Health Issues: Focus on Pregnancy

Shannon N. Buhs, PT and Catherine Rush Thompson, PhD, MS, PT

"For American women, being healthy is far more than getting a good checkup or being disease-free. Being healthy means both physical and emotional wellness and having a healthy family."

~ NATIONAL WOMEN'S HEALTH RESOURCE CENTER

Women's Health

The American Physical Therapy Association has a section devoted specifically to women's health created in 1977 by Elizabeth Noble, a leading women's health physical therapist. Once the section on obstetrics and gynecology, it is now the section on women's health, titled as such to represent the scope of practice including all health concerns of women: incontinence, pelvic/vaginal pain, prenatal and postpartum musculoskeletal pain, osteoporosis, rehabilitation following breast surgery, lymphedema, education, prevention, wellness, and exercise. While women's health issues often center on reproductive health, the top five medical conditions affecting adult women are heart attacks, depression, strokes, lung cancers, and *osteoarthritis* (joint inflammation commonly associated with "wear and tear" and aging), all conditions affecting men and women alike. Breast cancers and smokers' lung are sixth and seventh and, likewise, affect both men and women. Women's reproductive capabilities create additional health concerns that should be acknowledged during a screening.

Screening for Women's Health Issues

The National Women's Health Resource Center (NWHRC)[1] surveyed 1,005 women about their knowledge, attitudes, and perceptions of their health. Survey results indicated that women's perceptions of why their health improved or declined were strongly linked to lifestyle issues, such as changes in stress levels and exercise. Women reported that time management and reduced stress would most improve their health; however, only half reported reduced stress, and only 15% visited a mental health counselor. While 65% reported exercising more and 59% said they dieted, few women indicated they met their diet or weight-loss goals. These data suggest that health care professionals can more effectively use office visits to explain how wellness strategies, such as stress management and health screenings, can improve women's health. "The survey findings indicate a clear need for women and their health care professionals to do a better job of communicating about both physical and emotional wellness and how to achieve them."[1]

Additional findings indicated that many women lacked familiarity with their family's medical history: 33% of Caucasian women, 40% African-American, 49% of Latina, and 66% of Asian women report being unfamiliar with their family's medical history.[1] n addition, African-American women reported the greatest awareness about a broad range of guidelines for preventive medical screenings, and Asian women were less aware about preventative screenings, specifically those relating to their gynecologic health.[1] Physical therapists need to explore each individual's medical history and familiarity with preventive care. Questions on an intake form or by interview can elicit additional information, including the following:

1. Do you have any concerns about pregnancy or the use of contraceptives? An excellent resource for additional information about the various types of contraception, including the efficacy, advantages, and disadvantages of each, is available on the web.[2]
2. Do you have any concerns related to your risk for breast, uterine, or cervical cancer? Physical therapists should be mindful that women with a family history of cancer, particularly women over the age of 60, are at increased risk.[3,4]
3. How would you characterize your health behavior, including exercise, nutritional intake, mental health, and use of cigarettes, alcohol, or other substances? While emphasizing exercise as a key component of both physical and mental health, it is essential to address lifestyle behaviors that can lead to chronic illness.
4. Do you have any significant stressors in your life that may be affecting your health (including domestic problems, issues related to children, work-related stressors, or uncontrollable events causing stress)? Women play multiple roles in their personal and professional lives, leading to a variety of stressful situations. Stress management resources should be made readily available to women of all ages. The National Women's Health Information Center,[5] sponsored by the United States Department of Health and Human Services, provides helpful information on the web.
5. Are you feeling overly fatigued or experiencing any unusual pain?
6. Are you familiar with controllable risk factors for cancer, osteoporosis, and heart disease? Six times more women die of heart disease than breast cancer.[6] Women's risk of developing heart disease is generally delayed 10 to 15 years. This delay in disease development is generally attributed to the influence of female hormones believed to be cardioprotective.[7] Younger women, in particular, as less likely to have high levels or fatty plaque contributing to cardiovascular disease when compared to young men..[7] These gender differences may contribute to the differential effectiveness of diet and medications for the prevention of heart disease.

   Physical therapists need to advise all women of the benefits of exercise for preventing heart disease. The National Coalition for Women with Heart Disease offers a helpful information website describing "Healthy Heart Exercise Tips" that can guide women in fitness and nutrition for a healthier lifestyle.[8]
7. Are you having regular health screenings for risk reduction performed by your physician or other health care professional?

   Positive findings indicate the need for health education and a potential medical referral. Resources for women's health education are listed in Appendix C.

TABLE 8-1

SYMPTOMS OF BREAST CANCER

- A lump or thickening in the breast or armpit
- A change in the breast's size or shape
- A change in the color of the breast or the areola (area around the nipple)
- Any dimpling or puckering of the skin or change in the color or texture of the skin
- An abnormal discharge from the nipple
- Scaling of the nipple or nipple retraction

Adapted from National Cancer Institute. Understanding breast changes: a health guide for all women. Available at: http://www.cancer.gov/cancertopics/understanding-breast-changes. Accessed January 20, 2006.

Women should be reminded of the following screening guidelines recommended for maintaining and monitoring health status:

- The *breast self-examination* includes both feeling for lumps as well as looking at the breasts carefully to detect any changes in shape or size, any dimpling, puckering, changes in the color of the skin, or changes in the nipple. Table 8-1 lists symptoms of breast cancer[4] that should be reported immediately to a physician.
- A *pap smear test* is used to identify precancer cells lining the cervix. Infections, including a

virus called human papillomavirus (HPV), may lead to such changes, requiring an additional pap smear or HPV testing. Certain types of HPV infections related to sexual contact cause genital warts and increase the risk of cervical cancer. Additional risks factors for cervical cancer include diethylstilbestrol (DES) exposure before birth, HIV infection, and a weakened immune system due to organ transplant, chemotherapy, or chronic steroid use. Symptoms of cervical cancer that require a medical referral for more extensive testing include abnormal vaginal bleeding or discharge, bleeding after intercourse, or painful intercourse.[9]

- The *cervix, uterus, ovaries, fallopian tubes, and rectum* should be monitored. A speculum is inserted into the vagina so that the doctor can see the upper part of the vagina and cervix for possible abnormalities.[10]

Exercise and Lifestyle for Women

Exercise and healthy lifestyle habits offer many benefits to women but must be monitored because cyclic hormonal changes affect women from puberty to postmenopause. Physical therapists should be aware of these changes and their impact on physical activity.

Premenstrual syndrome (PMS) is a constellation of physical and psychological symptoms seen among women of reproductive age. While all women may experience some discomfort prior to menstruation, women with PMS have such severe symptoms that they interfere with the individuals' lives. Approximately 75% of women have some symptoms of PMS; 30% to 40% have impairments from PMS; and 3% to 8% have severe PMS affecting their functional abilities.[11] Monthly symptoms are both psychological and physical, including irritability, anxiety or depression, diminished self-esteem, difficulty concentrating, sleep problems, appetite changes, low energy, bloating, headache, and breast swelling and tenderness. While the type and intensity of symptoms may vary among women, all can be distressing.[12] Management of PMS includes lifestyle and stress management, dietary restrictions (salt or carbohydrate), diuretics, prostaglandin inhibitors (such as Motrin), progesterone (hormone treatment), ovulation inhibitors, vitamins (pyridoxine), lithium, and antidepressants.[11] Aerobic exercise may reduce stress associated with premenstrual syndrome and improve mood;[12] however, health habits during PMS may attenuate the symptoms commonly limiting engagement in regular exercise. The following suggestions may reduce the impact of PMS on women engaged in regular physical activity[12]:

- Eat smaller meals or snacks throughout the day. Snack suggestions include plain yogurt, unsalted nuts, unsalted sunflower seeds, unsalted popcorn, whole wheat bread with peanut butter, pumpkin, zucchini or banana bread, graham crackers, unsalted whole grain crackers, bran or oatmeal muffin, raw vegetables, apple slices, celery with peanut butter, apple sauce, raisins, dates, dried apricots or prunes, grapes, banana, grapefruit, or orange slices.
- Eliminate or reduce caffeine. Coffee, tea, colas, and chocolate all contain varying amounts of caffeine. Caffeine can make breast symptoms (ie, swelling and tenderness) and headache symptoms worse.
- Reduce salt. Excess salt intake may worsen water retention symptoms.
- Reduce alcohol intake.
- Perform relaxation techniques. Relaxation exercises reduce the mood symptoms of PMS and are particularly helpful for women who are able to identify their stressors.[13]

The Female Athlete Triad

Women should exercise to maintain general health-related fitness, including preventing changes in body function secondary to hormonal changes across the lifespan. While weight-bearing exercise is heralded for reducing the risks of osteoporosis, increased physical activity, especially increased female participation in organized athletics, has revealed a triad of medical conditions resulting from the hormonal shifts and lifestyle habits altering female regulatory systems. The female athlete triad includes (1) *anorexia nervosa* and *bulimia* (eating disorders/disordered eating behavior), (2) *amenorrhea/oligomenorrhea*, and (3) decreased bone mineral density (*osteoporosis and osteopenia*) and requires intervention by a multidisciplinary team, including prevention, assessment, and intervention by physical therapists.[14] Female athletes who must maintain a certain body type or weight class are at the highest risk of developing eating disorders. Young female gymnasts and dancers are classic examples of athletes whose bodies are ideally lean and muscular. To maintain this ideal body weight, girls and women will limit healthy eating or will binge on food, then purge the meal to avoid weight gain.

- *Anorexia nervosa* is an eating disorder involving limited eating and weighing at least 15% less than the ideal weight. *Bulimia nervosa* is an equally unhealthy eating disorder that involves binge eating or eating large quantities of food at one sitting, regardless of hunger, often followed by vomiting or purging the food. Disordered eating can result in decreased athletic performance, increased morbidity, and occasional mortality.[13] Interventions include psychological counseling, encouraging healthy lifestyle habits, and hormone replacement therapy, as needed to manage or stop the condition.[13]

- *Amenorrhea* occurs when a woman of childbearing age fails to menstruate. There are two types of amenorrhea: primary amenorrhea and secondary amenorrhea. *Primary amenorrhea* is often associated with delayed puberty and commonly occurs in girls who are very thin or very athletic. The normal puberty-related rise in body fat responsible for triggering the initial onset of menstruation is absent.[15] In some cases, the lack of menstruation may have other causes than body fat. *Secondary amenorrhea* is a condition in which a previously menstruating woman fails to menstruate for three consecutive months.[15] Secondary amenorrhea is naturally caused by pregnancy, breast feeding, and menopause (the normal age-related end of menstruation); however, other conditions related to genitourinary or endocrine system pathology may cause this condition. Other preventable causes include obesity, frequent strenuous exercise, rapid weight loss, or stress, either emotional or physical.[15] Amenorrhea affects 2% to 5% of all women of childbearing age in the United States. The incidence of menstrual irregularities is much higher in activities where a thin body is required for better performance. Female athletes, especially young women, may be more likely to have amenorrhea.[15] While exercise or physical activity itself does not cause amenorrhea, it is more likely to occur in women who exercise very intensely or who increase the intensity of exercise rapidly. Women who engage in sports associated with lower body weight, such as ballet dancing or gymnastics, are more likely to develop amenorrhea than women in other sports are.
- *Oligomenorrhea* is the term used to describe infrequent or very light menstruation in a woman with previously normal periods.[15] Oligomenorrhea can also be caused by emotional and physical stress, chronic illnesses, tumors that secrete estrogen, poor nutrition, and eating disorders such as anorexia nervosa. Female athletes often develop oligomenorrhea secondary to their restricted diets, the use of anabolic steroid drugs, and strenuous exercise.[15] Oligomenorrhea can be caused by a hormonal imbalance.[15] For both amenorrhea and oligomenorrhea, individuals should be encouraged to eat a healthy diet, exercise moderately, use healthy stress management resources, and balance lifestyle to reduce unnecessary emotional stress.
- *Osteoporosis* may result when the bone-maintaining properties of estrogen are compromised whenever menstrual cycles are altered. Of particular concern in female athletes is the increased risk for stress fractures from repetitive forces transferred to the bone either through muscle fatigue or from the tensile forces generated by forceful muscle contractions.[16] Female athletes experiencing amenorrhea and increased fracture risk may benefit from decreases in both the intensity and duration of training as well as increases in calcium intake (1200 to 1500 mg/day) and reduced use of oral contraceptives. The dietary alterations could be accomplished by adding three glasses of skim milk per day to the diet.[16] A program of resistance training designed to increase both muscle strength and mass may improve the skeletal profile of these athletes as well as protect against soft tissue injuries. Estrogen replacement therapy (ERT) may be considered by those unwilling to make changes in their diet and exercise regimen.[16]

Perimenopausal, Menopausal, and Postmenopausal Changes

Menopause marks the physiological aging process after which a woman no longer menstruates. Menopause, typically commencing when a women turns 50 years old, results from hormone alterations affecting not only reproductive capabilities, but other body systems as well.[17] Symptoms of *perimenopause* (the period prior to menopause as the woman's body transitions into menopause) and menopause that women may experience include the following[17]:

- Hot flashes and skin flushing
- Night sweats
- Insomnia
- Mood swings including irritability, depression, and anxiety
- Irregular menstrual periods
- Spotting of blood in between periods
- Vaginal dryness and painful sexual intercourse
- Decreased sex drive
- Vaginal infections
- Urinary tract infections

Of particular interest to physical therapists are bone loss and eventual osteoporosis, changes in cholesterol levels, and greater risk of heart disease. Factors that reduce the age of onset of menopause include smoking, hysterectomy, and living at high altitudes.[17]

Various studies indicate that exercise, proper diet, and if advisable, hormone therapy can help prevent or minimize many of the problems associated with menopause.[17,18,19] Since both the quantity and the quality of bone decline during perimenopause, it is particularly important to address changes as early as possible. Furthermore, identification of women at high risk for fracture *postmenopause* (after the onset of menopause) through bone scans is important[18] while encouraging healthy lifestyle habits, including eating a diet with sufficient calcium and vitamin D, regular weight-bearing activities, measures to reduce fall risk, smoking cessation, and moderation of alcohol intake.[20] Certain pharmacologic agents containing biphosphates and selective estrogen receptor modulators may increase bone mass and reduce fracture risk.[20]

Changes With Pregnancy

More than 6 million women will become pregnant in the United States this year.[21,22] Women tend to seek out health care more often than men, so it is highly likely that physical therapists will treat women who are pregnant or who have been in the past. Therefore, it is crucial that therapists understand the effects of pregnancy on the female body. The musculoskeletal system, for example, undergoes incredible changes to accommodate the growth of the fetus and to prepare for childbirth.

Anatomical and Physiological Effects of Pregnancy

From conception to birth, a pregnant woman's body undergoes significant changes. Each system within the body uniquely adapts to support and sustain the growing fetus as well as prepare for the childbirth process. Although these changes are vital for the process of pregnancy, oftentimes, the woman will develop discomfort because of them. For example, in order to create more room for the enlarged uterus, the rib cage actually expands, allowing the diaphragm to elevate up to 4 cm.[23] As a result, there is increased stress where the ribs articulate with the thoracic spine, leading to potential back pain. Furthermore, the elevated hormone levels responsible for the increased laxity within her joints often do not return to baseline for several months after the baby is born.[23] These musculoskeletal changes create the need for physical therapy if body function is disturbed. Understanding how each body system specifically adapts during pregnancy will help therapists optimally treat these women's complaints and differentiate among various clinical diagnoses.

During pregnancy, the levels of estrogen, progesterone, and relaxin drastically change, causing increased softening of ligaments, growth of breast tissue, and retention of fluid.[24] Relaxin is responsible for much of the relaxation that occurs in the ligaments, symphyses, and fibrocartilage of the pelvis, as well as in peripheral joints.[24] Relaxin also begins to affect tissues right after conception, reaching its peak around 3 months and then either remaining at a constant level or dropping 20% to 50% for the remaining months of pregnancy.[25] Due to this laxity, the sacroiliac joints, in particular, can become hypermobile and lead to pain with activities such as bed mobility, transfers, gait, and stair negotiation. If a woman chooses to breast feed her child, her hormone levels may continue to remain elevated well after delivery, a key consideration for the postpartum woman.

Altering hormonal levels are also responsible for the mood changes, periods of fatigue, increased metabolism, and the decreased tolerance to heat that women develop, whether pregnant or menstruating, often contributing to the inability to adhere to an exercise program.[25]

The musculoskeletal system uniquely adapts to support the growth of a pregnant woman's uterus. Unfortunately, the changes that take place within the musculoskeletal system often contribute to various discomforts. Although these physiological changes are common with pregnancy, the discomfort or dysfunction that may result is not something to be ignored. Physical therapists are experts in the treatment of musculoskeletal impairments and can often provide the relief that many women need. Table 8-2 lists musculoskeletal changes associated with pregnancy.[25]

Many of these anatomical changes are a direct result of the weight gain that occurs with pregnancy. The American College of Obstetricians and Gynecologists (ACOG) recommends an average weight gain of 27.5 pounds unless the woman was under- or overweight prior to becoming pregnant.[26] As the abdomen enlarges, her center of gravity shifts forward, causing an increased *lumbar lordosis* ("swayback") and eventually a more pronounced *thoracic kyphosis* ("humpback"). The shift in gravity, in addition to the *diastasis recti*, or separation of the rectus abdominus muscles, leads to decreased back stability and oftentimes pain.[25] An abdominal support binder often relieves this pain during functional activities. Due to the increase in breast tissue, added stress is placed upon the thoracic spine. In order to prevent discomfort, women should wear supportive undergarments. Specific back stretches and stabilization exercises may help, as well.[25] In addition to lumbar pain, pregnant women often develop *sacroiliac dysfunction,* which can lead to sciatica or pain directly in the low back. These symptoms usually flare up with activity, especially asymmetrical movements, such as bed mobility, transfers, and stair negotiation.[25] Wearing a sacroiliac belt can often bring women symptom relief in combination with a back stabilization program. If these strategies completely alleviate the symptoms, she may benefit from manual techniques to improve the alignment of the joint itself.

Pubic symphysis separation occurs around 2 to 32 weeks gestation as the pubic symphysis widens to approximately 4 to 7 mm to prepare the pelvis for a vaginal delivery.[27] Because of the attachments of both the abdominal and pelvic floor muscles to this area, some women may develop pain as their muscles stretch. Others may develop a "waddling gait" because of the separation, potentially leading to back pain. Wearing a sacroiliac belt will help provide added stability during gait and transfers; exercises that stress the adductor muscles should be avoided.

Round ligament pain results from the stretch of ligaments suspended from the lateral aspects of the uterus to the labia majora during pregnancy. Oftentimes, this considerable stretching causes sharp pain in the woman's groin and/or vagina. Commonly, pain is experienced after prolonged periods of standing or walking, although some women report sharp pains in this region when transferring out of a chair or bed. Limited weight bearing activities and/or wearing an abdominal support binder can limit excessive stretching. Some women may even find relief from simply lifting their abdomen with their hands when they have one of these sharp pains.

Pelvic muscle weakness results from the added pressures on the pelvic floor muscles during pregnancy. Pelvic floor muscles, located at the base of the pelvis, have three major roles: sphincteric, supportive, and sexual, the "three S's."[28] These muscles connect the pubic bones to the sacrum by forming a "sling." When at their optimal strength and length, pelvic floor muscles have the ability to perform the following three functions: (1) control the passing of urine, feces, or gas, (2) support the pelvic organs (bladder, bowel, and uterus), and (3) facilitate enhanced sexual pleasure.[18] As the uterus increases in size throughout pregnancy, added pressure is placed upon the pelvic floor muscles, causing them to stretch and possibly weaken. If they are not strong enough to withstand this force, bladder and bowel control may be impaired, resulting in incontinence.[25]

TABLE 8-2

Musculoskeletal Issues Associated With Pregnancy

- Increased lumbar lordosis
- Posterior shift/increased kyphosis of the thoracic spine
- Rib cage expansion to accommodate growth
- Diastasis recti (thinning of the linea alba, causing separation of the rectus abdominus muscles)
- Rounded shoulders due to increasing weight of breasts
- Sacroiliac joint hypermobility
- Pubic symphysis separation (4 mm in nuliparas women, 4.5 to 8.0 mm in multiparas women)
- Round ligament pain
- Pelvic floor muscle weakness/incontinence
- Increased subtalar joint pronation
- Increased knee hyperextension
- Nerve compression (carpal or tarsal tunnel syndrome, thoracic outlet syndrome)
- Swelling or lymphedema issues

When a woman's bladder becomes full, stretch receptors within the bladder send a message to the brain that it is time to find a bathroom. If the woman is not near a bathroom, a message is sent from the brain to the pelvic floor muscles to "hold it" or contract. The contraction of the pelvic floor muscles causes the smooth muscle lining of the bladder (the *detrusor muscle*) to relax and continue to hold the urine. Once she is ready to void, she relaxes her pelvic floor muscles, causing the detrusor to contract, and urine then flows out. If a woman's pelvic floor muscles are weak, they may not be able to sufficiently contract. This can lead to insufficient closure of the urethral sphincter, causing leakage of urine. There are three common types of incontinence associated with pregnancy: (1) *stress incontinence* (leakage of urine during an event of increased intra-abdominal pressure, such as sneezing, coughing, laughing, or lifting), (2) *urge incontinence* (leakage of urine due to an inability to delay a strong, sudden urge to urinate [ie, "overactive bladder syndrome"]), and (3) *mixed incontinence* (a combination of both stress and urge incontinence).[29] Due to these pelvic floor issues, it is crucial that physical therapists help educate woman about the importance of pelvic floor strengthening. This is a topic not only for the pregnant population but also for all women. Age, hormonal changes, and the effects of gravity and certain

TABLE 8-3

HEALTHY BLADDER HABITS

1. Normal voiding frequency is to urinate every 2 to 5 hours if one is drinking 6 to 8 glasses of water per day. Total voiding in a 24-hour period should be approximately 6 to 8 times. "Normal" nocturnal voiding should be 0 to 1 times a night for children and adults under 65 years of age and 1 to 2 times a night for adults over 65 years of age. Going to the bathroom "just in case" is not recommended because it may train the bladder to empty before it is sufficiently full.
2. Avoiding bladder irritants, such as caffeinated or decaffeinated coffees/teas/sodas, fruit juices high in acidity, alcohol, chocolate, spicy foods, nicotine, and various medications, can decrease bladder urgency and frequency.
3. The stream of urine should last at least 8 seconds from start to finish and should be steady, not exceedingly slow or fast.
4. It is important to use proper hygiene after going to the bathroom by wiping the perineum from front to back. This ensures that feces from the anus are not introduced to the vaginal region.

Adapted from DukeMedNews. Duke health brief: healthy bladder habits. Available at: http://dukemednews.duke.edu/news/article.php?id=8479. Accessed January 28, 2006.

physical activities all contribute to pelvic floor muscle weakness and the potential for incontinence or even *pelvic organ prolapse* (the descent of an organ within the pelvic cavity). Table 8-3 lists healthy bladder habits for females.[30]

A pregnant woman's feet take quite a toll during pregnancy. With more weight to support, the arches begin to fall and a resulting pronation occurs.[25] The equal and opposite ground reaction force is then altered, causing added stress on the knees, hips, and once again, low back. Due to these issues, it is very important that pregnant women wear supportive shoes and try to avoid standing with their knees hyperextended.

By the end of pregnancy, most women retain an extra three liters of fluid.[25] With more time spent in weight-bearing positions, fluid tends to pool in the lower extremities, causing discomfort. Wearing supportive hose can often improve lower extremity circulation and help decrease this discomfort. This additional fluid within their connective tissues can also lead to various *nerve compression syndromes.* Due to the postural changes that pregnant women develop and the amount of fluid they retain, nerves can often become compressed. Some of the more common nerve compression syndromes are *carpal tunnel syndrome, tarsal tunnel syndrome, thoracic outlet syndrome, lateral femoral cutaneous nerve entrapment, ilioinguinal nerve compression, intercostal neuralgia,* and *peroneal nerve compression.*[25] Oftentimes splints, supportive garments, postural education and instruction on various stretches, and nerve mobilization can help women with these complaints.

The respiratory system goes through incredible changes to accommodate the demands of pregnancy. "Oxygen consumption alone increases by 14% (half going to the fetus and placenta and the other half going to the uterine muscle and breast tissue)."[31] Due to the increase in overall tidal volume, women may develop dyspnea or hyperventilation.[25] Hyperventilation helps with the diffusion of carbon dioxide from the fetus to maternal circulation.[31] As stated earlier, the diaphragm elevates up to accommodate the enlarged uterus. This diaphragmatic elevation causes the mother's breathing pattern to become more "chest breathing" than "abdominal breathing." Due to all of these changes within the respiratory system, the overall pulmonary function of the mother is not impaired.[31]

Like each of the other body systems, the cardiovascular system uniquely adapts to meet the needs of the growing fetus. Blood volume increases by 40% to 50%, causing an eventual increase in overall cardiac output to 50% above nonpregnant values, leading to increases in stroke volume and heart rate.[31] It is important to note that a pregnant woman's resting heart rate will be higher than it was prepregnancy. Some say that being pregnant is exercise in and of itself because of this. Overall blood pressure, however, decreases throughout pregnancy. This decrease in blood pressure is primarily due to the smooth muscle relaxation taking place within the blood vessel walls with increasing levels of progesterone.[31]

Exercise During Pregnancy

Although each system of the female body uniquely adapts to the physiological demands of pregnancy, it is still very important to take caution when advising someone on prenatal exercise. Caution should be taken to not exceed the thresholds of the metabolic, respiratory, or cardiac thresholds.[31] The ACOG no longer suggests a specific heart rate for pregnant woman to stay under during exercise, rather they advise exercise within 60% to 75% of maximal heart rate, approximately 140 bpm for most women.[31] Since factors such as age, fitness level, and overall health affect a pregnant woman's ability to exercise, it is always important to first consult with the involved

TABLE 8-4

BENEFITS OF EXERCISE DURING PREGNANCY

- Increased muscle tone
- Increased endurance/energy level
- Decreased tension/stress
- Decreased swelling
- Improved posture and body mechanics
- Improved circulation
- Improved pelvic floor muscle strength
- Decreased discomfort/pain
- Better sleep patterns
- Preparation for the intensity of labor and delivery
- Quicker return to prepregnancy shape
- Improved self-esteem
- Networking with other pregnant women

Adapted from American College of Obstetricians and Gynecologists. Exercise during pregnancy and the postpartum period. ACOG Technical Bulletin 189. Washington, DC: American College of Obstetricians and Gynecologists; 1994.

physician before initiating an exercise program. Table 8-4 lists the benefits of exercise during pregnancy, and Table 8-5 provides the ACOG guidelines for exercise during pregnancy.[32]

The pregnant woman should be educated about signs and symptoms to monitor while exercising. Certain clinical manifestations suggest potential problems needing medical attention, such as pain, vaginal bleeding, persistent dizziness, numbness or tingling, faintness, shortness of breath, generalized edema, severe headache, or severe calf pain, swelling, or redness. These and other problematic clinical manifestations are listed in Table 8-6.[32]

The physical therapist should be familiar with the client's medical history and exercise tolerance, recognizing relative and absolute contraindications to exercise in pregnancy. Tables 8-7 and 8-8 list the absolute and relative contraindications to exercise.[32]

Exercises for pregnancy are designed to address the issues that are precipitated by the various anatomical and physiological changes that occur during the months preceding delivery. The most familiar exercises are the Kegel exercises, known to strengthen the pelvic floor muscles and prevent incontinence.

The principle behind Kegel exercises is to strengthen the muscles of the pelvic floor, thereby improving the urethral and rectal sphincter function. The success of Kegel exercises depends on proper technique and adherence to a regular exercise program.[33]

TABLE 8-5

ACOG'S GUIDELINES FOR EXERCISE DURING PREGNANCY

- Exercise regularly (3 times/week minimum).
- Avoid ballistic movement, quick changes in direction, or any exercise that requires extreme ranges of joint motion.
- Warm up prior to exercise and cool down after exercise.
- Avoid anaerobic exercise.
- Avoid exercising in the supine position after the first trimester to avoid "supine hypotension syndrome."
- Strenuous exercise should be limited to 15- to 20-minute intervals to avoid overheating.
- Avoid exercising in environments of high heat, humidity, or pollution.
- Avoid prolonged periods of motionless standing, especially in the third trimester.
- Modify the intensity of exercise according to signs of overexertion.
- Do not exercise to levels of exhaustion.
- Resting in a left side-lying position, after an adequate cool down, may improve cardiac output.
- Increase caloric intake to 500-kcal/day if regularly exercising.
- Consume plenty of water before, during, and after exercising to avoid dehydration.
- To avoid gastrointestinal discomfort, avoid eating less than 1.5 hours before exercising.
- Do not go by "no pain, no gain" when exercising during pregnancy.
- Avoid valsalva maneuvers by low-resistance and high-repetition exercise principles.
- Non-weight-bearing exercises, such as aquatic exercise, are favored over weight-bearing exercises.
- Stop exercising immediately if any unusual symptoms develop.

Adapted from American College of Obstetricians and Gynecologists. Exercise during pregnancy and the postpartum period. ACOG Technical Bulletin 189. Washington, DC: American College of Obstetricians and Gynecologists; 1994.

Some people have difficulty identifying and isolating the muscles of the pelvic floor. Care must be taken to learn to contract the correct muscles. Typically, most people contract the abdominal or thigh muscles while not even working the pelvic floor muscles. These incorrect contractions may even worsen pelvic floor tone and incontinence.[33]

TABLE 8-6

SIGNS AND SYMPTOMS TO STOP EXERCISE AND CONTACT A PHYSICIAN

- Pain
- Vaginal bleeding
- Uterine contractions that are <15 minutes apart or are not affected by rest or a change in position
- Persistent dizziness, numbness, or tingling
- Visual disturbances
- Faintness
- Shortness of breath
- Heart palpitations or tachycardia
- Persistent nausea and vomiting
- Leakage of amniotic fluid
- Decreased fetal activity
- Generalized edema
- Severe headache
- Severe calf pain, swelling, or redness

American College of Obstetricians and Gynecologists. Exercise during pregnancy and the postpartum period. ACOG Technical Bulletin 189. Washington, DC: American College of Obstetricians and Gynecologists; 1994.

TABLE 8-7

ABSOLUTE CONTRAINDICATIONS TO EXERCISE IN PREGNANCY

- Pregnancy-induced hypertension (BP >140/90 mm Hg) or preeclampsia (toxemia: increased blood pressure, excessive edema [especially in hands and face] rapid weight gain, and protein in the urine)
- Diagnosed cardiac disease
- Premature rupture of membranes
- Abruptio placentae
- Preterm labor or history of preterm labor prior to 37th week of gestation
- History of recurrent miscarriage (may be allowed to exercise after first trimester)
- Persistent vaginal bleeding
- Fetal distress
- Intrauterine growth retardation
- Incompetent cervix
- Placenta previa
- Toxemia
- Polyhydramnios (amniotic fluid volume >2000 mL)
- Oligohydramnios (abnormally low volume of amniotic fluid)

American College of Obstetricians and Gynecologists. Exercise during pregnancy and the postpartum period. ACOG Technical Bulletin 189. Washington, DC: American College of Obstetricians and Gynecologists; 1994.

Additional details about the history of Kegel exercises, how to perform these exercises, techniques to identify the correct muscles, and how biofeedback is used to facilitate muscle contractions can be found on the web.[33]

Prenatal Care

In addition to concern about her own body during pregnancy, a pregnant woman is concerned about her unborn child's health. A physical therapist can remind women to practice healthy lifestyle habits to promote her unborn child's good health at birth. Embryological and fetal development are generally predictable in terms of structures that develop from one month to the next; however, environmental factors, such as the mother's diet, smoking habits, use of alcohol, or other risky behaviors, can significantly impact the normal development and function of these structures. After the first 8 weeks following conception, the fetus' developing organs mature throughout the remainder of gestation for full function at birth, yet are continually susceptible to the mother's lifestyle habits. Maternal factors that can negatively impact a developing embryo and fetus include exposure to infections (rubella, syphilis, genital herpes, AIDS, cytomegalovirus), inadequate nutrition, high levels of stress, advanced age, use of drugs, alcohol, metabolic disorders, placental inadequacy, and pre-eclampsia.[34] One of the most feared mutagens, and teratogens, or toxic agents to the fetus, in current times, is radiation exposure.[35] Health care providers should obtain complete occupational and medical histories and discuss risk of exposure with pregnant clients.

Prenatal undernutrition has permanent effects on cardiovascular risk factors. Infants exposed to famine during gestation have an increased risk of coronary heart disease in later life. Either maternal or fetal metabolic disorders can alter normal growth patterns in the developing fetus. Phenoketonuria is a hereditary enzymatic defect that results in an accumulation of phenyalanine in the body and its conversion to abnormal metabolites.[36] If this condition continues unrecognized, the child may appear normal at birth but, within a year, can develop progressive mental retardation.

Preeclampsia is another common condition that some women experience in the second half of pregnancy.[37] The condition is more common during the first pregnancy and in women who are over 40, teenage mothers, and mothers who are carrying multiple babies. Clinical manifestations of preeclampsia include high blood pressure and continuous swelling. Additional signs and symptoms include severe headaches, vomiting blood, excessive swelling of the feet and hands, decreased urine output, bloody urine, rapid heartbeat, excessive nausea, drowsiness, fever, double vision, and ringing in the ears.[36] Preeclampsia can prevent the placenta from providing sufficient blood to the fetus. This deprivation can cause low birth weight and other problems for the baby.

It is recommended that all pregnant women be screened for gestational diabetes, a carbohydrate intolerance that starts or is first recognized during pregnancy.[38] An oral glucose tolerance test between the 24th and 28th week of pregnancy is commonly used to detect this type of diabetes, and nearly 40% of women diagnosed with DM develop persistent diabetes up to 10 years following the initial diagnosis.[38] Risk factors for developing gestational diabetes include the following:[38]

- Race: African or Hispanic
- Overweight
- Atypical previous birth: baby weighing over 9 pounds, or unexplained death of fetus or newborn
- Recurrent infections
- Older age

Maintaining blood glucose levels within normal limits during the duration of the pregnancy can improve the mother's health as well as that of the fetus.[38]

If any prenatal health risks are suspected, the physical therapist should advise the mother to seek medical attention to address maternal problems contributing to fetal injury. Prenatal care should be continually encouraged throughout the pregnancy.

TABLE 8-8

RELATIVE CONTRAINDICATIONS TO EXERCISE IN PREGNANCY

- Multiple gestation (twins, triplets, etc)
- Renal or cardiac transplant
- Cigarette smoking
- History of back pain
- Fever
- Obesity
- Unwilling or unable to exercise
- Chronic hypertension
- Asthma
- Physically strenuous employment
- Hot, humid environment
- Acute infectious illness

Adapted from American College of Obstetricians and Gynecologists. Exercise during pregnancy and the postpartum period. ACOG Technical Bulletin 189. Washington, DC: American College of Obstetricians and Gynecologists; 1994.

Summary

Women have special health needs, particularly during pregnancy, that are commonly addressed by physical therapists. With the increasing risk of heart disease, along with problems with osteoporosis, incontinence, pelvic/vaginal pain, and prenatal and postpartum musculoskeletal pain, physical therapists play an essential role in preventive care. Physiological and anatomical changes during pregnancy and competition by women athletes warrant particular attention and should be carefully monitored. In addition, preventive care for an unborn child should be considered whenever working with women of childbearing age.

References

1. National Women's Health Resource Center. National survey reveals critical barriers to improving women's health. News from the NWHRC. May 4, 2005.
2. Omnia M, Samra O, Johnson R. Contraception. Emedicine. Available at: http://www.emedicine.com/med/topic3211.htm. Accessed January 28, 2006.
3. Bondy ML, Lustbader ED, Halabi S, Ross E, Vogel VG. Validation of a breast cancer risk assessment model in women with a positive family history. *J Nat Cancer Inst.* 1994;86(8):620–625.
4. National Cancer Institute. Understanding breast changes: a health guide for all women. Available at: http://www.cancer.gov/cancertopics/understanding-breast-changes. Accessed January 20, 2006.
5. The National Women's Health Information Center. US Department of Health and Human Services. Available at: http://www.4woman.gov/faq/stress.htm. Accessed February 6, 2006.
6. Heart disease and stroke statistics 2004 Update. Dallas, Tex: American Heart Association; 2003.

7. Burke AP, Farb A, Malcom GT, Liang Y, Smialek J, Virmani R. Effect of risk factors on the mechanism of acute thrombosis and sudden coronary death in women. *Circulation.* 1998;97:2110–2116.
8. Kohatsu W. Healthy heart exercise tips. National Coalition for Women with Heart Disease. Available at: http://www.womenheart.org/information/fitness_wellness.asp#Anchor-Health-54930. Accessed February 6, 2006.
9. American Association for Clinical Chemistry. Pap smear. Lab tests online. Available at: http://www.labtestsonline.org/understanding/analytes/pap/test.html. Accessed January 28, 2006.
10. University Health Center at the University of Georgia. Pelvic exam. Available at: http://www.uhs.uga.edu/sexualhealth/women/pelvic_exam.html. Accessed January 28, 2006.
11. Bhatia S, Bhatia S. Diagnosis and treatment of premenstrual dysphoric disorder. *Am Fam Phys.* 2002;77:7.
12. Prior JC, Vigna Y, Sciarretta D, et al. Conditioning exercise decreases premenstrual symptoms: a prospective, controlled 6-month trial. *Fertil Steril.* 1987;47(3):402–408.
13. Goodale IL, Domar AD, Benson H. Alleviation of premenstrual syndrome symptoms with the relaxation response. *Obstetr Gynecol.* 1990;75(4):649–655.
14. Birch K. The female athlete triad. *Brit Med J.* 2005;330:244–246.
15. Otis CL. Exercise-associated amenorrhea. *Clin Sports Med.* 1992;11:351–362.
16. Hobart U, Smucker D. The female athlete triad. *Am Fam Phys.* 2002;61:11–13.
17. Centers for Disease Control. Department of Health and Human Services. Women's reproductive health: menopause. Available at: http://www.cdc.gov/reproductivehealth//WomensRH/Menopause.htm. Accessed January 28, 2006.
18. Borer KT. Physical activity in the prevention and amelioration of osteoporosis in women: interaction of mechanical, hormonal, and dietary factors. *Sports Med.* 2005;35(9):779–830.
19. Green JS, Stanforth PR, Rankinen T, et al. The effects of exercise training on abdominal visceral fat, body composition, and indicators of the metabolic syndrome in postmenopausal women with and without estrogen replacement therapy: the HERITAGE family study. *Metabolism.* 2004;53(9):1192–1196.
20. Keenan NL, Mark S, Fugh-Berman A, Browne D, Kaczmarczyk J, Hunter C. Severity of menopausal symptoms and use of both conventional and complementary/alternative therapies. *Menopause.* 2003;10(6):507–515.
21. United Nations (UN) Department of Economic and Social Affairs, Population Division. *The Sex and Age Distribution of the World Populations: The 2002 Revision.* New York, NY: UN; 2003.
22. United Nations (UN) Department of Economic and Social Affairs, Population Division. *US Bureau of the Census, Statistical Abstract of the United States, 2003.* 123rd ed. Washington, DC: US Bureau of the Census; 2003.
23. Hall C, Thein L. *Therapeutic Exercise—Moving Toward Function.* Philadelphia, Pa: Lippincott Williams & Wilkins; 1999.
24. Novak J, Danielson LA, Kerchner LJ, et al. Relaxin is essential for renal vasodilation during pregnancy in conscious rats. *J Clin Invest.* 2001;107(11):1469–1475.
25. Stephenson R, O'Connor L. *Obstetric and Gynecologic Care in Physical Therapy.* Thorofare, NJ: SLACK Incorporated; 2000.
26. Stotland N, Haas J, Brawarsky P, et al. Body mass index, provider advice, and target gestational weight gain. *Obstet Gynecol.* 2005;105(23):633–638.
27. Ritchie J. Orthopedic considerations during pregnancy. *Clin Obstet Gynecol.* 2003;46(2):456–466.
28. Nishimoto T. How fit is your pelvic floor? *Denver Physical Therapy Women's Corner.* 1998;4:1.
29. Bauman B, Frahm J, Hakeem F, McDonald G, Wallace K. *Incontinence: A Physical Therapist's Perspective.* Alexandria, Va: American Physical Therapy Association; 2005.
30. Duke Health Brief. Healthy bladder habits. Available at: http://dukemednews.duke.edu/news/article.php?id=8479. Accessed January 28, 2006.
31. Wang T, Apgar B. Exercise during pregnancy. *Am Fam Phys.* 1998;57:8.
32. American College of Obstetricians and Gynecologists. Exercise during pregnancy and the postpartum period. ACOG Technical Bulletin 189. *Int J Gynaecol Obstet.* 1994;45(1):65–70.
33. Medline Plus. Kegel exercises. Medical Encyclopedia. Available at: http://www.nlm.nih.gov/medlineplus/ency/article/003975.htm. Accessed February 6, 2006.
34. Emedicine. Psychosocial and environmental pregnancy risks. Available at: http://www.emedicine.com/med/topics3237.html#selection~introduction. Accessed October 31, 2004.
35. Hall C. The fetal and early life origins of adult disease. *Indian Pediatrics.* 2003;40:480–502.
36. Anderson PJ, Wood SJ, Francis DE, et al. Neuropsychological functioning in children with early-treated phenylketonuria: impact of white matter abnormalities. *Dev Med Child Neurol.* 2004;46(4):230–238.
37. Odegard RA, Vatten LJ, Nilsen ST, Salvesen KA, Austgulen R. Pre-eclampsia and fetal growth. *Obstetr Gynecol.* 2000;96(6):950–955.
38. Medline Plus. Gestational diabetes. Medical Encyclopedia. Available at: http://www.nlm.nih.gov/medlineplus/ency/article/000896.htm. Accessed February 6, 2006.

Prevention Practice for Older Adults

Ann Marie Decker, PT, MSA, GCS; Gail Regan, PhD, PT;
and Catherine Rush Thompson, PhD, MS, PT

"If I'd known how old I was going to be, I'd have taken better care of myself."

~ADOLPH ZUKOR
on approaching his 100th birthday

Our National Treasures

Older adults are our "national treasures"[1] and, as such, deserve considerable attention, particularly in the area of health and wellness. As they adjust to retirement, they shift from the stresses of maintaining a vocation, in many cases, to exploring a new avocation. This adjustment includes realigning their financial resources to manage their health and livelihood. Oftentimes, older adults can focus more of their energies on their personal relationships, allowing new opportunities to rediscover the unique qualities of their spouses and others. Many maintain active lifestyles and remain engaged in various social roles in their community. According to Erikson, the final stage of psychosocial development presents the challenge of accepting one's whole life and reflecting on it in a positive manner versus sensing despair, fearing death, and reflecting negatively on the final years of life.[2] Choices of the older adult may reflect this "relatively" positive or negative view of the aging process. Physical therapists should recognize the unique value of each older adult and support continued engagement in the community to the fullest extent possible. Physical therapists are uniquely positioned to identify problems in the older adult that, over time, lead to decreased independent function and to provide education to seniors, making them more aware and knowledgeable about maintaining their own health in their "golden years."

While aging is commonly associated with declines and changes in body systems, current evidence strongly suggests that genetic predisposition to illness and individual lifestyle behaviors significantly impact the aging process; the decline of the human body, once thought to be an inevitable consequence of aging, is as much related to the long-term consequences of lifestyle choices as to an individual's chronological age. It has been estimated that by the year 2030, the United States population over 65 years will number 70 million, with the fastest growing segment of the population being those 85 and older.[3] More women than men live well into old age, with almost half of women aged 65 and older widowed.[3] Difference in life expectancy is not purely a gender difference but rather a gender-related combination of genetic, hormonal, and social influences. Extended lifespan is not only attributable to good health but also is related to technological advances in keeping people alive. In developed countries, there is an interest in slowing or reversing the aging process. Nutritional status and activity level, especially physical activity, are considered two important factors in influencing the rate and extent of physiological and cognitive changes in the aging process.[4]

People age in different ways and at different rates, although there is some consensus as to normal aging and what may be termed "successful aging." On the simplest level, chronological age may determine whether an individual is classified as an older adult. Many sources categorize people as older adults, or "senior citizens," if 65 or older; some further distinguish between the *young-old* (those between 65 and 74 years), *old* (those between 75 and 84 years), and *old-old* (those 85 and older). The *frail elder* is described in the literature as the older adult with problems in multiple domains or who is vulnerable, fragile, and lacking resilience. Frail elders are generally over the age of 65 and present with deficiencies in at least two of the following domains: physical, cognitive, nutritive, and sensory. The frail older adult has less physiologic reserve upon which to draw, and, therefore, is at increased risk of disability. It is important to note that frailty can result from the synergistic effects of aging, disease, malnutrition, disuse, and/or abuse.

What was once thought to be "normal aging" is now viewed as "typical aging," and further study is helping elucidate "successful aging." While a segment of the population may escape most chronic disease and disability until later life, statistics suggest that it is much more common for individuals to experience a chronic illness or loss of function over time.[3] "Typical" aging results in highly variable changes in the function and overall health status of older adults. Exercise tolerance, strength, and balance frequently experience a decline with age, yet regular activity and exercise have been shown to preserve these functions over time and, in some cases, reverse the usual decline.

Anatomical and Physiological Changes With Aging

Muscle Strength

Muscle strength and postural alignment are critical to efficient and effective function in the older adult. Loss of isometric and dynamic strength has been documented in individuals as young as 50 to 59 years old.[5] This decline in strength is closely associated with increased age, loss of type II muscle fibers, and loss of muscle mass. Normal changes in the aging musculoskeletal system, including reduced muscle mass and loss of bone density, can be compounded by physical inactivity. Generally, within 2 weeks of discontinuing resistance training, more than 5% of the benefits gained are greatly diminished.[5] Not only can physical inactivity accelerate the physiologic decline associated with aging, it can also hamper the ability to cope with acute physiologic stressors. If older persons are forced by illness or injury to spend days or weeks exclusively on bed rest, muscle strength as well as aerobic capacity swiftly decline; muscle strength is lost at approximately twice the rate it takes to regain. Less muscle mass leads to increased rate of disability.

The concept of threshold values for strength necessary for independent function is an interesting one. For example, there is a threshold value for quadriceps strength necessary to rise from a chair or toilet seat. At worst, when deterioration of function prevents an older adult from carrying out essential daily activities independently, professional assistance either in the home or a care center is warranted. On the other hand, a small strength gain may translate into considerable functional improvement. For example, an increase in muscle strength that allows one to transfer independently can make a substantial difference in quality of life and potential living possibilities. Numerous studies have suggested that loss of muscle strength may be slowed or reversed with progressive resistive exercise programs.[6] Though loss of muscle strength appears "typical" in older adults, regular strength training 3 times per week minimizes and, in some instances, reverses this loss. Physical therapists are well-equipped to screen for muscle strength in the older adult and make recommendations related to specific muscle strengthening exercise programs.

Changes in Bone and Joints

Age-related bone density differs from site to site. More peripheral sites, such as the radius, experience relative stability in density until menopause, while more central skeletal structures, such as the spine and the neck of the femur, show bone loss 5 to 10 years earlier.[7] Men and women age 65 years and older can reverse bone loss and reduce fracture risk through vitamin supplementation (500 mg of calcium and 700 international units of vitamin D). In addition, weight-bearing exercises minimize bone loss and, in some instances, diminish the decrease of bone density commonly seen with advancing age.[7]

Loss of joint fluid commonly associated with aging also adds to the "wear and tear" on the joint. Joint changes seem almost "inevitable" with advanced age, and in fact, osteoarthritis is one of the conditions nearly all 100-year-old persons experience.[7] Exercise and activities that promote optimal postural alignment and strength assist in reducing the occurrence of these changes until very late in life.

Changes associated with the spine are the primary reason behind the postural changes typically noted in the older adult. With aging, the intervertebral discs lose water, flatten, become porous, and undergo other deleterious changes at a cellular level.[7] These changes account for loss of disc height and compression of the spinal column, and hence, the inevitable height loss for all older adults. Spinal compression, combined with decrease in strength of intrascapular muscles, and gradual wedging of the thoracic vertebrae are contributing factors in increased thoracic spine *kyphosis* (rounding of the shoulders with a forward lean), commonly seen in the elderly.

Changes in Cardiopulmonary Function

Although aerobic capacity generally declines as one ages, the rate of decline can be diminished through physical activity.[8] *Maximum ventilatory uptake* (the maximum amount of oxygen the body inhales) usually drops between 5% and 10% per decade between the ages of 20 and 80 years.[8] Aerobic capacity, as measured by *maximal rate of oxygen consumption (VO_2 max)*, declines in sedentary and active people with aging; however, the rate may be modulated by exercise training. Because cardiorespiratory capacity declines with age, it becomes less important to measure peak or maximal aerobic capacity unless monitoring the effectiveness of a particular cardiorespiratory intervention. Decline in VO_2 max can be attributed to a decrease in maximum heart rate with aging and to decreased muscle mass and decreased muscle demands, requiring less oxygen.[8] The metabolizing tissue contributing to VO_2 max measurement is almost exclusively muscle tissue and, unless exercising to preserve muscle mass and strength, older adults experience a gradual loss of both. It appears that improving the lung's functional capacity and functional reserve are keys to slowing the rate of decline of VO_2 max.[8] It is possible for older adults to increase functional capacity with aerobic exercise training. Consistent physical activity over the course of one's life has been found to maintain ventilatory oxygen uptake at a higher level than in those who are inactive.[8]

Changes in Psychomotor and Psychological Functions

In general, there is a slowing in psychomotor performance in older adults. However, differences in cognitive processing during the aging process are also subject to individual differences related to intelligence, health, and years of formal education.[9] Cerebrovascular disease and coronary heart disease can negatively affect cognition. Examples of some of the commonly observed changes in cognition with aging are (1) a decrease in *choice reaction time* (where a decision has to be made between tasks or in sequencing) and (2) an increase in *processing time for working memory* for complex tasks, such as involved mental arithmetic and lengthy sentence comprehension. *Fluid intelligence,* or the ability to learn new information, is believed to decline with age, as opposed to *crystallized intelligence,* which reflects experiential learning.[9] Examples of crystallized intelligence, generally understood to be maintained or improved over the life span, are verbal knowledge and comprehension.

Exercise over the long term has been found to be positively correlated with delaying the age-associated slowing of cognitive processing, specifically simple, discrimination, or choice reaction time.[9] Age-related cognitive decline is variable in both rate and onset, as evidenced by cross-sectional and longitudinal studies. However, it has been observed that the reduction in cognitive efficiency seems to differentially affect knowledge-based and process-based abilities (also called *crystallized abilities* and *fluid abilities,* respectively).[9] While the process-based abilities appear more vulnerable to decline, there is no single definitive mechanism to explain that observation. Sensory deficits, decreased attention, decreased processing speed, impaired neurotransmitter function, and impaired frontal lobe function are all possible contributing factors to change in fluid abilities with age.[9] Alzheimer's disease, stroke, and Parkinson's syndrome are the most prevalent of brain pathologies with obvious cognitive impairments affecting older persons. While physical activity may preserve functional independence to a point and promote oxygen delivery to the brain, claims cannot be made for it serving in a *direct* preventive manner against Alzheimer's disease and Parkinson's syndrome. These two health problems have more complicated etiologies than inactivity.

Physical activity can be used to reduce the risk of depressive disorders among adults as well as treat unpleasant symptoms of depression.[10] Exercise is a useful early intervention for mild to moderate depression, and chronic exercise has been associated with decreased depression. Unfortunately, only 34% of all adults with depressive symptoms are diagnosed and treated.[10] Especially in light of depression's prevalence, the importance of healthy preventive tactics cannot be overstated. In most adults, effects of depression include lethargy, slowing of thought processes, moderate to severe sadness, possible confusion, memory loss (or difficulty retrieving memories), appetite loss, and perhaps less commonly, restlessness and irritation.[10] Physical activity can help promote self-efficacy about the physical tasks of self-care and housekeeping.[10]

Mobility for Older Adults

Mobility is crucial to functional independence. There are several factors contributing to a slowing of walking speed, primarily decrease in leg strength, lack of confidence in mobility or fear of falling, and an increased response time to environmental stimuli. The gait pattern of older adults often reflects a decreased stride length, a decrease in velocity, and concomitant higher cadence. Decreased joint flexibility can add to the slowing of walking speed because it encourages a decreased stride length and may influence compromised balance. Walking should be encouraged for all older adults to maintain functional independence and stamina.

Successful Aging

Individuals who are at least 100 years of age, referred to as *centenarians,* are increasing in number, and many of these individuals live independently as well as participate in leisure and work activities. According to the New England Centenarian Study, individuals who live to be 100 years of age appear to escape some of the typical changes associated with aging; they have fewer instances of disease, hospitalization, and functional decline.[11] Eight percent had no incidence of life-threatening cancer and 89% were living independently at age 92.[11] A survey of approximately 900 licensed physical therapists living into their ninth decade indicated they experienced some declines in physical function and ambulation but less than those experienced by peers of the same age.[9] One might suspect that physical therapists possess the knowledge from their training about health and disease guiding their healthy lifestyle habits. While a debate remains regarding how much genetics controls longevity, current evidence suggests that engaging in regular exercise and maintaining a healthy weight contributes significantly to a longer and healthier life. The Harvard Alumni Health Study[13] followed a large group of men aged 45 to 84 beginning in 1977 to 1988 or until they reached the age of 90. The Harvard study strongly supports the physical exercise-longevity relationship. Essentially, it was found that the more active people were, the lower the risks of death from all causes between 1977 and 1988.[12]

Fitness and physical activity have been shown to positively influence cognitive functioning, working memory, risk and symptoms of depression, anxiety, positive self-concept, high self-esteem, mental well-being, and positive perceptions of health. There is a growing amount of evidence that the level of physical fitness, particularly cardiorespiratory fitness, is inversely related to the rate of cognitive decline.[13] The direct effects of physical activity include increased cerebral blood flow, increased glucose metabolism, neural efficiency, and increased production of neurotransmitters associated with memory storage and retrieval. While "typical aging" seems to result in the development of chronic health conditions and loss of function, individuals who experience "successful aging" maintain a higher quality of life and overall health than other older adults.

Common Health Problems of Older Adults

Osteoarthritis

Osteoarthritis, also known as degenerative arthritis, is a form of arthritis occurring mainly in older persons that is characterized by chronic degeneration of the cartilage of the joints. Osteoarthritis is by far the most prevalent condition among older adults. Estimates for those affected by osteoarthritis range as high as 8%.[14] Traditionally, health professionals have advised older adults with osteoarthritis to refrain from many types of exercise for fear that exercise would lead to joint destruction, increased pain, and possible further injuries. Fortunately, the National Institutes of Health (NIH) and the American Geriatrics Society have both issued consensus statements supporting exercise in prevention and treatment of osteoarthritis.[14] Regular exercise does not hasten disease progression but rather contributes to the reduction of pain, stiffness, and maintenance of range of motion in affected joints.[15] In addition to walking, more vigorous exercise such as fairly high intensity resistance training (60% to 80% of one repetition maximum weight) and stair climbing protect bone mass over time.[14] Not only does progressive resistance training assist in maintenance of bone mass, but it has been shown to lead to increases in muscle mass and strength, important contributors to fall prevention and overall functional independence.[14]

Although weight bearing generally is beneficial in terms of bone density, individuals prone to osteoarthritis may benefit from exercising at least 50% of the time in a nonweight-bearing or low-impact environment, such as aquatic exercise or bicycling. Exercise programs for persons who either have osteoarthritis or who are at high risk for osteoarthritis should be modified at the first mention of joint pain with exercise. Close attention to proper alignment and technique is also essential for safe completion of the recommended exercise program.

Cardiovascular Disease

Among the leading causes of death and disability of older adults are *cardiovascular disease (CVD),* stroke, and cancer.[15] Approximately 9% of adults age 70 and older are affected by strokes every year. Incidence of stroke was followed as part of the Harvard Alumni Health Study, and all but light intensity activities appeared protective of stroke for this group of approximately 11,000 men when data for stroke incidence were gathered in 1988 and 1990.[15]

Heart disease in older adults is commonly the culmination of life-long lifestyle habits, including exercise, diet, and stress management. Additional information about CVD is discussed in Chapter 13.

DIABETES MELLITUS

Diabetes mellitus (DM) is one of those common chronic diseases that causes mortality and complicates other health problems older adults experience. Risk factors for type 2 DM include advancing age (older than age 45 years), obesity, family history, and a history of gestational DM. Research examining the effectiveness of the Diabetes Prevention Program found that intensive counseling on effective diet, exercise, and behavior modification reduced their risk of developing diabetes by 71% in adults over age 60.[17] Additional information about the Diabetes Prevention Program and management of diabetes can be found at the National Diabetes Information Clearinghouse website.[16]

CHRONIC OBSTRUCTIVE PULMONARY DISEASE

Approximately 11% of older adults are affected by one form of chronic obstructive pulmonary disease (COPD) (eg, bronchitis, emphysema, or asthma). Exercise benefits the physical functioning, the ability to breathe, and the mood of adults with this condition, but it also offers cognitive benefits to older adults. In a study of older adults with COPD (mean age = 67.8 + 74 years), acute aerobic exercise for 20 minutes was associated with improved cognitive functioning, including improved verbal fluency and verbal processing.[17] This study further supports the benefits of physical activity to reduce pathology and improve mental health, particularly in the older adult population. Additional information about COPD is provided in Chapter 13.

Screening Older Adults for Health, Fitness, and Wellness

After screening the older adult for past medical conditions, prior treatment, use of medications, current complaints, and general health, more specific questions can address the areas that are often at risk in the older adult: mental, psychological, and physical function. While an in-depth examination of these three areas of function is beyond the scope of this text, recognizing the comprehensive nature of screening is critical for identifying and addressing the health needs of the older adult.

Older adults who are isolated with minimal interaction have been shown to experience more depression and perceive their life has a lower quality than individuals who report more regular interactions with family and friends. Increasing numbers of seniors are being identified as having problems associated with addiction to alcohol or drugs. Estimates of alcohol abuse are listed from 2% to 17% with most experts agreeing the incidence will increase as the generation known as the "baby boomers" enter their sixth decade.[18]

The older adult dependent upon family or health care organizations for any daily living activities is particularly vulnerable to abuse; the incidence of elder abuse varies widely from 450,000 to 1.5 to 2 million.[19] Screening procedures by physical therapists should include information related to the signs and symptoms of elder abuse. Information about red flags for elder abuse and appropriate referrals are discussed in Chapter 10.

Recognizing signs and symptoms of abuse and taking appropriate steps to report the information is critical to promoting basic safety and security for older adult clients.

NUTRITION SCREENING FOR OLDER ADULTS

Good nutrition is essential for physical function and is often overlooked during a health screening. About 16% of elderly persons living in the community consume less than 1000 kilocalories per day, an amount that does not maintain adequate nutrition.[20] Individuals who are dehydrated or inadequately nourished can also experience dizzy spells contributing to falls.[20] The following screening tool can be used to identify older adults who may not be eating appropriate foods for optimal function:

Nutrition Screening

1. Does the individual appear dehydrated (dry lips, dry skin, parched mouth, difficulty speaking, frail skin)?
2. Does the individual take any vitamin or mineral supplements?
3. How many calories does the individual consume per day?

The Nutrition Screening Client Interview Form listed in Table 9-1 may prove useful in collecting additional information for a nutrition referral.[21]

TABLE 9-1
NUTRITION SCREENING CLIENT INTERVIEW FORM

Client's Name:_______________________________________ Date of Screening:______________________

Introduce self and purpose of visit: (I would like to ask you some questions so that we can assess your nutritional status.)

1. Have you experienced any changes in your weight in the last 6 months?
   - Weight loss of__________ lbs
   - Weight gain of __________ lbs
   - No change in weight__________
   - If weight loss, was it planned (trying to lose weight?)__________

2. What is your usual weight?________ lbs

   If weight loss calculate:

   % weight change = usual weight - current weight/usual weight x 100 = ______

   Evaluate significance of weight loss as follows:

Time	*Significant Weight Loss*	*Severe Weight Loss*
1 week	1% to 2%	>2%
1 month	5%	>5%
3 months	7.5%	>7.5%
6 months	10%	>10%

   Calculate: % usual body weight: current weight/usual weight x 100 = ________

   Enter % of usual body wt on screening form:__________

3. How would you describe your appetite? (circle one)

   Excellent Good Fair Poor* No appetite*

*4. Are you having any of the following problems? (check all that apply)

   ___difficulty chewing
   ___difficulty swallowing
   ___nausea
   ___vomiting
   ___constipation
   ___diarrhea
   ___mouth sores

5. Are there any foods that you are allergic to?

   ____

6. Do you have any food preference (likes or dislikes) you'd like to tell us about?

   ____

7. Have you been following any special diet at home? Are you currently taking any liquid supplements like Ensure or Sustacal? How often? Flavor preference?

   ____

8. Are you currently taking any vitamin, mineral, or herbal supplements? What kind?

   ____

Completed by:_______________________________________ Date: ______________________

*If patients are having any of the above problems, refer to dietitian.

Adapted from Laporte M, Villalon L, Payette H. Development and validity of a single malnutrition screening tool adapted to adult and elderly populations in acute and long term care facilities [abstract]. Dietitians of Canada Conference; 1998; Wolfville (NS). *Can J Diet Practice Res.* 1998;59:160.

MENTAL HEALTH FUNCTION

Mental health function is often referred to as psychological function or a person's mental and affective skills and abilities. While the complete examination and treatment of mental and affective function is outside of a physical therapist's area of practice, recognizing problems within these functional areas and making appropriate referrals is critical for long-term health and wellness of the individual. Common tests used for screening older adults' mental function status include the mini-mental status examination (MMSE) and the geriatric depression scale (GDS). The MMSE can identify problems with orientation, attention, immediate and short-term recall, language, and the ability to follow simple verbal and written commands.[22] The GDS is a short screening tool used to identify older adults at risk for depression or who are depressed when screened.[23] Individuals experiencing depression should be referred to the client's primary physician or a psychologist for a more comprehensive examination of presenting signs and symptoms.

PHYSICAL HEALTH

Because physiologic markers of fitness change as one ages, it becomes more important to measure physical fitness in the elderly in a way that does not use standards formulated with young persons. Relative improvements in oxygen uptake and utilization become more important with aging than absolute increases in maximal oxygen consumption. Physical mobility and gait are commonly measured with the same screening tools. Physical mobility may incorporate balance skills, transfer skills, and gait, as measured by the *Berg Balance Scale,* or may be focused on gait speed and the ability to stand up, as measured by the *Timed Up and Go Test.*[24] The *Tinetti Mobility Index* is another commonly used mobility scale, focusing primarily on balance and gait.[25]

SOCIAL FUNCTION

Understanding the role of social function is critical to the physical therapist. Healthy social function is a component of the healthy older adult. Attending to this area of function is critical for assuring the long-term health and wellness of the physical therapy client. Questionnaires and surveys associated with frequency of interactions with family and friends, frequency of trips outside the home, and schedule of activities for volunteer or work purposes provide some insight into an individual's social function.

COMPREHENSIVE SCREENING TOOLS

Many of these surveys or questionnaires are incorporated into more comprehensive screening tools, such as the SF-36. The recently updated *SF-36 (version 2)* has proven useful in surveys of general and specific populations, comparing the relative burden of diseases and differentiating the health benefits produced by a wide range of different treatments.[26] As a measure of perceived health, the SF-36 v 2 has greater face validity than the single-question self-ratings of health described above because it encompasses eight health concepts using multi-item scales plus one single item pertaining to change in perceived health during the last 12 months. General health perception (five items) is one of the eight scales of SF-36 v 2.[26] The other seven health concepts addressed by the multi-item scales are physical functioning (10 items), role limitations caused by physical health problems (four items), role limitations caused by emotional problems (three items), social functioning (two items), emotional well-being (five items), energy/fatigue (four items), and pain (two items).

The World Health Organization Quality of Life (WHOQOL-BREF) is another self-report questionnaire that can identify quality of life issues in older adults across multiple areas.[27] The 26-item questionnaire provides information in four domains: physical health, psychological health, social relationships, and environment. Used extensively in research, this questionnaire has been translated into 19 languages and serves as a useful tool for screening individuals from different cultures.[27]

Since older adults are at an increased risk for falls, many of the physical factors contributing to falls are screened using tools described in the multiple-dimension assessment of falls. Self-report questionnaires that combine measures of psychological, mental, and physical function are easily administered and provide valuable information. The Health Survey is a questionnaire updated to accommodate the special needs of older adults, providing a more consistent format and wording than earlier versions. The Health Survey is composed of 36 questions that address the physical components (physical function, physical role, bodily pain, and general health) and mental components (mental health, emotional role, social function, and vitality) of health.[28] This self-report tool yields an 8-scale profile of functional health and well-being scores as well as psychometrically based physical and mental health summary measures and a preference-based health utility index.

SCREENING FOR FALL RISK

The CDC National Center for Health Statistics estimates that by 2020, the health care costs for fall injuries among people over 65 will reach over 30 billion dollars per year.[29] Falls are a result of multiple factors, both intrinsic and extrinsic. Intrinsic, individual factors to consider include decreased

TABLE 9-2

SIDE EFFECTS OF GERIATRIC MEDICATIONS

Drugs Affecting Mobility	Adverse Drug Reactions
Tricyclic antidepressants	May cause postural hypotension, tremor, cardiac arrhythmias, or sedation.
Benzodiazepines and sedative hypnotics	May cause sedation, weakness, decreased coordination, or confusion.
Narcotic analgesics	May cause sedation, decreased coordination, or confusion.
Antipsychotics	May cause postural hypotension, sedation, or extrapyramidal effects.
Antihypertensives	May cause postural hypotension.
Beta-adrenergic blockers	May decrease ability to respond to workload.

Adapted from Young L, Koda-Kimble M. Chapter 101: Geriatric Drug Use and Rehabilitation. In: Koda-Kimble M, Young L, Kradjan W, Guglielmo BJ, Alldredge B. *Applied Therapeutics: The Clinical Use of Drugs*. 6th ed. Vancouver, Wash: Applied Therapeutics Inc; 1995.

sensory system function, decreased postural control and balance, increased reactions to single and multiple medications, musculoskeletal impairments, and decreased cognition. Extrinsic factors contributing to falls include the environment the individual resides in and equipment used for safety and mobility. Physical therapists are uniquely qualified to screen for both intrinsic and extrinsic factors that may place an individual at increased fall risk. Preventing or reducing falls in all elders should be of primary importance to the physical therapist. Early identification of high-risk individuals allows steps to be taken to decrease chances for future falls. Evidence suggests a prior fall places an individual at increased risk for future falls.[30] Therefore, simple questionnaires requesting information related to fall frequency and the factors surrounding the fall should include but not be limited to (1) the location of fall, (2) activity prior to fall, (3) loss of consciousness, (4) use of walking aids (eg, cane, walker) and/or protective devices (eg, hip protectors, helmet), (5) environmental conditions (eg, snow, ice), and (6) injuries that resulted from the fall.[30] It is helpful to know if anyone witnessing the fall can provide additional details about the circumstances.

SCREENING FOR VITAL SIGNS

Basic physiological functioning, measured by vital signs at rest and during exercise, helps to identify problems with blood pressure, respiration, or other body functions that may be compromised by acute illness or injury. For example, individuals with untreated hypotension are at increased risk of falling as they transition from one position to another, often a result of *orthostatic hypotension* (dropping blood pressure when positioned antigravity).

MEDICATIONS

In addition to questions related to fall history, a thorough history of current medications is needed when examining fall risk because certain medications can contribute to increased fall risk. It is particularly important to review current prescribed medications, over-the-counter medications, other dietary supplements, and recreational drugs (including alcohol) the individual may be using. Common side effects of drugs include drowsiness, confusion, dizziness, lethargy, sedation, changes in bladder or bowel function, impaired balance and reaction time, or hypotension. The use of multiple drugs, or *polypharmacy,* may further comprise motor function and lead to increased fall risk. Drug side effects commonly impair postural control and balance. Generalized sedation, postural hypotension, and impaired psychomotor abilities are common *associated drug reactions (ADRs)* that older adults experience with medication use. Limited evidence suggests multiple medications, as well as some specific classifications of medications, such as benzodiazepines (eg, Halcion), result in side effects that diminish an individual's balance ability.[31] In addition, medications for cardiovascular problems cause *hypotension* (a reduction in blood pressure of 20 mm Hg 1 or 3 minutes after moving between supine and standing). Orthostatic hypotension may place a client at an increased risk for falls if he or she has a recent history of one or more falls. Table 9-2 summarizes the side effects associated with commonly prescribed medications.[31] A careful medication history is critical to understanding and identifying an individual's fall risk.

SCREENING OF SENSORY SYSTEMS

A visual screening may help identify those at increased risk for falling. Using a Snellen chart, the physical therapist may determine visual acuity. Questions that are helpful for identifying visual problems include asking about current problems with poor visual acuity, problems related to a reduced visual field, impaired contrast sensitivity, and problems with depth perception. Note the date and results of the most recent eye examination. All older adults should be advised to have regular visual screening tests performed by their regular physician or an ophthalmologist. Vestibular dysfunction is also more common in older adults. Generally, individuals will complain of dizziness, difficulties with balance, or decreased tolerance to standing for long periods. Likewise, pain can alter overall posture leading to an increased risk for falls in older adults.

SCREENING UPRIGHT CONTROL AND BALANCE

Screening tools that examine upright control and balance tasks are recommended. While strength and range of motion contribute to overall functional gait and balance, assessing fall risk requires the examiner to attend to functional tasks associated with upright postural control and balance. The Timed Up and Go Test, Functional Reach Test, and Berg Balance Scale have all been shown to have limited predictive value of *future falls*.[32]

Falls are a complicated issue and usually *multi-factorial* in nature (ie, not purely the result of a single factor, such as poor balance). Used in combination, these screening tools and carefully crafted questionnaires and scales assist the physical therapist in identifying who would benefit from future follow-up from a physician, physical therapist, or other health care or social service provider. The older adult and their health care provider(s) should be provided with all information collected through the screening, including the physical therapist's recommendations. Physical therapists involved in identifying older adults at fall risk provide older adults, their families, and their communities with an important service. Even more importantly, this early identification allows the older adult an opportunity to modify fall risk through appropriate physical activity and exercise, environmental adjustment, and medical treatment. Recommendations for exercise to assist in prevention of falls usually include resistance training, aerobic exercise, and dynamic weight bearing exercise such as dance, Tai Chi, or sports, such as tennis and water exercise.[33]

ENVIRONMENTAL ASSESSMENT

An environmental assessment can often identify modifiable risk factors, such as rugs, floor mats, a lack of handrails in toilets, or clutter, potentially causing falls in older adults. For individuals with poor vision, nonglare surfaces on walls, floors, and stairs improve the ability to see potential obstacles. In addition, glare-free lighting enables a better view for walking. Often, wet floors or icy steps contribute to falls both inside and outside of the home. All individuals should be cautioned about venturing onto surfaces, such as freshly cleaned floors, that lack traction for safe walking.

Fall Prevention Programs for Older Adults

After performing the screening for falls, the physical therapist must determine if the risk factors are modifiable or nonmodifiable. Health education about the modifiable risk factors should be discussed in detail with resources for future reference. The American Physical Therapy Association provides a helpful booklet entitled "What You Need to Know about Balance and Falls" that can be easily obtained through their website.[34]

In addition, the National Institute on Aging offers advice for preventing falls and fractures because osteoporosis is one of the most common pathologies in older adults.[35] The website lists a number of suggestions for preventing falls and making the home safe.[35] The Home Safety Council, an organization whose mission is to educate and assist families in taking preventive action, lists similar information on its website.[36]

Since comprehensive fall prevention programs are the most effective efforts for reducing the risks of falls, the physical therapist should work with a team of health care professionals to reduce risk factors for older adults. Interventions for fall prevention include the following: (1) identification of individual risk factors that contribute to falls, (2) identification of the environmental factors that contribute to falls, (3) determining factors associated with the movement by the individual, such as reaching, lifting, walking, or turning, (4) properly managing medications and other health supplements, (5) improving physical mobility through exercise programs, balance and gait training, and appropriate use of walking aids, (6) educating family members about risk factors, (7) continence promotion and toileting programs, and (8) addressing any other factors that could potentially contribute to falls.[37] The most successful fall prevention programs are individualized to the unique needs of the senior after careful consideration of the areas listed above.

Health education is a key component of reducing risks of falls. The National Center for Injury Prevention and Control provides the following brochures free of charge: Check for Safety: A Home Fall Prevention Checklist for Older Adults (099-6156), Check for Safety (Spanish) (099-6590), What YOU Can Do to Prevent Falls (Spanish) (099-6589).[38]

Assessment of Physical Activity

Physical therapists are uniquely qualified to assess the physical activity of older adults. Physical activity, a complex behavior with no single standard measurement, has been shown to increase the quality and longevity of life. Current techniques include behavioral observation and diaries, physiological markers, electronic monitors, and self-report instruments. No one instrument meets all criteria of being valid, reliable, and practical. Over the course of one's life, physical activity may not always lead directly to favorable results, as indicated by the customary markers of physical performance and fitness, such as VO_2 max and body composition. There are now instruments, such as pedometers (devices that measure walking distance) and accelerometers (devices that measure body movement in three planes), as well as laboratory methods, such as *calorimetry*, which confines a person to a closed space in order to measure calorie expenditure. However, the most frequently used tools are self-reports covering a range of frequencies (one day to decades). The Minnesota Leisure-Time Physical Activity Questionnaire,[38] the Yale Physical Activity Survey for Older Adults,[39] and the Modified Baecke Questionnaire for Older Adults[40] are three well-validated, easily-administered activity assessments. The Minnesota Leisure Time Physical Activity Questionnaire is an interviewer-administered tool that covers the last 12 months and is completed in part by an interviewer.

Before initiating an exercise program, the older adult should be screened for possible signs and symptoms that need medical attention. The following clinical manifestations warrant a visit to the physician before initiating a standard exercise program: chest pain or pressure, shortness of breath, heart beat irregularities, blood clots, infections or fever, unplanned weight loss, foot or ankle sores that will not heal, a hernia, joint swelling, pain or trouble walking after a fall, a bleeding or detached retina, recent eye surgery or laser treatment, recent hip surgery, light-headedness or dizziness, difficulty with balance, or nausea. The fitness levels of older adults vary considerably based upon the physical activity and general health of the older adult. To obtain a complete picture of the health-related fitness of the older adult, one needs to assess cardiorespiratory function, muscular strength, muscular endurance, flexibility, and body composition.

There are several ways to assess cardiorespiratory fitness or estimated VO_2 max; however, for some elderly individuals, these tests can be taxing. The Rockport One-Mile Walk Test, involving a 1-mile walk at the fastest pace possible, is commonly used.[41] The Three-Minute Step Test is an alternative for estimating VO_2 max from postexercise recovery heart rate; however, it is not feasible for extremely deconditioned individuals or those with visual perception or balance deficits. If conducted properly, a submaximal VO_2 test provides a valid measure of cardiorespiratory fitness; however, it does not measure physical fitness in a broader sense.

Functional fitness refers to "the physical capacity of the individual to meet ordinary and unexpected demands of daily life safely and effectively."[42] A functional fitness test provides health-related fitness information that can be used to determine independent living in the later years. The focus of functional fitness assessments is on assessment of the individual's capacity to perform skills for daily activities and evaluation of the individual's routine. For those at risk for functional dependence, functional fitness tests are more sensitive than traditional measures of cardiorespiratory fitness.[42] Besides being a more holistic approach to fitness than strictly VO_2 max, a functional fitness test has a second practical value of potentially challenging elderly participants without pushing them to exhaustion. Since physical mobility problems contribute the most to lost functional independence,[42] it is prudent to rely on a functional test that assesses several mobility-related fitness parameters. Functioning testing can also identify risk factors or developing problems missed on self-report questionnaires. Functional measures have shown their utility in predicting outcomes, such as mortality or nursing center placement, as well as in assessing present mobility and independence in ADLs.[42] Another important consideration in the older adult population is that factors such as pain, visual deficits, and compromised balance may modify the association between strength and function. Conducting a functional fitness test enables the examiner to evaluate whether any of these aforementioned factors affect physical performance.

The Continuous Scale Physical Functional Performance Test (CS-PFP) examines upper body strength, lower body strength, flexibility, balance and coordination, and endurance and is composed of several tasks quantified by time, distance, or weight.[43] An example of a CS-PFP item in the lower body strength domain is timed performance of five repetitions of sit-to-stand movements. A limitation of this examination tool is the significant amount of time needed to instruct and observe each test item; however, it can be helpful in demonstrating clinical improvements in specific health-related areas.[43]

The Physical Performance Test (PPT) assesses multiple domains of function simulating activities of daily living: strength, mobility, and dexterity.[44] Meant to be administered in 10 minutes or less, there are two versions: one with nine items and one with seven. The abbreviated version does not entail stair climbing. Tasks are quite varied, ranging from writing a sentence to walking 50 feet, enabling the examiner to identify limitations in separate domains of function.

AAHPERD Test Battery for Older Adults was developed for the American Alliance for Health, Physical Education, Recreation and Dance (AAHPERD) as a sound, practical measure of fitness; however, there are two features that limit its use: the flexibility measure must be completed from a straight-leg position on the floor, and the test of aerobic endurance is quite challenging for many, as it is a half-mile walk.[45]

The *Senior Fitness Test* is a battery of performance tests designed to assess the physical parameters associated with functional mobility in older adults.[46] The motive behind the development of this functional test was to detect physical decline and address it, since some physical decline during aging is preventable and, to some extent, reversible. The 6-Minute Walk, a subtest of the Senior Fitness Test, has been used to effectively determine exercise capacity in older patients with congestive heart failure and has convergent validity with self-rated health and physical functioning. Development trials for the Senior Fitness Test show that lower extremity function subtests (the Chair Stand, the 8 Feet Up-and-Go, and the 6-Minute Walk) are strongly associated with walking, moving quickly when necessary, stair-climbing, dressing, and bathing. In older adults, if muscle weakness develops in the lower extremities, it may lead to the inability to perform fundamentally important activities, such as getting up from a seated position. The Chair Stand subtest is also helpful in identifying older adults who are more active.

It is important that functional fitness tests be administered by health professionals or professionals trained in exercise science not only to ensure safety of those participating in the test but also because of knowledge necessary to interpret the results. Baseline vital signs should be taken and closely monitored during and following more strenuous tests.

Fitness for Older Adults

The general recommendation of 30 minutes or more of moderate intensity exercise on most and preferably all days of the week applies to older adults who are not limited by serious health problems. One feature of this public health recommendation is the acknowledgment that intermittent, brief sessions of physical activity are appropriate for meeting the 30-minutes total.[46] Some examples are walking two miles in 30 minutes, shoveling snow for 15 minutes, and raking leaves for 30 minutes. Swimming laps at a moderate pace for 30 minutes burns about twice as many calories. Barbara Ainsworth of the School of Public Health at University of Minnesota, along with several exercise science colleagues, has developed a compendium of occupational, household, recreational, and sport physical activities.[47] The main impetus for developing this compendium was to develop comparable coding systems for physical activities across research studies. This resource lists activities by purpose and energy cost. There is a metabolic equivalent (MET) unit listed for each activity. Moderate intensity physical activities are generally 3 to 5 METs. Many older adult clients, however, are more attuned to energy expenditure in terms of kilocalories or time spent on an activity.

In light of the expected growth of the older segment of the population, increasing the knowledge about the relationships among physical fitness, physical activity, and health in the senior citizen has the potential to positively influence overall health and wellness for this population. According to the Centers for Disease Control and Prevention, 28% to 44% of adults over the age of 65 are inactive[48] (ie, they participate in no leisure-time physical activity). Inactivity is more common in older people than in middle-aged men and women, and women were more likely than men to report no leisure-time activity. Since successful aging is largely determined by individual lifestyle changes, this portion of the population is at the greatest risk of developing pathology secondary to a sedentary lifestyle. Women who are inactive and nonsmoking at the age of 65 have 12.7 years of active life expectancy compared to active, nonsmoking women, who have 18.4 years.[48] Estimates for 2000 indicate that only 13% of individuals between ages 65 and 74 reported engaging in vigorous physical activity for 20 minutes 3 or more days per week, and only 6% of those 75 and older reported such exercise.[48]

By 2030, the number of older adults in the United States is expected to reach 70 million, and the total population aged 65 or older is expected to grow to 20%.[49] This growing population will place increasing demands on the public health system and on medical and social services. "Lack of physical activity and poor diet are the major causes of an epidemic of obesity that is affecting the elderly as well as middle-aged and younger populations. An estimated 18% of adults over age 65 in the United States are obese, and another 40% are overweight, putting them at substantially increased risk for diabetes, high blood pressure, heart disease, along with other chronic diseases."[49] Being inactive also affects balance, as a result of loss in muscle strength, and increases the risk of falls. Every year, fall-related injuries among older people cost the nation more than $20.2 billion. By 2020, the total annual cost of these injuries is expected to reach $32.4 billion.[49] Preventing chronic illness and injury in older adults should be cause enough to engage in regular physical activity. Older adults can benefit physically, cognitively, and psychosocially from physical activity performed on a regular basis. For this reason, increased physical activity in older adults should be promoted on a local, state, and national level.

Substantial health benefits occur with a moderate amount of activity (eg, at least 30 minutes of brisk walking) on 5 or more days of the week. Brief episodes of physical activity, such as 10 minutes at a time, can be beneficial if repeated. Sedentary persons can begin with brief episodes and gradually increase the duration or intensity of activity. One review of the literature revealed that programs to build muscle strength, improve balance, and promote walking significantly reduced falls in older persons. Experts recommend that older adults should participate at least 2 days a week in strength training activities that improve and maintain muscular strength and endurance.[50] Older adults are sensitive to the effects of physical activity, and even small amounts of activity are healthier than a sedentary lifestyle. Water exercises and low-impact exercises can be complemented by strength-training exercises. Exercise programs that involve tai chi have been shown to help enhance balance while yoga can improve flexibility.[51]

A recent study found that only half of all adults were asked about their exercise habits by their health care provider; older patients were asked less often than younger patients, and individuals who had been asked reported being more active than those who were never asked.[52] Collecting information from older clients about their activity level is a critical step all physical therapists should undertake in the overall management of the geriatric client. Physical therapists should assist their older clients in setting activity and fitness goals and recommend individually tailored physical activity regimens. Physical therapists also need to have knowledge of community resources of benefit to the older adult interested in improving overall health, wellness, and fitness.

Summary

Older adults are a diverse population with significant needs in the area of long-term health, wellness, and fitness. Physical therapists are in a unique position to provide optimal screening, referrals, education, and recommendations to assist the older adult in maintaining or improving overall health. Perhaps more so than any other age group, older adults experience a wide variety of changes in the body and abilities due to their unique genetic make-up, lifestyle, and environment. Identifying each individual's opportunities for optimal health and wellness through the entire lifespan is an important role for the physical therapist.

References

1. Kentucky Cabinet for Health and Human Services. Celebrate long-term living during Older Americans Month. Available at: http://chfs.ky.gov/news/Older+Americans+Month+1.htm. Accessed February 6, 2006.
2. Erickson E. *Erikson on Development in Adulthood: New Insights from the Unpublished Papers*. London, England: Oxford University Press Inc; 2002.
3. Centers for Disease Control and Prevention. *Unrealized Prevention Opportunities Reducing the Health and Economic Burden of Chronic Disease*. Atlanta, Ga: CDC, National Center for Chronic Disease Prevention and Health Promotion; 1997.
4. Rosenberg IH, Miller JW. Nutritional factors in physical and cognitive functions of elderly people. *Am J Clin Nutr.* 2000;55:1237S-1243S.
5. Nelson ME, Fiatarone MA, Morganti CM, Trice I, Greenberg RA, Evans WJ. Effects of high-intensity strength training on multiple risk factors for osteoporotic fractures: a randomized controlled trial. *JAMA*. 1994;272:1909-1914.
6. Slovik DM. Osteoporosis. In: WR Fronters, ed. *Exercise in Rehabilitation Medicine.* 3rd ed. Champaign, Ill: Human Kinetics; 1999:313-348.
7. Turner CH, Robling AG. Designing exercise regimens to increase bone strength. *Exerc Sport Sci Rev.* 2003; 31:45-50.
8. Spirduso WW. *Physical Dimensions of Aging.* Champaign,Ill: Human Kinetics; 1995.
9. Gucionne A. *Geriatric Physical Therapy.* 2nd ed. St. Louis, Mo: Mosby, 2000.

10. Churchill JD, Galvez R, Colcombe S, Swain RA, Kramer AF, Greenough WT. Exercise, experience and the aging brain. *Neurobiology of Aging.* 2002;23:941-955.
11. Dellara T, Wilcox M, McCormick M, Perls T. Cardiovascular disease delay in centenarian offspring. *The Journals of Gerontology Series A: Biological Sciences and Medical Sciences.* 2004;59:M385-M389.
12. Lee IM, Hsieh CC, Paffenbarger RS. Exercise intensity and longevity in men. The Harvard Alumni Health Study. *JAMA.* 1995;273(15):1179-1184.
13. Colcombe S, Kramer AF. Fitness effects on the cognitive function of older adults: a meta-analytic study. *Psychol Sci.* 2003;14(2):125-130.
14. American Geriatrics Society Panel on Exercise and Osteoarthritis. Exercise prescription for older adults with osteoarthritis pain: consensus practice recommendations. a supplement to the AGS Clinical Practice Guidelines on the management of chronic pain in older adults. *J Am Geriatr Society.* 49:808-823.
15. American Heart Association. *Heart and Stroke Statistical Update.* Dallas, Tex: American Heart Association; 2002.
16. National Diabetes Information Clearinghouse. The Diabetes Prevention Program and management of diabetes. Available at: http://diabetes.niddk.nih.gov/dm/pubs/preventionprogram/.
17. Berry MJ, Rejeski WJ, Adair NE, Ettinger HH Jr, Zaccaro DJ, Sevick MA. A randomized, controlled trial comparing long-term and short-term exercise in patients with chronic obstructive pulmonary disease. *J Cardiopulmon Rehabil.* 2003;23:60-68.
18. Williams GD, Stinson FS, Parker DA, Harford TC, Noble J. Demographic trends, alcohol abuse and alcoholism, 1985-1995 [Epidemiologic Bulletin No. 15]. *Alcohol Health & Research World.* 1987;11(3):80-83,91.
19. Reed R, Mooradian A. Treatment of diabetes in the elderly. *Am Fam Phys.* September 1991.
20. PDR Health. Dietary targets for your senior years. Available at: http://www.pdrhealth.com/content/nutrition_health/chapters/fgnt20.shtml. Accessed February 12, 2006.
21. Laporte M, Villalon L, Payette H. Development and validity of a single malnutrition screening tool adapted to adult and elderly populations in acute and long term care facilities [abstract]. Dietitians of Canada Conference; Wolfville (NS). *Can J Diet Practice Res.* 1998;59:160.
22. Folstein MF, Folstein SE, McHugh PR. Mini-mental state: a practical method for grading the state of patients for the clinician. *J Psychiatric Research.* 1975;12:189-198.
23. Brink TL, Yesavage JA, Lum O, Heersema P, Adey MB, Rose TL. Screening tests for geriatric depression. *Clin Gerontol.* 1982;1:37-44.
24. Steffen TM, Hacker TA, Mollinger L. Age- and gender-related test performance in community-dwelling elderly people: Six-Minute Walk Test, Berg Balance Scale, Timed Up and Go Test, and gait speeds. *Phys Ther.* 2002;82(2):128-137.
25. Tinetti ME, Williams TF, Mayewski R. Fall risk index for elderly patients based on number of chronic disabilities. *Am J Med.* 1986;80(3):429-434.
26. Friedman B, Heisel M, Delavan R. Validity of the SF-36 five-item Mental Health Index for major depression in functionally impaired, community-dwelling elderly patients. *J Am Geriatr Soc.* 2005;53(11):1978-1985
27. World Health Organization. WHO QoL Study Protocol. WHO (MNH7PSF/93.9). 1993.
28. Medicare Outcomes Health Survey. RAND 36-Item Short Form Health Survey 1.0 (RAND SF-36). Available at: http://www.hosonline.org/surveys/hos/hosinstrument.asp. Accessed February 12, 2006.
29. National Center for Injury Prevention and Control. Falls and hip fractures among older adults. Available at: http://www.cdc.gov/ncipc/factsheets/falls.htm. Accessed February 12, 2006.
30. Allain H, Bentue-Ferrer D, Polard E, Akwa Y, Patat A. Postural instability and consequent falls and hip fractures associated with use of hypnotics in the elderly: a comparative review. *Drugs Aging.* 2005;22(9):749-765.
31. Young L, Koda-Kimble M. Chapter 101: geriatric drug use and rehabilitation. In: *Applied Therapeutics: The Clinical Use of Drugs.* Baltimore, Md: Lippincott, Williams, and Wilkins; 1995.
32. Thapa PB, Gideon P, Brockman KG, Fought RL, Ray WA. Clinical and biomechanical measures of balance as fall predictors in ambulatory nursing home residents. *J Gerontol A Biol Sci Med Sci.* 1996;51(5):M239-M246.
33. Li F, Harmer P, Fisher KJ, McAuley E, Chaumeton N, Eckstrom E, Wilson NL. Tai chi and fall reductions in older adults: a randomized controlled trial. *J Gerontol Med Sci.* 2005;60A(2):187-194.
34. American Physical Therapy Association. What you need to know about balance and falls. Available at: http://www.apta.org. Accessed February 12, 2006.
35. National Institute of Aging. Preventing falls and fractures. Available at: http://www.niapublications.org/engagepages/falls.asp. Accessed February 12, 2006.
36. Home Safety Council. Available at: http://www.homesafetycouncil.org. Accessed February 12, 2006.
37. The National Center for Injury Prevention and Control. Check for safety: a home fall prevention checklist for older adults (099-6156). Available at: http://www.cdc.gov/ncipc. Accessed February 12, 2006.
38. Folsom AR, Jacobs DR Jr, Caspersen CJ, Gomez-Marin O, Knudsen J. Test-retest reliability of the Minnesota Leisure Time Physical Activity Questionnaire. *J Chronic Dis.* 1986;39(7):505-511.
39. Dipietro L, Caspersen CJ, Ostfeld AM, Nadel ER. A survey for assessing physical activity among older adults. *Med Sci Sports Exerc.* 1993;25(5):628-642.
40. Buchheit M, Simon C, Viola AU, Doutreleau S, Piquard F, Brandenberger G. Heart rate variability in sportive elderly: relationship with daily physical activity. *Med Sci Sports Exerc.* 2004;36(4):601-605.

41. Pober DM, Freedson PS, Kline GM, McInnis KJ, Rippe JM. Development and validation of a one-mile treadmill walk test to predict peak oxygen uptake in healthy adults ages 40 to 79 years. *Can J Appl Physiol.* 2002;27(6):575-589.

42. Blair SN, Cheng Y, Holder JS. Is physical activity or physical fitness more important in defining health benefits? *Med Sci Sport Exerc.* 2001;33(6 Suppl):S379-S399.

43. Cress ME, Buchner DM, Questad KA, Esselman PC, deLateur BJ, Schwartz RS. Continuous-scale physical functional performance in healthy older adults: a validation study. *Arch Phys Med Rehabil.* 1996;77(12):1243-1250.

44. Falconer J, Hughes SL, Naughton BJ, Singer R, Chang RW, Sinacore JM. Self report and performance-based hand function tests as correlates of dependency in the elderly. *J Am Geriatr Soc.* 1991;39(7):695-699.

45. Clark BC. Test for fitness in older adults, AAHPERD fitness task force. *JOPHERD.* 1989;60:66-71.

46. Reuben DB, Valle LA, Hays RD, Siu AL. Measuring physical function in community-dwelling older persons: a comparison of self-administered, interviewer-administered, and performance-based measures. *J Am Geriatr Soc.* 1995;43(1):17-23.

47. Ainsworth BE, Haskell WL, Leon AS, Jacobs DR Jr, Montoye HJ, Sallis JF, Paffenbarger RS Jr. Compendium of physical activities: classification of energy costs of human physical activities. *Med Sci Sports Exerc.* 1993;25(1):71-80.

48. Centers for Disease Control and Prevention. Prevalence of health care providers asking older adults about their physical activity levels—United States, 1998. *Morbidity and Mortality Weekly Report.* 2002;51(19):412-414.

49. Center for Disease Control and Prevention. Cost of injury. Available at: www.cdc.gov/ncipc/pub-res/cost_of_injury/intro-ch1.pdf. Accessed February 12, 2006.

50. Brown M, Sincacore DR, Host HH. The relationship of strength to function in the older adult. *J Gerontol - Biologicl Med Sci.* 1995;50:A55-A59.

51. Shephard RJ, Cox M. Step test predictions of maximum oxygen uptake before and after an employee fitness programme. *Can J Appl Sport Sci.* 1982;7(3):197-201.

52. Coups EJ, Gaba A, Orleans CT. Physician screening for multiple behavioral health risk factors. *Am J Prev Med.* 2004;27(2 Suppl):34-41.

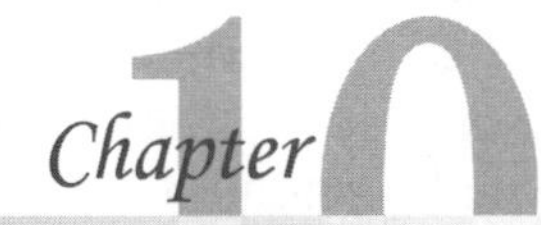

Resources to Optimize Health and Wellness

Martha Highfield, PhD, RN, AOCN and Catherine Rush Thompson, PhD, MS, PT

"The contemporary disarray in health affairs in the United States is a result of history. It is the cumulative result of inattention to chronic disabling illness."

~DANIEL FOX
President of the Milbank Memorial Fund

Prevalence of Chronic Illness

According to the Centers for Disease Control and Prevention (CDC), chronic illness affects approximately 90 million people or approximately 1 in 3 persons in the United States.[1] The CDC further states the following[1]:

> *...chronic diseases, such as cardiovascular disease (primarily heart disease and stroke), cancer, and diabetes, are among the most prevalent, costly, and preventable of all health problems. Seven of every ten Americans who die each year (more than 1.7 million people) die of a chronic disease. The prolonged course of illness and disability from such chronic diseases, such as diabetes and arthritis, results in extended pain and suffering and decreased quality of life for millions of Americans. Chronic, disabling conditions cause major limitations in activity for more than one of every ten Americans, or 25 million people.*

More than 60% of the nation's medical care costs are attributed to chronic diseases.[1]

Common Impairments Encountered With Chronic Pathology

Impairments often encountered when working with individuals with chronic pathology include single system impairments, such as muscle weakness or decreased cardiovascular endurance, or multi-system impairments with compounded physical impairments, such as metastasized cancer or diabetes. Generally, individuals with chronic health conditions develop decreased musculoskeletal flexibility, reduced strength, and compromised cardiovascular endurance from decreased activity. *Hypokinesia* (abnormally decreased motor function or activity)[2] is a major contributor to the chronic health problems leading to disability resulting from multi-system deconditioning. Other health concerns associated with chronic illness include altered psychological status, changes in social interactions, altered sleep habits, unhealthy nutritional habits, changes with digestion and elimination, reduced balance and coordination, altered cognitive status (often secondary to medications), and concurrent use of several drugs that may pose additional health risks.

Any chronic condition can trigger depression, but the risk increases with the severity of illness and the degree of life disruption it causes. While depression alone can limit functional abilities, it can also aggravate signs and symptoms of pathology, including fatigue, lethargy, and pain, as well as lead to social withdrawal. While the risk of becoming depressed is approximately 10% to 25% for women and 5% to 12% for men in the general population, the risk increases for individuals with chronic illness.[3] Table 10-1 lists the risk of depression with common medical conditions.

Denial, anger, and frustration commonly accompany the realization that a chronic illness may be incurable. While coping with the changes diseases impose on lifestyle, those with chronic illness need to restore a sense of control in their lives. Providing information about pathological conditions, suggesting support groups, and directly addressing modifiable factors are all methods to help clients regain control of their lives. Emotional management of chronic illness includes regular exercise, maintaining daily activities, connecting with family and friends, as well as a support group on a regular basis, pursuing personal hobbies, maintaining a positive attitude, and seeking professional help from a psychologist when depression becomes evident.

Clients with chronic illness and their caretakers often have new demanding schedules that incorporate regular medical visits, specific medical regimens, prescribed diets, and extra time required for self-care activities. These changes in lifestyle require time management skills to meet the multiple time demands of clients with chronic illness. Additionally, these clients must maintain some flexibility to best adapt to their new lifestyles and uncertain futures. Recognizing the unique stresses caused by chronic illness, physical therapists can help clients and their caretakers focus on functional activities and time management skills to optimize time and effort required for daily activities. Routines can be established that help clients manage healthy habits of grooming, regular exercise, and eating appropriate foods; tracking their health status; attending to proper administration of medications, maintaining the home, and financial management. The physician should be contacted whenever progression of the pathology is apparent. The priority of health care is optimizing each individual's quality of life.

TABLE 10-1

DEPRESSION RISK WITH CHRONIC ILLNESS

The risk of depression accompanying chronic illness is listed for each of the following:

- Depression with no other medical condition – 5.3% (3.6% for men and 6.9% for women)
- Asthma – 50% (ranging from 25% for those with infrequent attacks to 87.5% for those with frequent attacks)
- Arthritis – 33% (greater depression is evident with increasing symptoms)
- Cancer – 25% to 50% (depending on the type of cancer)
- Cardiovascular disease – 16% (depression associated with smoking increases the likelihood of developing heart disease)
- Cerebrovascular accident (stroke) – 10% to 27% (strokes affecting the left hemisphere have a higher incidence; depression is associated with increased stroke morbidity and mortality)
- Diabetes – up to 25%
- Myocardial infarction (heart attack) – 40% to 65%
- Multiple sclerosis – 42%
- Obesity – 50%
- Parkinson's disease – 47%

Adapted from:
Chapman D, Perry G, Strine T. The vital link between chronic disease and depressive disorders. *Prev Chron Dis.* 2005;2(1): A14.
Hasin DS, Goodwin RD, Stinson FS, Grant BF. Epidemiology of major depressive disorder: results from the National Epidemiologic Survey on Alcoholism and Related Conditions. *Arch Gen Psych.* 2005;62(10);1097–1106.
Chwastiak L, Ehde D, Gibbons L, et al. Depressive symptoms and severity of illness in multiple sclerosis: epidemiologic study of a large community sample. *Am J Psych.* 2002;159:1862–1868.
Weintraub D, Moberg P, Duda J, et al. Recognition and treatment of depression in Parkinson's disease. *J Geriatr Psych Neurol.* 2003;16(3):178–183.

Making Lifestyle Changes

Many recommendations for intervention, while proven effective in reducing the risk of disease, are unheeded. The United States Preventive and Services Task Force (USPSTF)[4] recommends the following steps for helping individuals change poor health habits:

1. Identify an individual's beliefs about specific behaviors, and adjust advice to the individual's lifestyle.

2. Provide the rationale for each recommendation, and develop a realistic time frame for achieving results. As the individual achieves small successes, propose larger but achievable goals.
3. Add new behaviors. Adopting good habits is often easier than discarding bad ones.
4. Link positive behaviors with the daily routine. Have the individual explain how the behavior will be integrated into daily activities.
5. Sub-specialists in many chronic diseases have trained teams that can educate patients far more effectively than individual health care providers can. Another form of referral is sending novice patients to talk with successful patients.
6. According to research findings, a call from a health professional to inquire about progress is very effective in changing a behavior.

Ideally, unhealthy behaviors should be prevented before they develop into lifestyle habits. Unfortunately, unhealthy behaviors often develop in response to the inability to react to the many stresses individuals encounter across the lifespan. To best manage stress, it is important to understand what stress is and how it is most effectively managed.

Stress Management

Stress is a description of how an individual reacts (physically and emotionally) to change. Stress can be positive (*eustress*) or negative (*distress*). Behavior is influenced by daily stresses experienced in performing daily activities of living. Certain stresses may be desirable (eg, a job promotion), while other stressful situations create distress (eg, loss of a loved one). Neutral stress (*neustress*) has neither harmful nor helpful effects on the mind or body. While one situation may be very stressful for one individual, another individual may feel no stress from the situation.

Common sources of stress include employment or job issues, money problems, family issues, housework, health problems, and child care issues. These individuals need resources to manage their stress to avoid developing negative stress-related behaviors. Some physical distress symptoms include toe jiggling or foot tapping to reflect impatience or irritability; tight or rounded shoulders signaling anxiety, fear, or embarrassment; tightly folded arms suggesting disapproval; sagging or sloping shoulders reflecting fatigue or feeling burdened; nail biting conveying worry or tension; jutting the jaw showing apprehension or tension; clenched fists or tight fingers indicating anxiety; or a furrowed brow indicating worry, fatigue, or depression.[5] If stress is not well managed, stress can lead to chronic over-stimulation of body organs, leading to possible organ failure. Chronic stress-related illnesses include migraine headaches, tension headaches, psoriasis, panic attacks, ulcers, colitis, gastritis, cancer, noncardiac chest pain, heart attacks, dizzy spells, low back pain, rheumatoid arthritis, and high blood pressure. Behavioral consequences of chronic stress include overeating or a loss of appetite, smoking, alcohol abuse, sleeping disorders, and emotional outbursts, as well as violence and aggression.

Steps for managing stress include the following:

1. Identifying the stressor
2. Using a relaxation or coping strategy to relieve the stress
3. Seeking solutions for avoiding or controlling the stress
4. Being as fit and healthy as possible
5. Changing a way of thinking, as needed

Healthy nutrition and adequate rest, using relaxation techniques, time management, a positive attitude, and physical activity have all been shown to effectively reduce stress. For all types of stress management programming, interventions should be targeted to the individual; they should be behaviorally based, and they should be integrated into lifestyle behaviors through practice and reinforcement. The remainder of this chapter will offer various options for reducing or managing stress as well as resources for improving mental, spiritual, and emotional health and wellness.

Nutrition

Good nutrition involves receiving and using the optimal nutrients to manage variations in health and disease.[6] Signs of good nutrition include a toned and well-developed body, ideal body weight for body composition, smooth skin, clear and bright eyes, glossy hair, and an alert facial expression.[6] While other factors contribute to these healthy features, good nutrition is essential for optimal health. *Undernutrition* refers to a diet that lacks a full complement of healthy nutrients.[6] Individuals who are undernourished are limited in their physical work capacity, their immune function, their mental activity, and their ability to recover from illness and injury. *Malnutrition* occurs when nutritional stores are depleted and the body lacks sufficient nutrients for the demands of daily living.[6] While malnutrition is commonly reported in distressed and impoverished conditions, individuals with chronic disease may also lack sufficient stores of nutrients for their daily needs. *Overnutrition,* while literally referring to an overabundance of nutrients exceeding health guidelines, may mask malnutrition in severely obese individuals.[6] Certain lifestyle habits affect the body's ability to absorb and process nutrients appropriately. For example, those who drink alcohol heavily or smoke inhibit the body's ability to absorb vitamins B6, B12, A, and D; thiamin; folic acid; and niacin.[6] Table 10-2 provides a list of typical signs and symptoms that indicate the nutritional status of an individual.[6]

Popular Diets

Vegetarian diets, while limited in animal sources for protein and relying primarily on plant sources of protein, vary according to underlying philosophies or dietary needs of the individual. *Lacto-ovo vegetarians* exclude red meats, while allowing dairy products, eggs, and in some cases, fish and poultry.[6] *Lacto-vegetarians* accept dairy products and plant sources of proteins but do not allow meat, fish, or poultry.[6] The *vegan diet* is strictly limited to plant sources of proteins, including whole or enriched grains, legumes, nuts, and seeds.[6] The underlying need of vegetarians is to ensure adequate amino acid balance through well-planned diets. It is important to ask clients if they are getting adequate vitamin B12 and zinc in their diet if they are strict adherents, as these two deficiencies are often noted.[6] *Lactose intolerance* suggests that the individual has intolerance to milk and some dairy products.[6] For these individuals, it is important to encourage adequate calcium and vitamin D through other supplementation.

Some individuals eat *vitamin-enriched diets* through fortified cereal and other prepared foods. These individuals should be cautioned about taking more than 100% RDA for each nutrient—especially niacin, pyridoxine, and vitamins A, D, and E.[6] *Low carbohydrate diets* have proven effective for short-term weight reduction but are controversial. Physical therapists should be able to screen for possible nutritional deficits or conditions that pose nutritional risks for their clients and make proper referrals to the client's physician or a registered dietitian. Any dietary recommendations should be made by the individual's physician or a registered dietitian.

Certain metabolic conditions put individuals at increased risk for illness, including problems with water and electrolyte imbalances. Dehydration is one of the most preventable dietary problems but is also one of the most common. The CDC recommends the following tips to prevent dehydration,[6] especially during summer months: (1) the average adult should consumer at least eight 8-ounce glasses of fluid daily; (2) fluids with added sodium or flavoring should be avoided; and (3) caffeinated drinks and alcohol increase dehydration and should be avoided. A balanced diet is essential for growth, development, and healing; however, it is important to recognize common food allergies (cow's milk, eggs, nuts, wheat, corn, and seafood) and the common hypersensitivity reactions to foods that may be allergens. These reactions include eyes itching, wheezing, and the feeling of the throat tightening. If food allergies are suspected, medical attention should be immediate. Individuals who are prone to food allergies often carry medications to reduce the threat of an extreme allergic reaction.

The Importance of Physical Activity and Good Nutrition

Much of the chronic disease burden is preventable. Physical inactivity and unhealthy eating contribute to obesity, cancer, cardiovascular disease, and diabetes. Together, these two behaviors are responsible for at least 400,000 deaths each year.[1] Only tobacco use causes more preventable deaths in the United States. People who avoid unhealthy behaviors that increase their risk for chronic diseases can expect to live healthier and longer lives.

The Obesity Epidemic

Obesity has reached epidemic proportions; nearly 59 million adults are obese.[1] Moreover, the epidemic is not limited to adults; the percent age of young people who are overweight has more than doubled in the last 20 years. Of children and adolescents aged 6 to 19 years, 15%—about 9 million young people—are considered overweight.[1] The estimated annual cost of obesity and overweight people in the United States in 2000 was about $117 billion. Promoting regular physical activity and healthy eating and creating an environment that supports these behaviors are essential to reducing this epidemic. Only about one-fourth of adults in the United States eat the recommended five or more servings of fruits and vegetables each day. In addition, in the last 30 years, calorie intake has increased for both men and women.[1] Poor eating habits are often established during childhood. Only 21% of young people eat the recommended five or more servings of fruits and vegetables each day.[1] Because obesity is caused by a complex and interrelated set of individual and community factors, state obesity prevention programs are testing interventions that focus simultaneously on nutrition and physical activity among individuals and on related community and environmental issues.

TABLE 10-2
CLINICAL SIGNS OF NUTRITIONAL STATUS

Body Area	Signs of Good Nutrition	Signs of Poor Nutrition
Appearance	Alert, responsive	Listless, apathetic, *cachectic* (appearing "wasted" and emaciated)
Posture	Erect posture, arms and legs straight	Sagging shoulders, sunken chest, humped back
Weight	Normal for height, age, and body build	Overweight or underweight (special concerns if underweight); reduced circumferential measurements
Cardiovascular System		
Endurance	Good endurance, energetic, sleeps well, vigorous	Easily fatigued, no energy, falls asleep easily, looks tired, apathetic
Heart rate and blood pressure	Normal heart rate and rhythm, no murmurs, normal blood, pressure for age	Tachycardia, enlarged heart, abnormal rhythm, elevated blood pressure
Peripheral circulation	No swelling in extremities	Swelling in hands and legs
Endocrine System		
Neck (glands)	No enlargement	Thyroid enlargement
Integumentary System		
Face and neck	Skin color uniform, smooth, pink, healthy appearance, not swollen	Greasy, discolored, scaly, swollen, skin dark over cheeks and under eyes, lumpiness or flakiness of skin around nose and mouth
Hair	Shiny, lustrous, firm, not easily plucked, healthy scalp	Stringy, dull, brittle, thin, and sparse; depigmented; can be easily plucked; premature gray
Lips	Smooth, good color, moist, not chapped, not swollen	Dry, scaly, swollen, or angular lesions at corners of the mouth or fissures
Nails	Firm, pink	Spoon-shaped, brittle, ridged
Skin (general)	Smooth, slightly moist, good color	Rough, dry, scaly, pale, pigmented, irritated, bruises, petechia, rash, easily bruised
Gastrointestinal System		
General function	Good appetite and digestion, normal regular elimination	Anorexia, indigestion, constipation, or diarrhea
Gums	Good pink color or deep reddish in appearance, not swelling or bleeding	Spongy, bleed easily, marginal redness, inflamed, gums receding
Mouth and oral membranes	Reddish pink mucous membranes in oral cavity	Swollen, boggy oral mucous membranes
Stomach, liver, spleen	No palpable organs or masses	Liver and spleen enlargement
Tongue	Good pink color or deep reddish in appearance, not swollen or smooth, surface papillae present, no lesions	Swelling, scarlet and raw, magenta color, beefy, hyperemic and hypertrophic papillae, atrophic papillae
Teeth	No cavities, no pain, bright, straight, no crowding, well-shaped jaw, clean, no discoloration	Unfilled cavities, absent teeth, worn surfaces, mottled, malpositioned

(continued)

TABLE 10-2 *(continued)*

CLINICAL SIGNS OF NUTRITIONAL STATUS

Body Area	Signs of Good Nutrition	Signs of Poor Nutrition
Musculoskeletal System		
Legs, feet	No weakness	Weakness
Muscles	Well developed, firm, good tone; some fat under skin	Flaccid, poor tone, underdeveloped, tender, "wasted" appearance, cannot walk properly
Skeleton	No malformations	Bowlegs, knock-knees, deformity of chest wall, abnormally shaped ribs, prominent scapula, bone tenderness, joint pain
Neurological System		
Nervous control	Good attention span, not irritable or restless, normal reflexes, psychological stability	Inattentive, irritable, confused, weakness and tenderness of muscles
Reflexes	Normal reflex responses	Decrease or loss of ankle and knee reflexes
Sensation	Normal sensation	burning and tingling of hands and feet, loss of position and vibratory sense
Vision	Bright, clear, shiny, no sores at corner of eyelids, membranes moist and healthy pink color, no prominent blood vessels or amount of tissue or sclera, no fatigue circles beneath	Eye membranes pale, redness of membrane, dryness, signs of infection, redness and fissuring of eyelid corners, dryness of eye membrane, dull appearance of cornea, impaired night vision

Adapted from:
Merck Manual. Signs and symptoms of nutritional deficiency. Available at: http://www.merck.com/media/mmpe/pdf/Table_002-1.pdf. Accessed February 6, 2006.
Guigoz Y, Lauque S, Vellas BJ. Identifying the elderly at risk for malnutrition. The mini nutritional assessment. *Clin Geriatr Med*. 2002; 18(4):737–757.

Dental Health

Another key issue described in *Healthy People 2010* is the need for increased dental care. Data from the third National Health and Nutrition Examination Survey (NHANES III) indicates that 30% of all adults have untreated dental decay and 85% have experienced *dental caries (cavities)*. More than 37% of persons aged 65 years or older in the United States with teeth had at least one decayed or filled root surface.[7] Physical therapists can encourage their clients to take good care of their teeth to avoid potential disease and difficulties eating. While public health policies encourage the fluoridation of water to prevent cavities, regular brushing and flossing must be encouraged to prevent caries. In addition, physical therapists need to remind individuals to wear protective mouth gear when engaging in sports. Teeth protection may also be needed for individuals who tend to exhibit *bruxism* (grinding of the teeth). A dentist can determine the need for special guards to protect the teeth from excessive stress that can wear down dental surfaces. All individuals should have their teeth examined annually for potential dental problems resulting from injury, disease, poor hygiene, or teeth grinding.

Overall, managing one's physical health through a well-rounded, nutritious diet and maintaining dentition for healthy eating habits contribute to general health and stress management across the lifespan. In addition, regular physical activity works in conjunction with a healthy diet to ensure physical fitness.

Sleep

Individuals need adequate sleep to function normally. Sleep allows the body to repair and restore itself; over 70% of the body's daily dose of growth hormone is circulated during sleep.[8] Sleep is also an important time for the regeneration of the immune system, so missing sleep reduces the body's ability to resist and fight infection. Sleep is essential for mental ability and concentration. The ability to undertake useful mental work declines by 25% every 24 hours without sleep; in shift work, this can lead to a much higher possibility of accidents.[8] Studies suggest that sleep loss leads to sleepiness and lethargy during the day and contributes to more than 100,000 highway crashes, causing over 71,000 injuries and more than 1,500 deaths each year in the United States alone.[8]

Recent students have examined the effects of sleep deprivation on healthy volunteers. These studies show that sleep loss has an adverse effect on the body's ability to metabolize sugar. In one week of severe sleep deprivation (sleep limited to four to five hours per night), a healthy, lean, fit volunteer fell into a prediabetic state.[8] In addition, sleep deprivation has been associated with obesity and weight gain.[8] Nearly 12% of the population in the United States experiences *insomnia* (difficulty falling asleep, sleeping too lightly, being easily disrupted with multiple spontaneous awakenings, or early morning awakenings with an inability to fall back asleep).[8] Approximately one-third of all Americans have sleep disorders at some point in their lives. Increasing age predisposes individuals to sleep disorders (5% in persons aged 30 to 50 years and 30% in those aged 50 years or older).[8] Older individuals commonly experience a decrease in total sleep time with more frequent awakenings during the night. Oftentimes, older adults need to take medications on a regular schedule throughout the night, leading to sleep disruption. Physical therapists should ask their clients about sleep difficulties and locate resources for sleep management. Medications may be useful in managing insomnia. Surgery may be indicated to correct some underlying medical conditions causing insomnia, such as palate surgery in some cases of sleep apnea.

Relaxation Techniques

If sleep is a chronic problem, physical therapists may offer techniques to help reduce stress and induce relaxation. Relaxation techniques have been widely used to reduce stress in a variety of populations, including patients with mental and physical health conditions. Herbert Benson coined the term relaxation response, referring to the body's natural response to restore homeostasis in the body.[9] According to Benson, the relaxation response is the body's homeostatic mechanism designed to attenuate the effects of stress or "overstress."[9] The stress-sensitive sympathetic nervous system activates body systems to fight or flight any perceived threat, while the parasympathetic response restores the body to a more restful state, characterized by a lower heart rate and slowed breathing. The relaxation response, reflecting the role of the parasympathetic nervous system in restoring homeostasis, calms the overactive sympathetic nervous system and restores the body to a healthier state of natural equilibrium.[9]

Various relaxation techniques enable individuals to self-manage stress. Relaxation techniques are discussed in the sections that follow.

Progressive Muscle Relaxation

Progressive muscle relaxation is a relaxation technique commonly used by physical therapists to reduce symptoms of stress, anxiety, insomnia, and certain types of chronic pain. The technique of progressive muscle relaxation was described by Edmund Jacobson in the 1930s and involves simple isometric contractions of one muscle group at a time followed by a release of the tension.[10] The muscle contraction and relaxation technique is performed on a succession of muscles from the lower extremities and progressing toward the head, ending with contractions of facial muscles. The progressive relaxation may be facilitated by verbal directions, either in person or on audiotape: "Tighten the muscles in your feet and hold it for 5 seconds...1...2...3...4...5... now relax." The technique may be performed when sitting comfortably on a supportive surface or when lying in a relaxed posture. Each muscle group is contracted for 5 to 8 seconds, then relaxed. After relaxing for approximately 30 seconds, the next set of muscles may be contracted and relaxed. Once all muscle groups have been contracted and relaxed, the individual may rest in this posture as long as possible to achieve complete relaxation. This technique may be augmented by visual imagery, as described below.

Visual Imagery

Visual imagery is the practice of using one's imagination to create mental pictures in a way that promotes relaxation and helps relieve pain. A combination of relaxation and imagery is effective in improving the sleep of critically ill adults but may be contraindicated for individuals with mental illness who may become agitated by visual images.[11] Physical therapists should screen their patients for good mental health prior to using visual imagery for relaxation purposes, recognizing the benefits for individuals free of mental illness.

Meditation

Meditation, one of the most common mind-body interventions, is a conscious mental process that induces a set of integrated physiological changes termed the relaxation response.[12] The two most popular forms of meditation in the United States include transcendental meditation, characterized by repeating a mantra (a single word or phrase), and mindfulness meditation, focusing one's attention on moment-by-moment thoughts and sensations. Meditation has been shown in one study to produce significant increases in left-sided anterior brain activity, which is associated with positive emotional states, as well as increased antibody titers to influenza vaccine, suggesting potential linkages among meditation, positive emotional states, localized brain responses, and improved immune function.[12] Meditation has not only a relaxing effect but possibly the ability to augment the body's immune response.

AUTOGENIC TRAINING

The autogenic training procedure uses visual imagery and body awareness to elicit a relaxation response. The individual self-regulates the body by focusing on specific areas needing relaxation, including the limbs, lungs, heart, diaphragm, and head. The individual attempts to induce the following physiological responses through concentration: increased muscle relaxation, increased peripheral blood flow, lowered heart rate, lowered blood pressure, slower and deeper breathing, and reduced oxygen consumption. In separate meta-analyses examining the effects of autogenic training, researchers revealed a significant reduction in patients' tension and migraine headaches, decreased blood pressure for clients with mild-to-moderate essential hypertension and coronary heart disease, reduced asthma symptoms, reduced symptoms associated with somatoform pain disorder (unspecified type), decreased symptoms of Raynaud's disease, reduced impairments from anxiety disorders, reduction of mild-to-moderate depression, and improvement in sleep for patients with functional sleep disorders.[12]

BIOFEEDBACK

Biofeedback is a technique employing feedback from body functions to increase the person's awareness of internal body workings. Body function is measured with electrodes and displayed on a monitor that both the participant and his or her practitioner can see. The monitor thereby provides feedback to the participant about the internal workings of his or her body. Biofeedback is an effective therapy for many conditions, but it is commonly used to treat tension headaches, migraine headaches, and chronic pain.[12]

MASSAGE

Massage involves the manipulation of soft tissues for the purpose of reducing muscle tension or normalizing other soft tissue structures. There are various types of massage including *relaxation massage* (to promote general relaxation, improve circulation, enable full range of movement, and relieve muscular tension), *therapeutic massage* (to restore function to injured soft tissue or move abnormal fluids from one body compartment to another), *sports massage* (to enhance sports performance and recuperation postinjury), *acupressure massage* (involving pressure at particular acupressure points associated with visceral structures), and *Oriental massage therapies* (such as acupressure and shiatsu, designed to treat points along the acupressure meridians, aiming to ease discomfort).[12]

Essentially, all types of massage can provide several benefits to the body, including increased blood flow, reduced muscle tension and neurological excitability, and increased well-being.[12] Massage techniques include *petrissage* (kneading or rubbing with force to manipulate tissues and muscles), *effleurage* (characterized by light or heavy stroking of the skin designed to improve flow to the circulatory and lymphatic systems), and friction massage or, more specifically, *deep transverse friction massage* (using firm finger pressure in soft tissue to treat muscles, tendons, ligaments, and joint capsules).

FLUID EXERCISE

Tai chi and yoga, as discussed in Chapter 4, can also contribute to mental health and relaxation.

ADDITIONAL SUGGESTIONS

Additional suggestions for stress management and relaxation techniques are listed on the web (Appendix C). While these various techniques can all contribute to stress reduction and relaxation, none are guaranteed. It is important to provide individuals with a list of stress resources ranging from relaxation techniques to psychological referral sources for an evaluation, as appropriate.

Time Management

Certain factors contribute to increasing levels of stress[13]:

- Average working times over the last decade have increased by 20%.
- Leisure time has decreased by 32%.
- Forty-three percent of people find it difficult to delegate.

- Seventy-five percent work more than 40 hours each week.
- Eighty-one percent of managers suffer stress at least once per week.
- Managers, on average, spend three hours each day on interruptions, up to three hours each week looking for things on their desk and 11 hours a week in meetings.
- Today, 600% more information has to be managed than 20 years ago.

Time management is a universal problem, and difficulties with time management contribute significantly to stress. Many people spend their days in a frenzy of activity but achieve very little because they are not concentrating on the right things. To concentrate on results, the individual must establish priorities and devise a plan to optimize strengths while downplaying weaknesses. The following process helps the individual determine strengths and weaknesses, identify goals to accomplish, and prioritize those goals for a concerted effort to accomplish each one.

ESTABLISH PRIORITIES

Generally, what the individual enjoys doing should be the highest priority and centers on that person's unique strengths and attributes. One way to determine an individual's strengths and weaknesses is to do a SWOT analysis.[14] The analysis asks the following questions:

Strengths: What advantages do you have? What do you do well? What relevant resources do you have access to? What do other people see as your strengths?

Weaknesses: What could you improve? What do you do badly? What should you avoid? Do other people seem to perceive weaknesses that you do not see? Are others doing any better than you?

Opportunities: Where are the good opportunities facing you? What are the interesting trends you are aware of? (Note: Useful opportunities can come from such things as changes in technology and markets, changes in government policy related to your field, changes in social patterns, population profiles, lifestyle changes, and local events.) Do personal strengths open up any opportunities? Alternatively, consider how opportunities increase by eliminating weaknesses.

Threats: What obstacles are you facing? What is threatening to you? Are the required specifications for a job, products, or services changing? Is changing technology threatening the position? Do you have bad debt or cash-flow problems? Could any of your weaknesses seriously threaten your roles in life?

This SWOT analysis can be helpful in pointing out what needs to be done and in putting problems into perspective. Overall, the SWOT analysis is a framework for analyzing strengths and weaknesses as well as the opportunities and threats the individual faces. This analysis helps the individual prioritize and focus on strengths, minimize weaknesses, and take advantage of opportunities while keeping in mind what could threaten the person's future.

MONITOR AND ANALYZE CURRENT TIME USE

Track the schedule of time spent the past seven days (where can time be spent more, and where can time be spent less). Time can be kept on a schedule that highlights how much time is spent on priorities versus nonprioritized activities. Many computer programs offer individuals electronic calendars for listing daily activities and tasks. In addition to listing tasks, the individual should note the times when fatigue, energy, or other emotions emerge throughout the day. Also, important health habits, such as eating well, having adequate sleep, and exercising on a regular basis, should be noted.

The individual needs to analyze how time is spent and determine if the time spent matches personal priorities. Is the current schedule affording adequate time to accomplish desired goals? Does the current schedule allow time for healthy eating, sleeping, and exercise behaviors? Does the current schedule incorporate time for socializing with family and friends?

SETTING GOALS

The next step is to develop a plan, listing activities based on priorities. The plan should also be based on what the individual desires for the long term rather than what must be done from one moment to the next. What goals does the individual want to accomplish in the next 10 years? These goals need to be broken down into achievable tasks that can be accomplished within reasonable time frames. The plan should realistically incorporate activities that emphasize strengths while reducing time that relies on areas of weakness. A simple "to do" list can be used to list the individual's tasks in order of priority and importance. Tackling the most important tasks will ensure that long-term goals are not overlooked.

Personal goals may be focused on particular areas; however, long-term goals probably address the multifaceted aspects of life including artistic goals, attitudinal goals, career goals, educational goals, family goals, financial goals, physical or athletic goals, recreational goals, and public service goals. Once these goals are determined, they need to be prioritized and broken down into short-term, achievable goals.

Delegate Tasks

The final step is to determine what can be delegated to others and what can be most easily managed by the individual. It is logical to consider delegating those tasks that are areas of weakness or responsibilities that do not directly contribute to the long-range plan the individual envisions.

Overview

Overall, time management can be a very useful stress management tool as well as a means of accomplishing personal goals in a meaningful time frame. The individual should always allow some time for unexpected or uncontrollable events; this flexibility allows the plan to stand the test of time.

Coping

Coping is the art of constantly changing cognitive and behavioral efforts to manage specific internal and/or external demands appraised as taxing or exceeding the resources of the person.[15] When experiencing stress, the individual needs to appraise the situation to determine whether the stressor justifies concern and, if so, what resources are available to manage the stressor. Coping resources include exercise, self-talk skills, problem-solving skills, communication skills, social support, material resources, and community services.

The Schafer Coping Model[15] offers three options for coping with stress:

1. Altering the stressor (eg, pacing life's demands in a more realistic manner)
2. Avoiding the stressor (eg, making changes that reduce its presence)
3. Adapting to the stressor (eg, using self-talk to resolve conflict or alter perception of the stressor; using health buffers like exercise, nutrition, and sleep; and controlling physical stress responses through relaxation and breathing)

Additional methods for adapting to a stressful situation include avoiding maladaptive health behaviors (alcohol, smoking, overeating, spending money, blaming others, escapism, or unloading difficult issues on others [ie, "dumping on others"]). Seeking coping resources, including social support, money, community services, and a belief system, can provide a buffer to potential stressors. Finally, controlling one's personal actions can have a positive impact on adapting to stressors. Being assertive, using effective communication (especially listening), and sharing concerns with others can often deter further complications.

Locus of Control

Locus of control is the way in which one attributes success or difficulty to either internal factors (such as personal effort) or to external factors (such as fate or others' behaviors). An *internal locus of control* (ie, under one's own personal control) can be a mediating factor of actions taken to prevent health problems. Individuals with a perceived internal locus of control showed a reduced cortisol response ("stress response") to an experimental stressor if they believe that they have some control over the stressor. Furthermore, studies have shown that *psychological hardiness* (a personality style consisting of commitment, control, and challenge) can help buffer the negative impact of stressors and can enhance personal development.[16] It is crucial that clients take control of their lives, recognizing healthy lifestyle behaviors and choices responsible for mitigating the impact of disease and injury.

Emotional Health

Many positive traits promise to improve the quality of life and mitigate distress, ultimately preventing pathology. These traits include optimism, hope, wisdom, creativity, future-mindedness, courage, spirituality, responsibility, and perseverance. Positive psychology, a newer branch of psychology, examines how optimism and hope affect health. The ultimate goal of positive psychology is to make people happier by understanding and building positive emotion, gratification, and meaning.

According to Abraham Maslow's theory of development, individuals become self-actualized as they experience personal growth.[16] When the individual takes responsibility and utilizes personal strengths, that person becomes more free, powerful, happy, and healthy. People with good emotional health are aware of their thoughts, feelings, and behaviors. They have learned healthy ways to cope with the stress and problems that are a normal part of life. They feel good about themselves and have healthy relationships. Those in emotional distress may not be in touch with their thoughts, feelings, and behaviors. The following are physical signs that an individual's emotional health may be out of balance: back pain, changes in appetite, chest pain, constipation or diarrhea, dry mouth, extreme tiredness, general aches and pains, headaches, high blood pressure, insomnia, lightheadedness, palpitations, sexual problems, shortness of breath, stiff neck, sweating, upset stomach, and weight gain or loss.[17] If an individual presents with these physical health problems, emotional problems should not be ruled out. A referral to a psychologist is appropriate, especially if the individual expresses emotional distress or feeling depressed.

Maintaining a Balance Between Work and Play

Frequently, stress mounts when life is out of balance. Too often, work demands crowd out more leisurely or playful activities. Play is generally engaging in activity voluntarily with the reward being intrinsic and a sense of freedom from life's demands. In order to restore a sense of balance and wellness to one's life, play is essential. In particular, laughter can play a key role in releasing stress. More rigorous and theoretically informed research is needed before firm conclusions can be drawn about possible health benefits of humor and laughter.

Spirituality and Religion

Both the Joint Commission for Accreditation of Healthcare Organization's standards and the American Physical Therapy Association Code of Ethics indicate that an individual's beliefs, values, and practices should be respected. Physical therapists are required to "recognize, respect, and respond to individual and cultural differences with compassion and sensitivity,"[18] including each individual's spirituality. Spirituality can be defined as a search for meaning and connectedness with others, nature, the self, and a greater power. All persons experience this search as longings and needs for forgiveness, hope, life purpose, and giving and receiving love and support. To the extent that these longings and needs are met, the person moves toward wellness. Those whose spiritual needs are met will have a sense of peace, describe life as meaningful, and experience supportive, caring relationships. For these individuals, spiritual values provide a sense of hope and that life and health problems are manageable. To the extent that they are not met, the person moves away from wellness. These individuals may experience conflicting values, loss of purpose in life, few or no trusting relationships, anger, inner conflicts regarding beliefs and values, and a sense of emptiness. The physical therapist must be aware of similar or conflicting spiritual values to ensure that their clients are able to maximize their own health promoting spiritual resources and possibly facilitate access to new resources. These efforts require ongoing self-assessment and developing competence.

Religion is complementary to and different from spirituality. It may be defined as those individual and community values, beliefs, and practices through which individuals meet their spiritual needs, and research suggests that religious involvement may be health promoting. Religious involvement has been associated with lower morbidity and mortality, shorter hospital stays, less depression, improved blood pressure, lower substance abuse, improved pain control, and other indicators of positive physical and psychosocial health. Additionally, religious organizations and churches often provide emotional and material support for their members, a phenomenon particularly recognized among some minority communities. Recent data suggests that most clients are religiously involved. In 1999, Gallup and Lindsay found that in the United States, 69% are members of a church or synagogue, 40% attended a service in the previous 7 days, and 89% want their children to have religious training.[19] They note that for the past five decades, at least 50% have reported having a religious faith.[19]

Physical therapists should listen to how each client describes any involvement in religion and then identify how that client's framework may facilitate health promotion. For clients who do not consider themselves religious, involvement in other organizations addressing their needs for support, hope, and meaning may serve as the context for health promotion. Religious involvement can be unique to that individual, or it may be an organized world religion like Christianity or Islam. It may be more Western and focus on a personal God and on living life to the fullest, or it may be more Eastern and focus on relinquishing personal existence to become one with a nonpersonal greater power. More information on various religions can be found online at BeliefNet (http://www.beliefnet.com). Hospital chaplains may consult with both the client and the physical therapist about how to work effectively within a client's religious framework. If outside spiritual leaders are requested by the client, either the client should contact them, or the in-house chaplain should make the consultative call.

A national sample of persons with AIDS reported using several spiritual practices frequently for their own health promotion. Activities ranking among the top 10 complementary therapies used by this group included prayer (56%), meditation (46%), support groups (42%), and other spiritual activities (33%).[20] When practiced, such activities are often described by the self-identified religious client as religious and by the self-identified nonreligious client as spiritual.

Prayer

Providers should be aware that prayer may take many silent or vocal forms, including meditation, thankfulness for things received, requesting needs be met, reading written prayers, conversing with God, and expressing anger or emotion. Appropriate prayers of "meditation," "adoration," "invocation," and "celebration" from many faiths and cultures can found at The World Prayers Project. Regardless of recent controversies about the role of prayer in physical healing, most individuals (72%) pray daily.[21] Many seriously ill persons use prayer to promote relaxation, hope, and comfort; and some health care providers use prayer to deal with their concerns about particular clients. Many physical therapists may wish to seek an appropriate spiritual leader to assist a client when that client desires prayer, but sometimes, a client may ask the physical therapist personally to pray with or for them. The physical therapist may comply if comfortable with the request or a referral is appropriate while assuring respect for the client's practices.

Spiritual Meditation

Silence, prayer, music, or other practices may facilitate meditation. Clinicians should be aware of both the activities that conflict with the religious beliefs of some in addition to the meditative practices used or adapted by those of Hindus, Jews, and Christians to promote health.

Music

Music helps one to express deep spiritual feelings, is present in all religions, and can be calming or enlivening. Some of music's positive effects include relaxation, lower blood pressure, improved mood, enhanced cognitive function, relief of boredom, and pain control. Evidence also shows that music timed to the individual's biological rhythms like a heartbeat can have a soothing effect. Recordings of religious music are readily available in bookstores and online and may include nature sounds, calming and meditative Buddhist or Taize chants, classical works, traditional Christian hymns, or rock and roll.

Devotional Supports

Health-promoting devotion, "an act of prayer or private worship," may be facilitated by silence, music, prayer, devotional items, and readings.[21] Examples of devotional items may include a small Buddhist altar, rosary beads, a prayer card, religious jewelry, or a bead to protect against an "evil eye." If clients request such items, chaplains or other spiritual leaders can be of assistance. Devotional items can provide clues about spiritual practice to the observant physical therapist, opening the door to discussion of belief systems. Devotional readings may enhance hope, peace, and relaxation. Most people in the United States (80%) regard the Bible as inspired scripture, and almost all (93%) have some religious scripture book in their homes.[21] Multiple translations of audio and print scripture online resources are available, including the Koran, Sikh scriptures, the Bible, and Christian devotional e-books.

PLAN Model

If a client seems to be having difficulty with a particular spiritual need, such as forgiveness, hope, or supportive relationships, the physical therapist may find the PLAN model helpful when used along with specific resources. A modified version of PLAN includes giving Permission for the individual to express concerns, providing Limited information or Activating past-coping resources, and if the issue is beyond the physical therapist's time, comfort, or competence, referring the client to Non-physical therapy disciplines, such as social work, psychology, or clergy is appropriate. PLAN can be coupled with some of the information below.

Forgiveness

Forgiveness is "letting go of negative feelings" toward others in a way that restores and repairs relationships.[22] Clients may focus more on forgiving than on being forgiven because they realize their negative feelings toward another person cause harm to themselves. Physical therapists can facilitate this health-promoting process by listening empathetically to the client through four forgiveness stages of anger: (1) inability to forgive, (2) wondering if they should forgive, (3) letting go of negative feelings, but (4) not forgetting. Multiple resources are available on the web to aid in understanding the meaning and process of forgiveness and its relationship to health (see Appendix C). In particular, the International Forgiveness Institute website has definitions, books, courses, and links to other research centers.

Hope

Hope may be best evidenced by the person's ability to imagine and participate in the enhancement of a positive future. Hope has been associated with lower anxiety, higher functional status, and better physical health. The physical therapist can build an individual's hope by promoting client confidence that he or she is not alone. The physical therapist can share a vision for the client of a mutually established, achievable, positive future and by committing energy to helping the person achieve wellness goals.

Cognitive Reserve and Lifestyle

A lifestyle characterized by social and intellectual engagement may be a buffer to the stresses in life and, ultimately, pathologies affecting the brain. While social support can be a stress resource, the development of a *cognitive reserve,* formulated through years of life experience coupled with innate intellectual ability, may supply a reserve that can slow the cognitive decline in healthy older adults and may reduce the risk of dementia, including Alzheimer's disease. Risk factors for Alzheimer's disease include advanced age, lower intelligence, small head size, history of head trauma, and female gender.[23] Evidence from functional imaging studies indicates that individuals engaged in cognitively challenging activities can clinically tolerate more Alzheimer's disease pathology, suggesting that life experience can provide cognitive reserves that delay the onset of clinical manifestations of dementia.[23]

Complementary and Alternative Medicine

Nontraditional resources for health and wellness are being investigated by researchers funded by the National Institutes of Health and other public and private institutions interested in expanding options for health care. *Complementary and alternative medicine (CAM)* includes forms of treatment used in addition to or instead of standard or usual medical treatments. These practices cover a wide range of treatment approaches such as special diets, vitamins, herbs, acupuncture, massage therapy, magnetic therapy, spiritual healing, and meditation and their use is increasing, from 34% in 1990 to 42% in 1997.[24] In one study of a group of 453 cancer patients, 83% reported using at least one CAM, including special diets, psychotherapy, spiritual practices, and vitamin supplements. When psychotherapy and spiritual practices were excluded, 64% of patients used at least one CAM therapy in their cancer treatments.[25] Since many of the CAM therapies have not been subjected to the same strict scientific evaluation for safety and effectiveness as conventional therapies, they may pose some risk. The National Cancer Institute (NCI) and the National Center for Complementary and Alternative Medicine (NCCAM) are sponsoring and cosponsoring various scientific studies of complementary and alternative medicine to determine which CAM therapies interfere with standard treatment or may be harmful when used with conventional treatment.

Summary

There is an incredible range of resources for managing health and wellness to prevent disease or to reduce the impact of pathology on the quality of life. While maintaining a balanced lifestyle is important, certain stressors in life can present barriers to good health and wellness. In 1950, only 8% of the population lived to the age of 65 or over; 20% are expected to live to 65 or over in this century.[25] Using resources wisely for health and wellness promises to prolong healthy living and, hopefully, enrich the quality of life throughout the life span.

References

1. Centers for Disease Control and Prevention. Profiling the leading causes of death in the United States: heart disease, stroke, and cancer. Available at: http://www.cdc.gov/nccdphp/publications/factsheets/ChronicDisease/west_virginia.htm. Accessed February 6, 2006.
2. Merck Manual. Dorland's Medical Dictionary. Available at: http://www.mercksource.com/pp/us/cns/cns_hl_dorlands.jspzQzpgzEzzSzppdocszSzuszSzcommonzSzdorlandszSzdorlandzSzdmd_h_22zPzhtm. Accessed February 6, 2006.
3. Chapman DP, Perry GS, Strine TW. The vital link between chronic disease and depressive disorders. *Prev Chronic Dis* [serial online]. Available at: http://www.cdc.gov/pcd/issues/2005. Accessed January 2005.
4. Block G, Wakimoto P, Metz D, et al. A randomized trial of the Little by Little CD-ROM: demonstrated effectiveness in increasing fruit and vegetable intake in a low-income population. *Prev Chronic Dis* [serial online]. Available from: http://www.cdc.gov/pcd/issues/2004/jul/04_0016.htm. Accessed July 2004.
5. Missouri Department of Mental Health. Anxiety disorders. Available at: http://www.dmh.missouri.gov/cps/facts/anxiety.htm. Accessed February 6, 2006.
6. Katz, D. *Nutrition in Clinical Practice: A Comprehensive, Evidence-Based Manual for the Practitioner.* Baltimore, Md: Lippincott Williams & Wilkins; 2000.
7. Centers for Disease Control and Prevention, Health Resources and Services Administration, Indian Health Service, National Institutes of Health. Healthy people 2010. Oral health. Available at: http://www.healthypeople.gov/Document/pdf/Volume2/21Oral.pdf. Accessed February 6, 2006.
8. Kowalenko T, Kowalenko J, Gryzbowski M, Rabinovich A. Emergency medicine resident related auto accidents—Is sleep deprivation a risk factor? *Acad Emerg Med.* 2000;7(10):1171.
9. Benson H, Beary JF, Carol MP. The relaxation response. *Psychiatry.* 1974;37:37–45.

10. Wilk C, Turkoski B. Progressive muscle relaxation in cardiac rehabilitation: a pilot study. *Rehabilitation Nursing.* 2001;26(6):238–242.
11. Sultanoff BA, Zalaquett CP. Relaxation therapies. In: Novey DW, ed. *Clinician's Complete Reference to Complementary and Alternative Medicine.* St. Louis, Mo: Mosby; 2000:114–129.
12. Bonadonna R. Meditation's impact on chronic illness. *Holistic Nursing Practice.* 2003;17(6):309–319.
13. Total Success. Stress management training. Available at: http://www.tsuccess.dircon.co.uk/stress_management.html. Accessed February 6, 2006.
14. Kyle B. SWOT analysis—strengths, weaknesses, opportunities, and threats. How much for just the spider? Strategic website marketing for small budget business. Available at: http://www.marketingprofs.com/login/join.asp?adref=rdblk&source=/3/kyle1.asp.
15. Rahe RH, Taylor CB, Tolles RL, Newhall LM, Veach TL, Bryson S. A novel stress and coping workplace program reduces illness and healthcare utilization. *Psychosom Med.* 2002;64(2):278–286.
16. Maddi SR. On hardiness and other pathways to resilience. *American Psychologist.* 2005;60(3):261–262.
17. Backman CL. Occupational balance: exploring the relationships among daily occupations and their influence on well-being. *Can J Occup Ther.* 2004;71(4):202–209.
18. APTA. Code of Ethics. Available at: http://www.apta.org/AM/Template.cfm?Section=Ethics_and_Legal_Issues1&CONTENTID=14343&TEMPLATE=/CM/ContentDisplay.cfm. Accessed February 6, 2006.
19. Adherents.com. Affliates. Available at: http://www.adherents.com/Na/Na_5.html. Accessed February 6, 2006.
20. MacIntyre RC, Holzemer WL. Complementary and alternative medicine and HIV/AIDS. Part II: selected literature review. *J Assoc Nurses AIDS Care.* 1997;8(2):25–38.
21. Thomas G. God MD: new studies examine prayer and healing. Available at: http://www.garythomas.com/resources/articles/god_md.html. Accessed February 6, 2006.
22. Younger J, Piferi R, Jobe R, Lawler, K. Dimensions of forgiveness: the views of laypersons. *J Social Pers Relat.* 2004;21(6):837-855.
23. Scarmeas N, Stern Y. Cognitive reserve: implications for diagnosis and prevention of Alzheimer's disease. *Curr Neurol Neurosci Rep.* 2004;4(5):374–380.
24. Cassileth B, Chapman C. Alternative and complementary cancer therapies. *Cancer.* 1996;77(6):1026–1033.
25. Federal Interagency Forum on Aging and Related Statistics. Older americans: key indicators of well being. Available at: http://www.agingstats.gov/chartbook2000/population.html. Accessed February 6, 2006.

Chapter 11

Health Protection

Catherine Rush Thompson, PhD, MS, PT

"The scars of others should teach us caution."

~ SAINT JEROME

One of the major goals of Healthy People 2010 is to reduce the incidence of injury and infection across the lifespan through health protection strategies. As part of the health care team, physical therapists play an important role in injury prevention and infection control through screenings and health education. Currently, physical therapists have an opportunity to provide primary prevention in a variety of community settings through (1) comprehensive health screenings to identify injury or infection risk factors, (2) education to address risk factors, and (3) collaboration with others to provide health protection resources designed to reduce injuries and infection.

Infection Control

One of the main objectives of Healthy People 2010 is to "reduce or eliminate indigenous cases of vaccine-preventable diseases."[1] *Infectious diseases* are those diseases caused by microbes that can be passed to or among humans by several methods, including contact with infectious agents that gain entry to the body through a variety of portals, including the skin, the mouth, the nose, and body parts engaged in sexual contact. Many infections may be transmitted from person-to-person, but some cases involve infection transmission through shared objects (eg, drinking glasses) or infected animals (eg, infected rodents). Infectious diseases, many of which are preventable, are the leading cause of death in the world.[1] Epidemics, such as severe acute respiratory syndrome (SARS) that spread between 29 countries in 2003,[2] remind the public of the possible fatal outcomes of uncontrolled infections. The National Center for Infectious Diseases provides specific information about infectious diseases.[1] The World Health Organization website offers more information about the spread of infectious diseases,[4] and information about emerging infectious diseases can be found at the Centers for Disease Control and Prevention (CDC) website.[5]

The best prevention from infection is adopting a risk-free or low-risk lifestyle that includes protective devices, immunizations, and sanitary health habits. Physical therapists should remind their clients to use protection when engaged in activities that pose any risk of infection (eg, condoms when engaged in sexual activity). In addition, clients should be advised to maintain their immunizations for prevention. Up-to-date vaccination schedules that should be brought to the attention of the public are located on the Institute for Vaccine Safety website.[6] Finally, physical therapists should promote sanitary habits whenever working with clients. One example of increasing awareness of healthy sanitary habits is providing signage that encourages frequent hand washing and cleaning of

TABLE 11-1

RISK OF INJURY BASED ON GENDER

Male	Female
• Males are at least 4 times more likely to commit suicide than females. • Men are more than three-quarters more likely to be victims of school homicide. • High school men commit 3 times more suicides. • Men are twice as likely to sustain a traumatic head injury. • Men are 4 times as likely to sustain a spinal cord injury (SCI). • Male high school students are less likely to wear seat belts. • Male pedestrians have double the death rate of female. • Men suffer 80% more drownings than women. • Men 65 and older have the highest rate of suicide, are twice as likely to sustain a motor vehicle-related accident, and are 22% more likely to die of a fall.	• Women are more likely to attempt suicide. • 25% of women report being raped or physically assaulted by an intimate partner at some time in their lives, as compared to 8% of men. • One in three women injured during a physical assault or rape require medical care. • Women 65 years and older are hospitalized for hip fractures 3 times more often than men.

Adapted from Centers for Disease Control and Prevention. Injury and violence prevention. Healthy People 2010. Available at: http://www.healthypeople.gov/Document/Word/Volume2/15Injury.doc. Accessed November 10, 2004.

areas likely to spread infections through hand or mouth contact. Clients should be reminded that skin that is broken by abrasions, burns, or wounds is particularly vulnerable to infection and needs to be kept free of infection through cleanliness and appropriate medical precautions.

Injury Prevention

Healthy People 2010 provides health care professionals with a framework to collaboratively work toward injury prevention goals. These goals include reducing injuries and deaths ranging from head injuries, poisonings, and firearms to increasing the number of states that collect data on causes of injury.[1] Health care providers need to increase public education about health risks in a variety of settings, including schools and universities, occupational settings, and the home. The CDC recommends increasing health education in the areas of unintentional injury, violence, and suicide for youth and adults.

HEALTH EDUCATION FOR INJURY PREVENTION

The CDC collects data on the most common types of injuries based on gender, race, and age group.[3] Tables 11-1 through 11-4 provide a summary of the various populations and the key risks that each group faces.[3]

INJURY PREVENTION IN CHILDHOOD AND ADOLESCENCE

Physical therapists can screen for potential risks for injury using CDC data. For example, children are particularly vulnerable to motor vehicle accidents (MVAs). Parents of younger children should be asked questions about their awareness of these risks, the need for appropriate booster seats and infant seats in the car, and consistent seatbelt usage. Additionally, children under the age of 4 are particularly vulnerable to poisoning, and parents should be advised to remove or lock up any hazardous agents in the home. For the older child, helmets are more essential. Nearly one-third of bicyclists killed in traffic crashes are ages 5 to 14.[7] Through the United States Department of Transportation, the National Highway Traffic Safety Administration offers a helpful checklist on their website to ensure bicycle safety.[8]

It is also important to ask details about the children's level of physical activity and about potential risks at the playground. Particularly, those therapists working with children in health care or daycare settings should determine possible hazards that exist at

TABLE 11-2

RISK OF INJURY BASED ON RACE

African Americans	Hispanic Americans	American Indians and Native Alaskans
• More African American males aged 15 to 19 years die from homicide than from any other cause. • African Americans are among those at the greatest risk of injury from residential fires. • Pedestrian fatalities are twice the number of that for whites. • The drowning rate is 1.6 times as high as whites and 2.5 times as high for children ages 5 to 9 years. • The rate of SCI is higher among African Americans than among whites.	• Motor vehicle accidents (MVAs) are the leading cause of injury-related deaths for Hispanics. • Poisoning is the second leading cause of death. • Homicide is the second leading cause of deaths for Hispanics ages 15 to 34 years. • The pedestrian fatality rate for Hispanics is 1.77 times higher than for whites.	• American Indians and Native Alaskans are at the greatest risk for residential fires. • The pedestrian fatality rate is nearly 3 times higher than for whites. • Women in this group are more likely than any other group to report being raped or physically assaulted. • Suicide is the second leading cause of death for American Indians and Alaskan Natives ages 15 to 34 years.

Adapted from Centers for Disease Control and Prevention. Injury and violence prevention. Healthy People 2010. Available at: http://www.healthypeople.gov/Document/Word/Volume2/15Injury.doc. Accessed November 10, 2004.

TABLE 11-3

RISK BASED UPON AGE GROUP—UNDER AGE 15

Infants and Young Children	Children and Adolescents
• For children under the ages 1 to 4 years: o Motor vehicle accidents are the leading cause of death (nearly half were riding unrestrained). o Drowning is the second leading cause of injury-related death. • Half of all poisonings are among children under 5. • Head trauma, often caused by violent shaking, is the leading cause of death and disability among abused infants and children.	• For children 5 to 14: Motor vehicle accidents are the leading cause of death. • Only 6% of children 4 to 8 years ride in booster seats, as recommended. • Two-thirds of children 15 and younger who died in alcohol-related motor vehicle crashed were riding with a drunken driver. • For children ages 10 to 14, suicide is the third leading cause of death. • Between 1980 and 1997, the suicide rate increased 109%. • Nearly one-third of bicyclists killed in traffic crashes are ages 5 to 14.

Adapted from Centers for Disease Control and Prevention. Injury and violence prevention. Healthy People 2010. Available at: http://www.healthypeople.gov/Document/Word/Volume2/15Injury.doc. Accessed November 10, 2004.

the playground of their facility. Playground injuries are responsible for 200,000 admissions to the emergency room with 70% of those injuries related to falls on surfaces. More than one-third of all playground-related injuries are severe (fractures, internal injuries, concussions, dislocations, and amputations).[9]

Physical therapists working in early intervention should educate families about how to make the home environment as risk-free as possible for accidents. Several ways to "baby-proof" the home include blocking dangerous entrances (ie, place a fence in front of staircases) and keeping children away from

TABLE 11-4

RISK OF INJURY BASED ON AGE GROUP—OVER AGE 15

Teens and Young Adults	Older Adults (Over Age 65 years)
• Homicide is the second leading cause of death of Americans ages 15 to 19. • In 1997, 14% of high school students had been in a physical fight on school property at least once in the last year. • Suicide is the third leading cause of death for Americans ages 15 to 19. • The risk of motor vehicle crashes is greatest for teen drivers. • Only 35% of high school students report wearing a seatbelt. • In 1998, 21% of drivers ages 15 to 20 who died in motor vehicle accidents had blood alcohol concentrations of at least 10%. • The percentage of teens who wear bicycle helmets is close to zero. • More than half the people who sustain spinal cord injuries are between the ages of 16 and 30. • Among young males, alcohol is a major factor in 50% of drownings.	• Older adults have a higher crash rate than teens per miles driven. • The pedestrian death rate is higher than for any other age group. • Falls are the leading cause of injury-related death among this age group. • Hip fractures are among the most serious fall-related injuries. Half of older adults who suffer a hip fracture never regain their previous level of function. • Older adults are among those at greatest risk for injuries from residential fires. • Adults 65 and older account for nearly 20% of suicides. This age group has the highest suicide rate since 1933, when reporting such data began.

Adapted from Centers for Disease Control and Prevention. Injury and violence prevention. Healthy People 2010. Available at: http://www.healthypeople.gov/Document/Word/Volume2/15Injury.doc. Accessed November 10, 2004.

electrical outlets, cords, heaters, fans, and other electrical devices. The BabyCenter recommends additional measures to "baby-proof" the environment on their website.[10]

As children grow older, they become more engaged in activities outside of the home.

INJURY PREVENTION IN YOUNG ATHELETES

Physical therapists are often involved in providing services to young athletes. The unique knowledge, skill and expertise of the physical therapist complements the knowledge of others who may be involved in managing a team, including the athletic trainer, the coach, and the team physician. The American Physical Therapy Association and the Sports Physical Therapy Section provide valuable resources to guide physical therapists in providing current information for children and adults engaged in sports. Before engaging in any sport, it is important for each child or youth to have a thorough preparticipation physical examination. The American Academy of Family Physicians, the American Academy of Pediatrics, the American Medical Society for Sports Medicine, the American Orthopedic Society for Sports Medicine, and the American Osteopathic Academy of Sports Medicine have collaboratively developed a preparticipation form that requires a thorough physical examination by a physician.[11] The form includes demographic information (name, date of birth, gender), personal information (address, school, sports, emergency contacts), medical history, height, weight, percent body fat, vision (specifying correction, as needed), papillary status, and clinical observations of appearance, eyes, ears, nose, throat, lymph nodes, heart, pulses, lungs, genitals (males only), skin, neck, back, shoulder/arm, elbow/forearm, wrist/hand, hip/thigh, knee, leg/ankle, and foot. The musculoskeletal examination focuses on joints that may be stressed by the particular physical activity or sport. For example, the physician might examiner the shoulder joint of a pitcher more thoroughly than his ankle joint.

The American Heart Association (AHA) recommends that preparticipation cardiovascular screenings for high school and collegiate athletes are "justifiable and compelling, based on ethical, legal, and medical grounds."[11] According to recent studies, "Preparticipation screening by history and physical examination alone (without noninvasive testing) is not sufficient to guarantee detection of many critical cardiovascular abnormalities in large populations of young trained athletes." The prevalence of athletic field deaths nationally range from 1:100,000 to 1:300,000 high school age athletes and is disproportionately higher in males, with the majority of deaths associated with undetected congenital heart defects.[12] To reduce this risk of athletic field deaths, one study recommends a comprehensive cardiovascular history[13] addressing the following: "(1) prior occurrence of exertional chest pain/discomfort or syncope/near-syncope as well as excessive, unexpected, and unexplained shortness of breath or fatigue associated with exercise; (2) past detection of a heart murmur or increased systemic blood pressure; and (3) family history of premature death (sudden or otherwise), significant disability from cardiovascular disease in close relative(s) younger than 50 years old, or specific knowledge of the occurrence of certain conditions (eg, hypertrophic cardiomyopathy, dilated cardiomyopathy, long QT syndrome, Marfan syndrome, or clinically important arrhythmias). These recommendations are offered with the awareness that the accuracy of some responses elicited from young athletes may depend on their level of compliance and historical knowledge. Indeed, parents should be responsible for completing the history forms for high school athletes. The cardiovascular physical examination should emphasize (but not necessarily be limited to) (1) precordial auscultation in both the supine and standing positions to identify, in particular, heart murmurs consistent with dynamic left ventricular outflow obstruction; (2) assessment of the femoral artery pulses to exclude coarctation of the aorta; (3) recognition of the physical stigmata of Marfan syndrome; and (4) brachial blood pressure measurement in the sitting position."[11]

In addition to screening for health status, the physical therapist should monitor the use of protective gear appropriate for the client's sport of choice. For example, individuals engaged in soccer need shin guards and properly fitted soccer shoes. Nearly all sports recommend protective gear that should be required of participants to prevent or reduce injury. In addition, the physical therapist can use appropriate athletic taping and strapping to provide support and prevent sports injuries. In addition, warm-up and cool-down exercises, such as stretching and light jogging, may reduce the risk of tissue injury. Finally, protective sunscreen should be used for all outside sports. Any physical activity, particularly summer sports, can lead to heat-related illnesses. Adequate fluids should be made available at all times to prevent dehydration or deficient body fluids. Children are especially vulnerable to heat-related illness because their thermoregulatory system is not fully developed. Preventable heat-related illnesses include dehydration, *heat exhaustion* (characterized by nausea, dizziness, weakness, headache, pale and moist skin, heavy perspiration, normal or low body temperature, weak pulse, dilated pupils, disorientation, fainting spells), and *heat stroke* (characterized by headache, dizziness, confusion, and hot dry skin, possibly leading to vascular collapse, coma, and death).[13] Physical therapists should caution young athletes and children in sports to maintain adequate hydration and cease activity if they show signs or experience symptoms of heat-related illness. An excellent reference for prevention of sports-related injuries has been developed by the National Institute of Arthritis and Musculoskeletal and Skin Diseases.[14]

Certain sports pose specific risks to players; note the concerns that should be addressed for each of the following sports.

Football

Football tends to cause a large number of injuries, especially among males. The most common injuries in football include soft tissue injuries (sprains and strains) as well as damaged bones and internal organs. Knees and ankles are the most common injury sites.[15] To reduce the incidence of injuries, football players should be encouraged to use the proper equipment (helmet, mouth guard, shoulder pads, athletic supporter for males, chest pads, arm pads, thigh pads, shin guards, and the proper shoes for the play surface).

Basketball

The most common injuries in basketball include sprains, strains, bruises, fractures, dislocations, abrasions, and dental injuries. Females have a higher incidence of knee injuries secondary to their lower-extremity alignment; however, other vulnerable joints include the ankles and shoulders (eg, a *rotator cuff injury*—a tear or inflammation of the rotator cuff tendons in the shoulder).[16,17] Basketball players should wear protective gear, including eye protection, mouth guard, elbow and knee pads, mouth guard, basketball shoes, and athletic supporters for (males).[16,17]

Soccer

Soccer injuries include primarily abrasions, lacerations, and bruises. Proper attire includes soccer cleats, shin guards, and athletic supporters for males. Recent studies have indicated that "heading" the ball, or using the head to strike the ball, may cause head injury or concussion. Players with the highest lifetime estimates of heading had poorer scores on scales measuring attention, concentration, cognitive flexibility, and general intellectual functioning.[16] One suggestion for reducing the risk of head injuries from heading the ball is ensuring proper proportion of the ball to the player.

Baseball and Softball

Baseball and softball share common injuries that relate to sliding into a base or being hit by a ball, resulting in soft tissue injuries and possible fracture.[17] Recommended attire for baseball and softball include the following: batting helmet, mouth guard, elbow guards, shin guards, and athletic supporters for males.

Track and Field

The most common injuries from events such as running, jumping, and throwing events include sprains, strains, and abrasions from falls.[17] As with most sports, the proper shoes are needed, along with athletic supporters for males.

Injury Prevention for Adolescents and Adults

Sports and Recreation

Sports and recreation can provide much needed physical activity but can also pose a risk to those who exercise without the proper precautions and protective gear. Over 365,000 hospital emergency room-treated injuries for individuals 35 to 54 years of age were for the treatment of sports-related injuries.[18] The most common sports-related injuries in adulthood include bicycling, basketball, baseball/softball, exercise/running, skiing, weight lifting, football, golf, inline skating, soccer, swimming, volleyball, tennis, and snowboarding.[18] Wearing protective gear, such as helmets and teeth guards, and using proper techniques can help reduce these injuries in adults. An excellent resource for injury prevention and care for injured athletes is *Sports Medicine for the Primary Care Physician* by Richard Birrer and Francis O'Connor. This book offers pre-participation examination details, details of common injuries and their management, and resources for injury surveillance and prevention.

Fire and Burn Safety

Physical therapists often work with burn patients in acute care, but few offer prevention education to protect against burn injuries. Of all fire deaths, 79% occur in the home, and alcohol contributes to 40% of residential fire deaths.[19] Physical therapists can share these facts with their clients and suggest that fire detectors be placed in the home of their clients. In addition, therapists can teach the "stop, drop, and roll" technique to extinguish fires in case someone encounters flames. Educational media is readily available at local fire stations as well as the National Fire Protection Association, located on the web.[20]

Poisonings

Most poisoning deaths are caused by pills, alcohol, gases and fumes, and chemicals with more than 90% of exposures occurring at home.[21] "About 78,000 children under five years old visited United States hospital emergency rooms due to unintentional poisonings in 2003—about 1 every 7 minutes."[22] Medications should be checked each time before taking them, noting the correct name, dosage, and precautions on the label and avoiding alcohol use while using selected medications. Additional helpful tips for preventing poisonings from medications are listed on the poison prevention website[22] and the website for the Food and Drug Administration's Center for Drug Evaluation and Research (see Appendix C). Another helpful site is sponsored by the National Center for Complimentary and Alternative Medicine.[23] This site offers information about dietary supplements and other alternative treatments that may affect the effectiveness or toxicity of medications.

The CDC estimates that 76 million Americans get sick from food-related illness every year.[24] More than 300,000 end up hospitalized, and about 5,000 die each year from food-borne illness.[24] Infections with the bacteria *Salmonella* alone account for $1 billion yearly in direct and indirect medical costs.[24] One helpful resource, "Diagnosis and Management of Food-Borne Illnesses: A Primer for Physicians and Other Health Care Professionals," contains charts, scenarios, and a continuing medical education section and is free to health care professionals.[25] The primer was created though a partnership of the American Medical Association (AMA) and the American Nurses Association (ANA)—American Nurses Foundation (ANF) in conjunction with the CDC's Food Safety Office, the Food and Drug Administration's (FDA) Center for Food Safety and Applied Nutrition, and the US Department of Agriculture's (USDA) Food Safety and Inspection Service.

Botulism is a muscle-paralyzing disease caused by a toxin made by a bacterium called *Clostridium botulinum*. Botulism can become food-borne when a person ingests preformed toxin that leads to illness within a few hours to days. With food-borne botulism, symptoms begin within 6 hours to 2 weeks (most commonly between 12 and 36 hours) after eating toxin-containing food.[26] Symptoms of botulism include double vision, blurred vision, drooping eyelids, slurred speech, difficulty swallowing, dry mouth, muscle weakness that always descends through the body: first shoulders are affected, then upper arms, lower arms, thighs, calves, etc.[26] Paralysis of breathing muscles can cause a person to stop breathing and die, unless assistance with breathing (mechanical ventilation) is provided. If a client presents with these signs and symptoms, botulism should be suspected and the individual should seek immediate medical attention.

Tobacco Use

Cigarette smoking is the leading preventable cause of death in the United States, but the health consequences extend beyond smokers to nonsmokers involuntarily exposed to environmental tobacco smoke or secondhand smoke. Each year, an estimated 3,000 lung cancer deaths and 62,000 deaths from coronary heart disease in adult nonsmokers are attributed to secondhand smoke.[27] A helpful website to facilitate smoking cessation is jointly offered by the National Cancer Institute, the CDC, the National Institute of Health, the US Department of Health and Human Services, and FirstGov, providing an online guide to quit smoking.[28]

Pesticides

Pesticides are substances used to kill pests, *herbicides* are pesticides used to kill weeds, *insecticides* are pesticides used to kill insects, and *fungicides* are pesticides used for controlling disease on crops and seed. Farmers are relatively heavy users of pesticides, and they appear to experience an excess of certain types of cancer. Cancers more commonly seen in farmers include non-Hodgkin's lymphoma, soft tissue sarcoma, and cancers of the lip, stomach, brain, and prostate.[29] Non-Hodgkin's lymphoma and sarcomas are also increasing in the general population of the United States, suggesting that a common set of exposures may be involved.[30] Further research is needed to clarify the relationship between cancer and agricultural exposures, including pesticides. If exposed to pesticides, individuals should exercise caution and try to avoid direct contact between pesticides and the sites of body entry—the skin and eyes. A wide variety of toxins surround Americans daily, and physical therapists need to be acutely aware of the risks of these toxins, whether they are natural organisms or man-made agents designed to kill microorganisms or other pests. Using sanitary health habits can reduce the risk of toxicity when exposed to both natural and synthetic toxins.

Firearms

Many Americans have access to guns, increasing the risk of injury and death from firearms. Most unintentional firearm-related deaths among children occur in or around the home: 50% at the home of the victim and 40% at the home of a friend or relative. Therefore, the risk of unintentional firearm-related death among children (especially if the firearm is loaded and kept unlocked) increases if firearms are placed in a secure location and left unloaded.[31] Unfortunately, more than one-half of firearm owners keep their firearms loaded and ready for use some of the time. Even children as young as 3 years of age are strong enough to pull the trigger of many handguns.[31] Additional resources on firearm safety are located on the web.[32] Copies of relevant information may be shared directly with clients or provided in clinic waiting rooms or other public areas.

Drowning

An average of 12 people per day die of drowning, and more than 80% of drownings occur among males.[33] Physical therapists should advise their clients to swim under the supervision of a qualified lifeguard and avoid swimming under risky conditions. Parents of children should also be advised to continually supervise bathing and other water-related activities.

Swimming

Physical therapists, particularly those who practice aquatherapy, should keep these tips in mind when developing client regulations for their programs: (1) do not enter the water with diarrhea, (2) do not swallow the water, (3) wash hands and bottom thoroughly with soap and water after a bowel movement, and (4) notify the lifeguard if fecal matter is seen in the water or if someone changes diapers on nearby tables and chairs. These precautions can reduce preventable health hazards for community pools.

Sun and Heat

Reduced sun exposure can reduce the risk of skin cancer. Individuals are at the greatest risk when the sun's ultraviolent rays are strongest, generally between 10:00 am and 4:00 pm.[34] Individuals should be encouraged to wear long sleeves and pants and apply sunscreen and a protective lip balm with an SPF of 15 or higher whenever exposed to sunlight. Sunscreen and lip balm should be reapplied frequently when swimming.

Safety and Occupational Health

The Occupational Safety and Health Administration's mission is to assure the safety and health of America's workers by setting and enforcing standards; providing training, outreach, and education; establishing partnerships; and encouraging continual improvement in workplace safety and health.[35] According to 2004 statistics, workers in steel and iron foundries, hog and pig farmers, and equipment manufacturers and operators are the occupations that report the most days away from work due to injury or illness.[36] The most common injuries are sprains, strains, and tears, and the areas of the body most commonly injured are the back, upper extremities, lower extremities, and trunk. Physical therapists can play a key role in preventing injuries by educating the public about proper posture and body position. Work ergonomics is a burgeoning area of physical therapy practice that can contribute significantly to injury prevention. Additional information about safety and occupational health is discussed in Chapter 12.

Product Safety

Certain products must be recalled because of manufacturing flaws or design flaws that put the public at risk. The United States Consumer Product Safety Commission (CPSC) is charged with the following[37]:

> *...protecting the public from unreasonable risks of serious injury or death from more than 15,000 types of consumer products under the agency's jurisdiction. Deaths, injuries, and property damage from consumer product incidents cost the nation more than $700 billion annually. The CPSC is committed to protecting consumers and families from products that pose a fire, electrical, chemical, or mechanical hazard or can injure children. The CPSC's work to ensure the safety of consumer products—such as toys, cribs, power tools, cigarette lighters, and household chemicals—contributed significantly to the 30% decline in the rate of deaths and injuries associated with consumer products over the past 30 years.*

Physical therapists can help reduce the incidence of product injuries by keeping informed of product risks and not encouraging their use.

Motor Vehicle Accidents

In any given year, approximately 1% of the United States population will be injured in MVAs, or over 3 million injuries annually.[38] Simply encouraging individuals to "buckle up" when they leave the physical therapy setting can be a brief but helpful reminder that could reduce fatal MVAs. Since 3 in 10 Americans will be involved in an alcohol-related crash in their lifetime, clients should be reminded to avoid drinking and driving as well as ensure that they are physically capable of controlling a vehicle.[31] Mental-health difficulties such as post-traumatic stress, depression, and anxiety are problems survivors of severe MVAs may exhibit.[38] Physical therapists treating patients post-MVA need to be aware of the need for psychological counseling if their clients show signs of post-traumatic stress disorder, including depression, substance abuse, problems of memory and cognition, and other problems of physical and mental health. The disorder is also associated with impairment of the person's ability to function in social or family life, including occupational instability, marital problems and divorces, family discord, and difficulties in parenting. Physical therapists should encourage survivors of MVAs to maintain as much of their pre-accident lifestyle as possible, with as much support from family and friends as available. Such coping strategies appear to be linked with positive mental-health outcomes.[38]

Spinal Cord Injuries

Spinal cord trauma can be caused by any number of spinal cord injuries (SCIs) resulting from MVAs, falls, sports injuries (particularly diving into shallow water), industrial accidents, gunshot wounds, assault, and others. Individuals with rheumatoid arthritis or osteoporosis are vulnerable to even minor injuries to their compromised skeletal system. MVAs are responsible for many SCIs and are the leading cause of SCIs under the age of 65.[39] Over the age of 65, falls are the leading cause of SCIs. Males between 15 and 35 years old are most commonly affected.[39] Complications of SCIs include respiratory complications, urinary tract infections, spasticity, and scoliosis. Prevention includes health education about physical activities that increase the risk the SCIs, including participating in risky physical activities, not wearing protective gear during work or play, or diving into shallow water.

Traumatic Brain Injuries

Over 2% of all Americans live with disabilities resulting from traumatic brain injuries (TBIs).[40] TBIs cost the nation about $56.3 billion per year.[40] Precautions can help reduce the incidence of TBI caused by motor vehicles and bicycles.

> *Automobile air bags, seatbelts, and infant or child safety seats greatly reduce the risk for serious injury or death in an accident. Despite overwhelming evidence that seatbelts and safety seats save lives, an estimated 26% of the population neglects or resists using them, and others use or install them incorrectly.*[40]

Suggestions for preventing TBIs include use of seat belts, infant and car safety seats, avoiding driving while under the influence of alcohol or drugs, and driving the speed limit. Additional measures include ensuring that air bags are properly installed and functional. Physical therapists should remind their clients that the risk of TBIs and SCIs warrant special attention to use of their vehicles. Chapter 14 provides additional information about prevention practice for individuals with TBIs and SCIs.

Suicide

According to the CDC, more people die from suicide than from homicide.[41] Overall, suicide is the 11th leading cause of death for all Americans and is the third leading cause of death for young people aged 15 to 24.[41] Certain populations are at increased risk for suicide: (1) males are four times more likely to die from suicide than females; however, females are more likely to *attempt* suicide; (2) Caucasians account for over 90% of all suicides; however, the suicide rates for young Native Americans and African-American males are increasing; and (3) suicide rates increase with age and are highest among Americans aged 65 years and older. Risk factors for suicide among older persons differ from those among the young. Older persons have a higher prevalence of depression, social isolation, and a greater use of highly lethal methods. The majority of suicides for all ages are committed with firearms.[36]

Suicide Awareness Voices of Education (SAVE) provides updated statistics and educational materials for suicide prevention through public awareness and education in hopes of decreasing the incidence of suicide, eliminating the stigma associated with suicide, and serving as a resource to those touched by suicide.[41] According to SAVE, warning signs of suicide include (1) talking about suicide (eg, "I have nothing left to live for," "I won't be a burden on my family much longer," "I should just kill myself"); (2) statements about hopelessness, helplessness, or worthlessness; (3) preoccupation with death; (4) suddenly becoming happier, calmer; (5) loss of interest in things one cares about; (6) visiting or calling people one cares about; (7) making arrangements, or setting one's affairs in order; (8) giving things away; (9) stockpiling pills or obtaining a weapon; and (10) refusal to follow doctor-prescribed medications and/or special diet.[41] The physical therapist should be aware of these warning signs of suicide and immediately refer any clients presenting with these warning signs to a doctor or psychiatrist. It is important to explore suicidal thoughts with depressed individuals in a nonjudgmental manner and take thoughts of or plans for suicide seriously. If necessary, the physical therapist may choose to contact 911 if the client has a serious plan for committing suicide.

Bicycle-Related Injuries

More than 95% of bicyclists killed were not wearing helmets. Research exploring risk factors for various populations provides evidence that helmet use can prevent head injuries and strategies to increase helmet use among cyclists, particularly young children, while riding both on- and off-road.[42] As advocates for physical activity, it is important to help clients understand the risks of riding a bicycle in their community. A number of suggestions for making a community more bicycle-friendly are offered on the Internet.[43] Physical therapists should educate their clients about personal safety habits, including selecting safe routes and demonstrating safe bicycling behaviors, such as wearing a bicycle helmet, obeying traffic signals and signs, riding in a straight line, signaling turns, riding with traffic, using lights and reflective clothing at night, and being courteous with others sharing the rode. In addition, physical therapists can serve as community advocates for safer bicycling routes to reduce the risk of injuries.

Dog Bite Injuries

While seemingly minor, dog bites account for a large number of preventable injuries, including fatalities. A national estimate of 333,687 dog bite injuries are treated in emergency departments each year with approximately 17 deaths.[44] Almost $165 million is spent treating dog bites in the United States for the estimated 800,000 dog-bite related injuries requiring treatment each year. Seventy percent of dog bites occur on the owner's property.[44] For this reason, individuals encountering unfamiliar dogs need to be cautious when visiting homes with dogs. It is wise to ask dog owners to secure their dogs before any guests arrive and to protect visitors from injury as much as possible. Should a dog be loose, it should be left alone. If the dog is approaching, distract the dog by throwing an object across the way for retrieval. Do not run and do not yell loudly, further creating a threatening situation.[44]

Many individuals with disabilities own dogs that are trained to assist with mobility or to serve as "seeing-eye" dogs. Likewise, the owners of these dogs must be aware of the importance of cautioning others about potential risks of interacting with their dogs. An eating or sleeping dog should be left alone and not approached. It is important to recognize the risks posed by dogs and to encourage appropriate and respectful interaction with dogs to reduce injuries.

VIOLENCE ACROSS THE LIFESPAN

Violence is defined as "the intentional use of physical force or power, threatened or actual, against oneself, another person, or against a group or community either resulting in or having a high likelihood of injury, death, psychological harm, maldevelopment, or deprivation."[45,46] Violence may be directed at an intimate partner, a child, an older adult, or a community, such as a school or workplace. Additionally, some violence is motivated by hate and intolerance, such as racial bigotry and intolerance to sexual orientation. The physical therapists should be aware of risk factors that put individuals at risk for violence.

Intimate Partner Violence

Intimate partner violence affects women more than men and includes domestic abuse, spousal abuse, battering, domestic violence, courtship violence, marital rape, and date rape. Nearly 5.3 million intimate partner victimizations occur each year among United

States women ages 18 and older. This violence results in nearly 2 million injuries and nearly 1,300 deaths.[47] Certain factors put women at an increased risk for intimate partner violence. These individual vulnerability factors include (1) a history of physical abuse, (2) prior injury from the same partner, (3) having a verbally abusive partner, (4) economic stress, (5) partner history of alcohol or drug abuse, (6) childhood abuse, and (7) being under the age of 24. In addition, research has identified several "relational vulnerability factors" related to intimate partner violence, including: marital conflict, marital instability, male dominance in the family, and poor family functioning.[47] If these factors are suspected, the physical therapist should make an attempt to interview the woman separately from her partner to inquire about the woman's personal concerns and fears of domestic violence.

Sexual Violence

Sexual violence may be perpetrated by someone the individual does not know, such as rape by a stranger. "Of rape victims who reported the offense to law enforcement, about 40% were under the age of 18, and 15% were younger than 12."[48] Alcohol is reported as a contributing factor in half of all reported rapes. Physical therapists need to be aware of such violence and ask open-ended questions that allow their clients to share their intimate experiences.

Individuals of all ages are vulnerable to rape. Behaviors exhibited postrape may include, but are not limited to, chronic headaches, fatigue, sleep disturbances, recurrent nausea, decreased appetite, eating disorders, menstrual pain, sexual dysfunction, and suicidal behavior.[50] Individuals who present with unusual behaviors or factors that put them at risk for violence should be examined thoroughly by an appropriate health care professional—a physician, a social worker, or a psychologist.

If any type of violence against a child is suspected, the physical therapist must report the suspected abuse to the Child Protective Services (CPS) agency in the state in which the abuse occurred. The Childhelp USA National Child Abuse Hotline (1-800-4-A-CHILD) can help locate the appropriate agency for reporting suspected abuse or negligence.[50]

Abuse of Children

Children may be vulnerable to sexual violence and *sexual abuse* (ie, fondling a child's genitals, intercourse, incest, rape, sodomy, exhibitionism, and commercial exploitation through prostitution or the production of pornographic material) in addition to *physical abuse* (ie, infliction of physical injury as a result of punching, beating, kicking, biting, burning, shaking, or otherwise harming the child) and *neglect* (failure to provide for the child's basic psychological, medical, emotional, or physical needs).[49] Children at an increased risk for neglect include those with mothers who are angry, have a low self-esteem, lack confidence, are impulsive, and have unrealistic expectations.[49] Furthermore, mothers and children in disadvantaged communities may be at higher risk for child neglect.

Elder Abuse

Elder abuse is a term referring to any knowing, intentional, or negligent act by a caregiver or any other person that causes harm or a serious risk of harm to a vulnerable adult.[51] The National Center on Elder Abuse (NCEA), funded by the United States Administration on Aging, is a gateway to resources on elder abuse, neglect, and exploitation. According to NCEA, the laws for elder abuse vary from state to state, but generally include the following: (1) *physical abuse* (inflicting, or threatening to inflict, physical pain or injury on a vulnerable elder or depriving them of a basic need), (2) *emotional abuse* (inflicting mental pain, anguish, or distress on an elder person through verbal or nonverbal acts), (3) *sexual abuse* (nonconsensual sexual contact of any kind), (4) *exploitation* (illegal taking, misuse, or concealment of funds, property, or assets of a vulnerable elder), (5) *neglect* (refusal or failure by those responsible to provide food, shelter, health care, or protection for a vulnerable elder), and (6) *abandonment* (the desertion of a vulnerable elder by anyone who has assumed the responsibility for care or custody of that person).[51] The physical therapist should be alert to signs of elder abuse:[51]

1. Physical signs of abuse, neglect, or maltreatment, such as bruises, pressure marks, broken bones, abrasions, and burns. Bruises around the breasts or genital area can occur from sexual abuse.
2. Unexplained withdrawal from normal activities, a sudden change in alertness, and unusual depression may be indicators of emotional abuse.
3. Sudden changes in financial situations may be the result of exploitation.
4. Bedsores, unattended medical needs, poor hygiene, and unusual weight loss are indicators of possible neglect.
5. Behavior such as belittling, threats, and other uses of power and control by spouses are indicators of verbal or emotional abuse; frequent arguments between the caregiver and elderly person are a common sign.

In addition, individuals who are incapable of self-care may exhibit self-neglect or behaviors that indicate the need for intervention. These behaviors include, but are not limited to, hoarding; poor hygiene; confusion; wearing inappropriate clothing; leaving stoves, irons, or other devices unattended; poor housekeeping; and dehydration. Oftentimes, self-neglect is coupled with declining health, isolation, Alzheimer's disease or dementia, or drug and alcohol dependency.[52] For older adults at increased risk for elder abuse and self-neglect, the physical therapist is responsible for reporting suspected abuse or neglect. Reporting can be done through the police department (calling 911) for individuals who are at immediate risk. Local adult protective services can be reached through the Eldercare Locator by telephone (1-800-677-1116).[53]

Overview

Ideally, health care professionals should work together to prevent violence to all populations at risk. The American Academy of Pediatrics offers a website dedicated to the prevention of violence directed toward children that links to other anti-violence resources.[54] Another helpful website is sponsored by the Center for the Study and Prevention of Violence at the University of Colorado.[55] This site lists a variety of publications geared toward reducing violence against all populations.

Falls

In 2020, it is estimated that fall-related injuries will cost $32.4 billion. Every hour, an older adult dies as the result of a fall. While not all injuries are fatal, approximately 300,000 older adults suffer fall-related hip fractures each year that lead to decreased functional independence.[56] Chapter 9 discusses how physical therapists can help screen older adults who are at increased risk for falling. In addition, the National Center for Injury Prevention and Control offers a helpful web page listing tips for reducing falls in older populations.[46] These tips include exercising to increase strength and balance, reducing environmental risks, monitoring medications for side effects influencing balance, and checking vision regularly for potential changes that could influence balance.

According to National Safe Kids, "falls are the leading cause of nonfatal, unintentional injuries and emergency department visits for children younger than 15."[58] Each year in the United States, more than 120 fall-related deaths and 2.5 million emergency department visits are reported among this age group. "Children less than 5 years old account for more than 50% of both categories."[58] Interestingly, many infants fall while supervised by their caregiver. The age of the child dictates the most likely cause of falling: (1) infants tend to fall from furniture, stairs, or walkers; (2) toddlers more often fall from windows and balconies; (3) older children fall from their bicycles, skateboards, scooters, and playground equipment.[58] Parents should be especially vigilant when children learn how to climb furniture and explore their new freedoms at increased heights. The American Red Cross addresses falls in children on their website.[59]

Alcoholism

Alcoholism is a health risk to both the individual and to society. Individuals who are under the influence of alcohol are more likely to behave dangerously (eg, driving while under the influence of alcohol and increased violent behavior). Alcohol is involved in greater than 50% of motor vehicle deaths, 67% of drownings, 70% to 80% of fire-related deaths, and 67% of murders.[60] According to community surveys, over 13% of adults in the United States will experience *alcohol abuse or dependence* (also referred to as *alcoholism*) at some point in their lives.[60] The cause of alcoholism is not well established. There is growing evidence for genetic and biologic predispositions for this disease, but this research is controversial. Relatively recent research has implicated a gene (D2 dopamine receptor gene) that, when inherited in a specific form, might increase a person's chance of developing alcoholism.[61] Twice as many men as women are alcoholics and 10% to 23% of alcohol-consuming individuals are considered alcoholics.[61] Usually, a variety of factors contributes to the development of a problem with alcohol. Social factors such as the influence of family, peers, and society, the availability of alcohol, and psychological factors such as elevated levels of stress, inadequate coping mechanisms, and reinforcement of alcohol use from other drinkers can contribute to alcoholism. In addition, the factors contributing to initial alcohol use may vary from those maintaining it once the disease develops.

Ideally, individuals who are prone to alcoholism would avoid drinking alcohol; however, alcohol consumption and drug abuse are prevalent in society, and it is difficult to eradicate the source of the problem. The National Council on Alcoholism and Drug Dependence facilitates an ongoing process of "promoting the individual's, the family's, and the community's full personal growth and potential in order to reduce the likelihood of problems related to alcohol and/or drug abuse."[62]

> *Prevention activities may take a two-pronged approach: (1) a deliberate and constructive process designed to promote growth of individuals and communities toward full human potential, (2) the counteraction of harmful circumstances such as health and safety hazards, family stresses, job pressures, isolation, violence, economic hardship, and inadequate housing, medical services, or child care.*[62]

If alcoholism is suspected, an immediate referral to the physician or psychologist is necessary.

PREVENTING HEARING LOSS

According to the National Institute of Deafness and Other Communication Disorders (NIDCD), approximately 28 million people in the United States have some degree of reduced hearing sensitivity. Of this number, 80% have irreversible hearing loss.[63] One in three people older than 60 and half of those older than 85 have hearing loss. Hearing loss can be caused by a virus or bacteria, heart conditions or stroke, head injuries, tumors, and certain medicines. Additionally, some individuals lose their hearing slowly as they age because of *presbycusis* (a progressive, age-related hearing loss that may be caused by changes in the blood supply to the ear because of heart disease, high blood pressure, vascular conditions caused by diabetes, or other circulatory problems).[63] With presbycusis, sounds often seem less clear and lower in volume and higher-pitched sounds are difficult to distinguish. Another common cause is noise exposure. Avoiding loud noises or protecting the ears with foam-tip earplugs can help protect against hearing loss, especially for those individuals who use loud machinery (eg, lawn mowers or power tools) or firearms. Screenings for hearing loss can alert individuals of their hearing ability so proper treatment can be sought. Table 11-5 provides a list of questions that can help an individual recognize the onset of hearing loss.[63] If hearing loss is suspected, a medical referral should be made to an audiologist, an otolaryngologist, or the primary physician for further examination. Hearing aids can, oftentimes, be used to augment hearing in the case of hearing loss.

Since communication is so important in daily living, it is important to prevent the psychosocial isolation that can accompany hearing loss. The following suggestions are offered by NIDCD[63]:

1. Face the person who has a hearing loss so that he or she can see your face when you speak.
2. Be sure that lighting is in front of you when you speak. This allows a person with a hearing impairment to observe facial expressions, gestures, and lip and body movements that provide communication clues.
3. During conversations, turn off the radio or television.
4. Avoid speaking while chewing food or covering your mouth with your hands.
5. Speak slightly louder than normal, but do not shout. Shouting may distort your speech.
6. Speak at your normal rate, and do not exaggerate sounds.
7. Clue the person with the hearing loss about the topic of the conversation whenever possible.
8. Rephrase your statement into shorter, simpler sentences if it appears you are not being understood.
9. In restaurants and social gatherings, choose seats or conversation areas away from crowded or noisy areas.

TABLE 11-5

SCREENING FOR ADULT HEARING LOSS

- Do I have a problem hearing on the telephone?
- Do I have trouble hearing when there is noise in the background?
- Is it hard for me to follow a conversation when two or more people talk at once?
- Do I have to strain to understand a conversation?
- Do many people I talk to seem to mumble (or not speak clearly)?
- Do I misunderstand what others are saying and respond inappropriately?
- Do I often ask people to repeat themselves?
- Do I have trouble understanding the speech of women and children?
- Do people complain that I turn the television volume up too high?
- Do I hear ringing, roaring, or hissing sounds a lot?
- Do some sounds seem too loud?

Adapted from National Institute on Deafness and Other Communication Disorders. Hearing, ear infections, and deafness. Available at: http://www.nidcd.nih.gov/health/hearing. Accessed February 2, 2006.

Summary

As part of the health care team, physical therapists can contribute to the identification of risk factors and developing health problems resulting from inadequate protection from infections and injury. The success of Healthy People 2010 relies on the expertise of health care professionals to identify individual and community risk factors that potentially lead to preventable accidents and diseases. Physical therapists play an essential role in providing health education and screenings to their clients who are at increased risk for hazards that further jeopardize health and wellness. As advocates, physical therapists can work to improve communities by developing accurate health protection information, detecting risks, recognizing at-risk populations, and locating resources for transforming communities into healthy, safe living environments.

References

1. Healthy People 2010. Injury Prevention. Available at: http://www.safetypolicy.org/hp2010/hp2010.htm. Accessed February 4, 2006.
2. Lam WK, Zhong NS, Tan WC. Overview on SARS in Asia and the world. *Respirology.* 2003;Suppl:S2–S5.
3. Centers for Disease Control and Prevention. Injury and violence prevention. Healthy People 2010. Available at: http://www.healthypeople.gov/Document/Word/Volume2/15Injury.doc. Accessed November 10, 2004.
4. World Health Organization. Available at: http://www.who.int/en. Accessed February 4, 2006.
5. Centers for Disease Control and Prevention. Emerging infectious diseases. Available at: http://www.cdc.gov/ncidod/EID/index.htm. Accessed February 4, 2006.
6. Institute for Vaccine Safety. Recommended childhood and adolescent immunization schedule. Available at: http://www.vaccinesafety.edu/2006-schedule.htm. Accessed February 4, 2006.
7. Rivara F, Thompson D, Patterson M, Thompson S. Prevention of bicycle-related injuries: helmets, education, and legislation. *Annu Rev Public Health.* 1998;19(1):293–318.
8. National Highway Traffic Safety Administration. Bikeability checklist. US Department of Transportation. Available at: http://www.nhtsa.dot.gov/people/injury/pedbimot/bike/Bikeability/checklist.htm.
9. National SAFE KIDS Campaign (NSKC). *Falls Fact Sheet.* Washington, DC: NSKC; 2004.
10. Baby Center. Child-proofing your house. Available at: http://parentcenter.babycenter.com/refcap/bigkid/gsafety/65742.html. Accessed February 4, 2006.
11. Maron B, Thompson P, Puffer J, et al. Cardiovascular pre-participation screening of competitive athletes. *Circulation.* 1996;94:850–856.
12. National Athletic Trainers Association. What happens if your child is injured on the sports field? Press release. September 23, 1999.
13. American Academy of Family Physicians. Heat-related illness: what you can do to prevent it. Brochure. 1994.
14. National Institute of Arthritis and Musculoskeletal and Skin Diseases. Childhood sports injuries and their prevention: a guide for parents with ideas for kids. 2001. Available at: http://www.niams.nih.gov/hi/topics/childsports/child_sports.htm. Accessed February 6, 2006.
15. Requa R. The scope of the problem: the impact of sports-related injuries. In: *Proceedings of Sports Injuries in Youth: Surveillance Strategies.* Bethesda, MD: National Institute of Arthritis and Musculoskeletal and Skin Diseases, National Institutes of Health; 1991:19.
16. Messina DF, Farney WC, DeLee JC. The incidence of injury in Texas high school basketball. *Am J Sport Med.* 1999;27(3):294–299.
17. Powell, John W, Barber-Foss, Kim D. Injury patterns in selected high school sports: a review of the 1995–1997 seasons. *J Athletic Train.* 1999;34:(3):277–284.
18. US Consumer Product Safety Commission. Baby boomer sports injuries. 2000. Available at: http://www.cpsc.gov/library/boomer.pdf. Accessed February 4, 2006.
19. US Fire Administration. Special report underscores link between alcohol abuse and fatalities from house fires. Available at: http://www.usfa.fema.gov/about/media/2004releases/020904a.shtm. Accessed February 4, 2006.
20. National Fire Protection Association. Available at: http://www.nfpa.org. Accessed February 4, 2006.
21. Litovitz TL, Klein-Schwartz W, White S, et al. Annual report of the American Association of Poison Control Centers Toxic Exposure Surveillance System. *Am J Emerg Med.* 2000;19(5):337–396.
22. Poisonprevention.org. US Consumer Product Safety Commission. Available at: http://www.poisonprevention.org. Accessed February 4, 2006.
23. National Center for Complementary and Alternative Medicine. Are you considering using complementary and alternative medicine (CAM)? Available at: http://nccam.nih.gov/health/decisions. Accessed February 4, 2006.
24. National Institute of Allergy and Infectious Diseases. Foodborne disease. Available at: http://www.niaid.nih.gov/factsheets/foodbornedis.htm. Accessed February 4, 2006.
25. American Medical Association. Diagnosis and management of foodborne illnesses: a primer for physicians and other health care professionals. Available at: http://www.ama-assn.org/ama/pub/category/3629.html. Accessed February 4, 2006.
26. Hatheway C. Botulism: the present status of the disease. *Curr Top Microbiol Immunol.* 1999;195:55–75.
27. National Center For Chronic Disease Prevention and Health Promotion. Clean indoor air regulations fact sheet. Available at: http://www.cdc.gov/tobacco/sgr/sgr_2000/factsheets/factsheet_clean.htm. Accessed February 4, 2006.
28. Smokefree.gov. You can quit smoking now: online guide to quitting. Available at: http://www.smokefree.gov. Accessed February 4, 2006.
29. University of Iowa Hospitals and Clinics Patient Education. Pesticides. Available at: http://www.uihealthcare.com/topics/medicaldepartments/cancercenter/cancertips/pesticides.html. Accessed February 4, 2006.
30. Patlack M. Non-Hodgkin's lymphoma becomes more common, more treatable. US Food and Drug Administration. Available at: http://www.fda.gov/fdac/features/096_nhl.html#tracking. Accessed February 4, 2006.
31. Committee on Adolescence, American Academy of Pediatrics. Firearms and adolescents. *American Academy of Pediatric News.* 1992;1:20–21.

32. University of Michigan Health System. Safety: guns and kids. Available at: http://www.med.umich.edu/1libr/your-child/guns.htm. Accessed February 4, 2006
33. Centers for Disease Control and Prevention. Injury fact book: water-related injuries. Available at: http://www.cdc.gov/ncipc/fact_book/30_WaterRelated_Injuries.htm. Accessed February 4, 2006.
34. University of Texas MD Anderson Cancer Center. Protecting yourself against skin cancer. *OncoLog.* 2004;July–Aug:49.
35. US Department of Labor Occupational Safety and Health Organization. Case and demographic characteristics for work-related injuries and illnesses involving days away from work. Available at: http://www.osha.gov. Accessed February 4, 2006.
36. US Department of Labor Bureau of Labor Statistics. Industry injury and illness data. Available at: http://www.bls.gov/iif/oshsum.htm. Accessed February 4, 2006.
37. US Consumer Product Safety Commission. CPSC overview. Available at: http://www.cpsc.gov/about/about.html. Accessed February 4, 2006.
38. Buckley T. Traumatic stress and motor vehicle accidents. National Center for Traumatic Stress Disorder. Available at: http://www.ncptsd.org/facts/specific/fs_mva.html. Accessed January 29, 2006.
39. Drkoop.com. Spinal cord trauma. Available at: http://www.drkoop.com/ency/article/001066.htm. Accessed January 30, 2006.
40. NeurologyChannel. Traumatic brain injury. Available at: http://www.neurologychannel.com/tbi/prevention.shtml. Accessed February 6, 2006.
41. SAVE: Suicide Awareness Voices of Education. Facts about suicide. Centers for Disease Control. Available at: http://www.save.org/basics/facts.html. Accessed February 6, 2006.
42. Jacobson GA, Blizzard L, Dwyer T. Bicycle injuries: road trauma is not the only concern. *Aust N Z J Public Health.* 1998;22(4):451–455.
43. Pedestrian and Bicycling Information Center. Available at: http://www.bicyclinginfo.org. Accessed February 2, 2006.
44. National Center for Injury Prevention and Control. Hospitalizations for dog bite injuries. Available at: http://www.cdc.gov/ncipc/duip/hospital.htm. Accessed February 2, 2006.
45. Black DA, Schumacher JA, Smith-Slep AM, Heyman R. Partner, child abuse risk factors literature review. In: Allen C, ed. *National Network of Family Resiliency, National Network for Health* [online]. 1999. Available at: http://www.nnh.org/risk. Accessed August 2004.
46. National Center for Injury Prevention and Control. Youth violence: overview. Available at: http://www.cdc.gov/ncipc/factsheets/yvoverview.htm. Accessed February 2, 2006.
47. Centers for Disease Control and Prevention Injury Center. Incidence, prevalence, and consequences of intimate partner violence against women in the United States. Available at: http://www.cdc.gov/ncipc/pub-res/ipv_cost/03_incidence.htm. Accessed February 2, 2006.
48. Centers for Disease Control and Prevention. Health matters for women. Available at: http://www.cdc.gov/od/spotlight/nwhw/newsltr/02summ.htm. Accessed February 2, 2006.
49. Allen C. Risk factors for partner abuse and child maltreatment: a review of literature. CYFERNet. Available at: http://www.cyfernet.org. Accessed February 2, 2006.
50. Childhelp USA. Treatment and prevention of child abuse. Available at: http://www.childhelpusa.org. Accessed February 2, 2006.
51. National Center on Elder Abuse. Frequently asked questions. Available at: http://www.elderabusecenter.org. Accessed February 2, 2006.
52. Woolf L. Elder abuse and neglect. Webster University; 1998. Available at: http://www.webster.edu/~woolflm/abuse.html. Accessed February 2, 2006.
53. Department of Health and Human Services. Eldercare search. Available at: http://www.eldercare.gov/Eldercare/Public/Home.asp. Accessed February 2, 2006.
54. American Academy of Pediatrics. Children's health topics: violence prevention. Available at: http://www.aap.org/healthtopics/violprev.cfm. Accessed February 2, 2006.
55. Center for the Study and Prevention of Violence. Fact sheets. Available at: http://www.colorado.edu/cspv/publications/factsheets.html. Accessed February 2, 2006.
56. Centers for Disease Control and Prevention. Aging: falls among older Americans: CDC prevention efforts. Available at: http://www.cdc.gov/washington/testimony/ag061102.htm. Accessed February 2, 2006.
57. National Center for Injury Prevention and Control. Preventing falls among seniors. Available at: http://www.cdc.gov/ncipc/duip/spotlite/falltips.htm. Accessed February 2, 2006.
58. National Safekids Campaign. Community Safety: Injury Prevention. Fall prevention—children. Available at: http://www.tvfr.com/CS/ip/Falls/fallprev_children.html. Accessed February 2, 2006.
59. American Red Cross. Health and safety tips: protect your child from dangerous falls. Available at: http://www.redcross.org/services/hss/tips/healthtips/falls.html. Accessed February 2, 2006.
60. Medicine Consumer Health. Alcoholism: when to seek medical care. Available at: http://www.emedicinehealth.com/articles/18863-4.asp. Accessed February 2, 2006.
61. Noble EP. Alcoholism and the dopaminergic system: a review. *Addiction and Biology.* 1996;1(4):333–348.
62. Santa Barbara Alcohol and Drug Program. FAQ—about prevention. Available at: http://www.silcom.com/~sbadp/faqs/preventionfaq.htm. Accessed February 2, 2006.
63. National Institute on Deafness and Other Communication Disorders. Hearing, ear infections, and deafness. Available at: http://www.nidcd.nih.gov/health/hearing. Accessed February 2, 2006.

Chapter 12

Prevention Practice for Musculoskeletal Conditions

Amy Foley, DPT, PT; Gail Regan, PhD, PT; and Catherine Rush Thompson, PhD, MS, PT

A critical component of prevention is the emphasis on early diagnosis and prompt treatment of the likely consequences of advanced disease, thereby averting or delaying the logical sequence of the pathologic process and shortening its duration and severity. This component is particularly crucial in the treatment of individuals with musculoskeletal pathologies. The musculoskeletal medical conditions examined in this section are those included within the *Preferred Practice Pattern D:* impaired joint mobility, motor function, muscle performance, and range of motion associated with connective tissue dysfunction; *Preferred Practice Pattern E:* impaired joint mobility, motor function, muscle performance, and range of motion associated with localized inflammation; and *Preferred Practice Pattern F:* impaired joint mobility, motor function, muscle performance, range of motion, and reflex integrity associated with spinal disorders. These include such medical conditions as musculotendinous injuries due to cumulative, repetitive stress syndromes, chronic low back pain, and osteoarthritis.[1] Much of the screening for complications, prevention of secondary complications, and resources for health and wellness for these musculoskeletal disorders can be applied to other conditions included in Preferred Practice Patterns A, B, and C.[1]

Familiarity with the normal development of body systems, in particular the musculoskeletal system, helps the physical therapist make keen observations during screenings across the lifespan. For children under the age of 1, it is important to note the development of musculoskeletal and neurological systems that enable motor function. During the first 6 months of life, the infant's skeleton is exposed to dynamic muscle activity and gravitational forces needed to grow long bones and develop proper alignment of skeletal structures.[2] The skull grows with forces exerted by the developing brain, and teeth emerge from the mandible as early as 6 months. As the child develops head control, the primary curve in the cervical region develops; with developing sitting posture, the secondary curve is evident in the lumbar spine. Rapid growth and development of the skeleton continues from 7 to 12 months, sufficient to support the infant's weight on all fours and in standing.[2] Table 12-1 summarizes the musculoskeletal changes during the first year of life.[2]

Muscular Changes During the First Year

Skeletal muscle fibers grow by multiplication as the infant uses the body to explore the environment. The stress of skeletal growth elongates the muscles,

TABLE 12-1

MUSCULOSKELETAL CHANGES IN THE FIRST YEAR OF LIFE

	1 to 6 months	7 to 12 months
Skeletal muscles	• Muscle fibrils grow by multiplication. • Muscle length is stimulated by skeletal growth. • Muscle is growing in size by accumulating cytoplasm rather than growing in numbers (after fourth to fifth month).	
Cardiac muscle	• Cells of the visceral muscle increase in number and in size with growth. • Cardiac muscle also increases by enlarging existing muscle fibers.	
Facial muscles	• Muscles of the face and respiration are well developed at birth.	
Postural patterns and functional movement associated with muscle development	• The second month is characterized by decreased flexion and increased extension and asymmetry. • The third month is characterized by the beginning of symmetry, and the beginning of bilateral control of neck muscles. • By 6 months, the baby can extend the neck against gravity.	• By 7 months, the baby can pivot around in prone using symmetrical upper extremity movement. • By 8 months, the baby can creep as the primary means of locomotion. • By 12 months, the baby is capable of rising to stand by sole use of legs. • By 12 months, finger opposition is present.

Adapted from:
Kaywood K, Hetchell N. *Life Span Motor Development.* Champaign, Ill: Human Kinetics; 2001.
Linn JP, Brown JK, Walsh EG. Physiological maturation of muscles in childhood. *Lancet.* 1994;343:1386–1389.

and cellular changes after 4 to 5 months cause an increase in fiber size.[2] Likewise, cardiac muscle tissue grows in size, and the myocardium (heart muscle) increases in size as existing muscle fibers grow with increasingly stronger heart beats to match demands by physical activity. The normal resting heart rate for an infant is 100 to 160 beats per minute.[2] The muscles of the face and respiration are well developed at birth, enabling the infant to eat and cry for attention.

Muscular Changes in Years 1 to 6

In the first 3 years of life, the child increases muscle strength to support bipedal locomotion. The cardiac muscle subsequently increases in size, especially the left ventricle, to accommodate the increasing workload associated with the motor activity of an infant and toddler. Children from 1 to 10 years of age have resting heart rates of 70 to 120 beats per minute, slightly slower than those of newborn babies.[2] As the child develops sphincter control, the child may begin toilet training and eliminate the need for diapers. With continued motor activity, particularly weight-bearing activities like walking and running, the child increasingly develops the strength of foot intrinsic muscles that support the longitudinal arches of both feet. In addition, the child displays progressively more sophisticated reach and grasp patterns that enable prehension and manipulation of objects for play.

Strength from age 4 to 6 is dependent upon the child's body proportions but can generally be determined by the child's ability to perform functional activities that are normal for a specific age. Growth can be variable and rapid, sometimes contributing to "growth pains" that emanate from muscles being stretched on growing bones.[2] By age 5, the child has sufficient postural control and fine motor strength to begin handwriting activities. Table 12-2 provides a summary of muscular changes from age 1 to 6.[2]

TABLE 12-2

MUSCULAR CHANGES IN YEARS 1 TO 6

	1 to 3 years	4 to 6 years
Skeletal muscles	• Early in this stage, the muscular strength of the trunk and the lower extremities increase to support bipedal locomotion.	• Creatinine in urine increases as muscle mass increases. • Muscle fibers increase in diameter as strength increases. • Muscle strength increases as activity increases.
Cardiac muscle	• Muscles of the left ventricle of the heart grow more than the right to accommodate the increase in workload.	
Sphincter muscles	• Sphincter muscles develop to allow toilet training.	
Postural patterns associated with muscle development	• With continued weight bearing, the growth of intrinsic feet muscles causes the once fat, thick, and archless foot to become arched with the development of the longitudinal arch. • At 2 years of age the toddler displays a mature grasp pattern that enables prehension and the manual exchange of objects.	• Muscle strength depends upon body proportions—adult normative values are not accurate for children. • Children may experience growth pains as muscle growth accompanies bone growth. • By age 5, children have adequate manipulation skills to begin handwriting.

Adapted from Kaywood K, Hetchell N. *Life Span Motor Development.* Champaign, Ill: Human Kinetics; 2001.

Skeletal Changes in Years 1 to 6

Dramatic changes take place in the skeletal system as the body assumes an upright posture. The leg growth accelerates with the increased weight-bearing performed by the ambulating toddler, and height increases as much as 5 inches in the second year of life and 2 inches during the third year.[2] The structural changes of long bones are the greatest when the child is 2.5 years old. The skull is completely ossified at age 2, and dentition continues to emerge.[2] With growth and gravitational forces affecting postural alignment, the toddler commonly stands with slightly bowed legs (*genu varus*) that become knock-kneed (*genu valgum*) with the remodeling of the pelvis. Increased walking realigns the lower extremities, causing the feet to become more averted and the femoral neck to decrease its angle with the shaft from 160 degrees to 125 degrees.[2] Between the ages of 4 to 6, the primary ossification centers appear in the patella and are evident in the carpal bones of the wrists. Height continues to increase at a rate of approximately 2 to 3 inches per year. By age 6, the child has developed all the primary dentition and has some teeth replaced by secondary dentition (permanent teeth). Seventy-five percent of children with genus valgum at age 3 have no evidence of abnormally malaligned knees by age 7. See Table 12-3, listing changes from ages 1 to 6.[2]

Skeletal Changes During Preadolescence and Adolescence

At age 6, the child's posture is characterized by a protruding abdomen and lumbar lordosis that eventually evolves into normal postural alignment as growing muscles support the skeleton.[2] The abdominal muscles increase in strength, supporting the lower trunk and reversing the lordotic curve. The child's growth in height during preadolescence results from the ossification of cartilage at the end of long bones—cartilage that is vulnerable to injury in sports activities.

TABLE 12-3

SKELETAL CHANGES IN YEARS 1 TO 6

	1 to 3 years	4 to 6 years
Spine and extremities	• Leg growth accelerates in the toddler years. • Height increases 5 inches in the second year and 2 inches during the third year. • The structural changes of long bone are greatest at 2.5 years of age.	• Primary ossification centers appear in the patella and the carpal bones by age 3 to 3.5 years. • Height increases from 5 to 6 cm per year.
Skull	• All bones of the skull are ossified by age 2.	
Dentition	• At about 6 months of age, the mandibular incisors are the first primary teeth to erupt.	• By age 6, the child has developed the primary dentition and has had some teeth replaced by the secondary dentition (permanent teeth).
Skeletal alignment/curvature	• Toddler stands bow-legged (genu varus) at age 18 months and knock-kneed (genu valgum) at 3 years because of remodelling of the pelvis. With increased walking, the lower limbs realign, the feet evert, and the angle made by the neck of the femur with the shaft gradually decreases from about 160 degrees to the adult value of 125 degrees.	• At age 3, nearly 75% of children develop genu valgum which is resolved by age 6 to 7 years.

Adapted from Sinclair D, Dangerfield PH. *Human Growth After Birth.* London, England: Oxford Press; 1998.

As the child becomes an adolescent, posture resembles that of an adult. Rather than increasing in height, skeletal changes become more lateral and gender specific. Males tend to increase their shoulder width through growth of the clavicle, and females increase their pelvic width, which differentially becomes wider, shallower, and roomier for subsequent childbearing.[2] The facial features appear more adult, with the mature nose projecting to its adult length. Overall, the maximum skeletal growth occurs between the ages of 10 and 14 in females and between the ages of 12 and 14 in males.[2] In addition, skeletal growth occurs differently in African Americans and Caucasians, with skeletal growth occurring more rapidly in blacks than whites.[2] See the summary of musculoskeletal changes during preadolescence and adolescence in Table 12-4.[2]

Physical therapists play a key role in identifying skeletal problems through musculoskeletal screenings. By adolescence, the upper spine normally has a gentle rounded posterior curve (*normal kyphosis*) and the *lower spine* has the reverse curve (*normal lordosis*). Certain amounts of *cervical (neck) lordosis, thoracic (upper back) kyphosis,* and *lumbar (lower back) lordosis* are normally present and are needed to maintain appropriate trunk balance over the pelvis. Deviations from this normal alignment may reflect abnormal kyphosis or lordosis or, more commonly, scoliosis. Scoliosis refers to a lateral curvature of the spine or a side-to-side deviation from the normal frontal axis of the body. According to the Scoliosis Research Society, in over 80% of the cases, the cause of scoliosis is unknown and is referred to as "idiopathic scoliosis."[3] A comprehensive screening for scoliosis involves a thorough medical history, developmental history, and family history. The physical screening centers on assessing the spinal alignment and symmetry both when standing erect and when bending forward with both knees extended, noting muscular versus skeletal asymmetries. The spinal asymmetry may be accompanied by uneven shoulder height when standing erect, unequal leg length, or the presence of dimples, sinuses, hairy patches, and skin pigmentation changes. Suspected scoliosis should be reported to the family physician for further diagnostic testing.

TABLE 12-4

MUSCULOSKELETAL CHANGES DURING PREADOLESCENCE AND ADOLESCENCE

	Preadolescence	Adolescence
Overall posture	• Six-year-old silhouette is characterized by a protruding abdomen and lordosis. • By age 10, the spine is better aligned, the abdomen is flatter, and the body is generally more slender and long-legged.	• Posture resembles adult posture.
Cartilage	• Skeletal growth is primarily linear, increasing the child's height. • Cartilage is being replaced by bone at the epiphyses (at ends of long bones and wrists).	• Skeletal growth is more lateral. Males increase their shoulder width through growth of the clavicle (one of the last bones to stop growing), and females increase width of the pelvis, which differentially becomes wider, shallower, and roomier (presumably for child-bearing). • Facial features become more prominent as the profile becomes more mature with the nose more projecting.
Skeletal maximum growth (Note: Skeletal growth also occurs more rapidly in blacks than in whites.)	• Skeletal growth occurs earlier in females than in males. • Maximal skeletal growth occurs between ages 10 and 14 in females and ages 12 and 14 in males.	• Linear growth is complete. Lateral growth during the adolescent spurt is most evident.

Adapted from:
Kaywood K, Hetchell N. *Life Span Motor Development.* Champaign, Ill: Human Kinetics; 2001.
Linn JP, Brown JK, Walsh EG. Physiological maturation of muscles in childhood. *Lancet.* 1994;343:1386–1389.
Hay M, Levin M, Sondheimer J, Deterding R. *Current Pediatric Diagnosis and Treatment..* 17th ed. New York, NY: Lange Medical Books/McGraw Hill; 2005:4–5.

Typical Changes Associated With Aging in the Musculoskeletal System

MUSCLE STRENGTH

Muscle strength and postural alignment are critical to efficient and effective function in the older adult. Loss of isometric and dynamic strength has been documented in individuals as young as 50 to 59 years old.[4] The decline in strength is closely associated with age, loss of type II, fast twitch muscle fibers, and loss of muscle mass. Normal aging is characterized by loss of muscle mass (*sarcopenia*) and integrity of the skeletal system.[5] Changes in the aging musculoskeletal system can be compounded by physical inactivity. Generally, within 2 weeks of discontinuance of resistance training, more than 50% of the benefits gained are greatly diminished.[6] Not only can physical inactivity accelerate the physiologic decline that can be associated with aging, it can also hamper an individual's ability to cope with acute physiologic stressors.[7] If older persons are forced by illness or injury to spend days or weeks exclusively on bed rest, muscle strength as well as aerobic capacity swiftly decline. Following disuse due to injury or inactivity, muscle strength is lost at approximately twice the rate it takes to regain it.[8] Older women who do not exercise risk losing one-quarter pound of skeletal muscle per year from age 40 on.[9] Less muscle mass leads to increased rate of disability.[9]

The concept of threshold values for strength necessary for independent function is an interesting one. For example, there is a threshold value for quadriceps strength necessary to rise from a chair or toilet seat.[10] At worst, when deterioration of function prevents an older adult from carrying out essential daily activities independently, professional assistance either in the home or a care center is warranted. On the other hand, a small strength gain may translate to a considerable functional improvement. For example, an increase in muscle strength that allows one to transfer independently can make a substantial difference in quality of life, not to mention residential setting. When strength increases are achieved by previously deconditioned older adults, there is a corresponding improvement in physical function.[11] Numerous studies have suggested that loss of muscle strength may be slowed or reversed with progressive resistive exercise programs. For example, healthy older adults trained for 12 weeks using a universal gym experienced a 109% increase in their 1RM (repetition max).[12] Frail elders living in long-term care participated in a strengthening program 3 times per week, resulting in a 174% increase in strength and a 9% increase in muscle mass. Even less "strenuous" exercise programs have resulted in modest gains in strength in a variety of older adult populations.[13] Though loss of muscle strength appears typical in the older adult, regular strength training has been shown to minimize and, in some instances, reverse this common change associated with aging. Physical therapists are well-equipped to screen for muscle strength in the older adult and make recommendations related to specific exercise programs to address weakness in all muscle groups.

Skeletal System

Age-related bone density differs from site to site. More peripheral sites, such as the radius, experience relative stability in density until menopause, while more central skeletal structure, such as the neck of the femur, show bone loss 5 to 10 years earlier.[14] Recent research has demonstrated that bone loss may be reversed in men and women age 65 years and older. Researchers gave 500 mg of calcium and 700 International Units (IU) of vitamin D to both women and men more than 65 years of age. These individuals were also receiving calcium in their diets. At the end of 3 years, participants had a 3% increase in hip bone mineral density. More importantly, fractures were prevented. Weight-bearing exercise has also been found to minimize bone loss and, in some instances, halt the decrease on bone density commonly seen with advancing age.[15] Though decreases in bone density appear to be common in the older adult population, some research suggests that this trend can be reversed with appropriate nutritional/dietary changes and exercise. Loss of joint fluid commonly associated with aging also adds to the "wear and tear" on the joint. Joint changes seem almost "inevitable" with advanced age, and in fact, osteoarthritis is one of the conditions nearly all 100-year-old persons develop.[16] There appears to be support for the fact that, over time, wear and tear on the joints will result in some changes. Exercise and activity that promote optimal postural alignment and strength assist in suppressing the occurrence of these changes until very late in life.

Postural Changes

Changes associated with the spine are the primary reason behind the postural changes typically noted in the older adult. With aging, the intervertebral discs essentially lose water and undergo other deleterious changes on a cellular level. At the same time as the intervertebral discs are flattening, the bones of the spine become more porous. This accounts for loss of disc height and compression of the spinal column and, hence, the inevitable height loss for all older adults. Spinal compression, combined with decrease in strength of intrascapular muscles and gradual wedging of the thoracic vertebrae are contributing factors in increased thoracic spine *kyphosis* (rounding of the shoulders with a forward lean), commonly seen in the elderly.

Ergonomics: Prevention Practice in Adulthood

Ergonomics is the field of study devoted to how work is done, especially in terms of body position, motion, and equipment used in the workplace.[17] Ergonomics encompasses changes in job processes and equipment to allow for pain-free work.

A certain amount of fatigue is normal at the end of a physically demanding work day. Usually, normal fatigue dissipates with adequate rest. Fatigue or pain that is always present is a warning sign that an injury will probably or has already occurred. These types of warning signs are typical of injuries contributed to by less than sound ergonomic practices. Physical therapists have long been treating repetitive use injuries and addressing job-related injuries. However, the term "ergonomics" has not always been applied to this type of work. As is the case for other venues of physical therapy education/clinical work, ergonomics is not solely addressed by physical therapists. Exercise physiologists, occupational therapists, occupational safety "specialists," and specially trained businesspersons are among the professionals who may see clients or employees with work-related injury and/or pain problems. The main certification presently available, Certified Professional Ergonomist, is obtained from the Board Certification in Professional Ergonomics (BCPE), a nonprofit organization established in 1990.[17]

In the United States, the Occupational Health and Safety Administration (OSHA) is responsible for regulations of the workplace, ensuring the welfare of workers. OSHA's responsibilities include enforcing the laws governing employee safety and providing information to employers about how to interpret workplace legislation. Educational Resource Centers that are operated by the National Institute for Occupational Safety and Health furnish training and outreach services. Regional offices of OSHA also may be contacted regarding their free consultation services on ergonomic problems.

Especially in light of the ever-increasing use of computers and automated processes in the workplace and the home, it behooves physical therapists to apply principles of ideal posture and body mechanics to both educate people about injury prevention and to determine whether work spaces are configured properly to avoid strain or stress. The goal of an ergonomics program or an individual ergonomic assessment is to reduce *musculoskeletal disorders (MDs)* or what now may be termed *cumulative trauma injuries (CTIs)*. CTIs are caused by too frequent, uninterrupted, repetitions of an activity or motion, unnatural or awkward motions such as twisting the arm or wrist, overexertion, incorrect and sustained postures, or muscle fatigue. CTIs occur most commonly in the hands, wrists, elbows, and shoulders but are also present in the neck, back, hips, knees, feet, legs, and ankles.[18] These disorders are characterized by pain, tingling, numbness due in part to the end-range strains applied to the tissue, visible swelling or redness of the affected area, and the eventual loss of flexibility and strength. Over time, CTIs can cause temporary or permanent damage to the soft tissues in the body, such as the muscles, nerves, tendons, and ligaments, and compression of nerves or tissue. In addition, CTIs affect individuals who perform mechanical loading of tissues in a repetitive, imbalanced fashion. These clients typically perform such work-related tasks as assembly line work, meat packing, sewing, playing musical instruments, and computer work. The disorders may also affect individuals who engage in recreational activities, such as gardening and tennis.[18] CTIs may be precipitated by problems in three major areas: (1) posture, (2) repetitive motion, and (3) force or pressure (including vibration). To further expand on the three main causes of CTIs, posture may induce pain/stiffness when a position is either awkward or has to be maintained for a long duration. Some posture problems or challenges may be created by repeated twisting, bending, kneeling, reaching, or having to carry out motions with arms overhead. Repetitive motions occur a number of ways, such as from continual typing at a computer, working steadily on an assembly line, or doing a monotonous stocking job.

Muscles and tendons are especially stressed with repetitive motion, with severity of potential risk dependent on the frequency of the motion, its speed, and requisite force. Force or pressure exerted to complete a certain activity or job can involve sustained muscle contractions, application of pressure over long durations repeatedly, or having to hold onto vibrating equipment and maneuver it. Force is a factor in tasks such as heavy lifting but also controlling equipment or tools that are not necessarily heavy but require a precision grip. Even innocent things such as how a person sleeps and moves during exercise may play a role in CTIs. As is true for most physical and mental health issues, there is quite a wide variation in both capacity to perform work and one's ability to respond to external work factors. This variation is a composite result of factors such as gender, age, lifestyle, physique, and individual strength and flexibility.

One of the most common repetitive use injuries affecting the upper extremity is *carpal tunnel syndrome*.[19] This is a condition involving compression of the median nerve caused by swelling tendons in the carpal tunnel. The tunnel is bounded by the transverse carpal ligament on the palmar surface and the carpal bones on the dorsal surface. As a result or poor wrist position and/or repetitive motion, the tendons or the tendon sheath running through this tunnel may become inflamed. A common mechanism of injury is sustained flexion or extension while typing for many hours of the day. A preferred position is the wrist in neutral as much as possible. Signs may include *anesthesia* (numbness), *paresthesia* (tingling), pain, and increased temperature sensitivity. Too much pressure on the median nerve can limit movement and sensation in the thumb and fingers. Symptoms reported may be dropping things due to decreased strength/control, pain at night, and stiffness similar to osteoarthritis.

A *herniated spinal disk* is a condition in which part or all of the soft, gelatinous central portion of an intervertebral disk (the *nucleus pulposus*) is forced through a weakened part of the disk, resulting in back pain and leg pain caused by nerve root irritation.[19] A herniated spinal disk may also be referred to as a *ruptured disk, lumbar radiculopathy* (pain in the low back region), *cervical radiculopathy* (pain in the neck region), *a prolapsed intervertebral disk*, or a *slipped disk*.[19] *Tension neck* syndrome, also known as *costoscapular syndrome*, is characterized by muscle tightness, palpable hardening, and tender spots with pain on resisted neck lateral flexion and rotation.[19] *Sciatica* is a term used to describe pain along the sciatic nerve, a nerve that runs along the back of the leg.[19] When this nerve is irritated; it can result in decreased ability to flex the knee; decreased ability to move the foot and toes in certain directions; numbness, burning, or tingling in the leg; and pain in the lower back that may travel to the back of the thigh and calf.

Epicondylitis is a painful inflammatory condition of the muscles and soft tissues around an epicondyle or bony prominence.[19] "Tennis elbow" refers to lateral epicondylitis of the humerus and is characterized by elbow pain that gradually worsens, pain radiating from the outside of the elbow to the forearm and back of the hand when grasping or twisting, and a weakened grasp. This condition can result from any type of overuse of the upper extremity.[19]

Hand-arm vibration syndrome has also been referred to as *vibration-induced white finger, traumatic vasospastic disease, dead fingers,* and *spastic anemia.* It is a chronic and progressive disorder, which affects the vascular, sensor neural, and musculoskeletal structures of the hand. It can result in permanent, painful numbness and tingling in the finger and hands, damage to bones in hands and arms, painful joints, and muscle weakness. Prevalence increases with increasing exposure time and vibration intensity.[20]

Finally, CTIs can be very costly to treat and debilitating for the worker; work site evaluation with the goal of injury prevention is an efficient intervention approach and will be discussed later in the chapter. Potential costs avoided are not simply those of medical treatment and possible hospitalization but also worker's compensation benefits, the indefinite cost of disability, and replacement cost of a worker not able to do his or her customary job. Those on the business side of the workforce are concerned with implementation for an ergonomics program or work site improvement and medical management of injuries that do occur.

Prevention Practice for Back Pain and Back Injuries

Close to 35% of the population in the United States has musculoskeletal symptoms and impairments, with back pain being the most likely area of complaint.[21] The prevalence of low back pain tends to increase with age, reaching 50% in people over age 60.[21] A strong etiological factor in the occurrence of low back pain and extremity pain is repetitive motion. Back pain and back injuries are the most common CTIs. As the term implies, most back injuries are not caused by a single event but rather the *cumulative* effect of poor body mechanics or external factors imposing repetitive posture problems, force, or pressure. Keeping the back in anatomical position (natural curves) is best for spine health. Natural curves can be viewed as a concave "C" for the cervical and lumbar regions, and a convex "C" for the thoracic region. Lifting heavy objects while twisting is probably the most dangerous motion as far as injuries go. In general, lifting rather than pulling or pushing objects may be a potential problem. Weight that has to be moved with arms overhead is also dangerous, particularly with respect to spinal compression. Standing for the day or the shift, particularly when on concrete or surfaces equally unforgiving, such as tile, can cause lower back pain. That pain may be induced by not only the hard surface of the floor but by poor job design with infrequent changes in position. For less physically demanding jobs, posture while sitting or standing is equally important to prevent upper back and neck pain. Especially when typing or viewing a computer screen much of the day, it is important for the terminal to be at a height where the neck is in a neutral position and the keyboard is placed so the wrist is neutral position or slightly flexed, rather than extended. The work station should be neither too high nor too low.

Prevention Practice Using Screening Tools

To address the staggering number of clients with musculoskeletal symptomology due to repetitive motion or cumulative trauma, physical therapists must screen for impaired posture and improper arthrokinetics at adjacent joints, examine job analysis and redesign, assess ergonomic principles at home and work, and identify the psychosocial factors that complicate the care of the client with CTIs and potentially lead to chronic pain. Table 12-5 provides potential signs and symptoms of common work-related problems of the neck and upper extremities.

OSHA provides screening tools that address the major risk factors previously discussed: repetition, force, awkward or unnatural postures, and vibration.[18] General questions of the employee include items such as areas and level of pain, level of fatigue, and whether the fatigue is greater in one area of the body than another. If management permits, one approach for evaluating stresses and risk factors of a job involves replicating the physical job demands. This option may include photographing or videotaping people working as they customarily do for movement analysis and examination of the ergonomics.

TABLE 12-5

SYMPTOMS AND PHYSICAL SIGNS OF COMMON WORK-RELATED DISORDERS OF THE UPPER LIMB AND NECK

Common Disorders	*Signs and Symptoms*
De Quervain's teneosynovitis (irritation of the synovial membrane surrounding the tendon)	• Swelling secondary to inflammation caused by repetitive grasping, pinching, squeezing, or wringing of hands • Pain on the radial aspect of the hands related to irritation to the abductor pollicis longus and extensor pollicis longus tendons • Soreness on the thumb side of the forearm; pain may spread up the forearm or down into the wrist
Extensor tendinitis (inflamed tendon of the finger extensor)	• Pain on top of the hand near the wrist
Flexor tendinitis (inflamed tendon of the finger flexors)	• Pain in fingers, especially when gripping • Common with use of a computer mouse
Trigger finger (tendon becomes locked in the tendon sheath, resulting in thickening in the tendon and the formation of a nodule and/or thickening of the pulley ligament)	• May hear a "popping" sound as the tendon catches on the tendon sheath • Locking of finger in bent position • Clicking sensation when the finger or thumb is bent • Pain when the finger or thumb is bent; Pain usually occurs when the finger or thumb is bent and straightened • Tenderness usually at the bottom of the finger or thumb (where a nodule is formed)
Ganglionic cyst (a ruptured tendon sheath swells with synovial fluid, causing a bump)	• Bumps beneath the skin surface on top of the hand, above and inside the wrist, and around the nails and knuckles • Achiness and weakness of the hands
Lateral epicondylitis (also known as tennis elbow—tendon inflammation of the muscles attaching to the lateral epicondyle of the elbow [outer elbow])	• Inflammation of the tendon • Pain and tenderness at the lateral epicondyle (outside aspect of the elbow) that worsens with movements associated with wrist extension or holding objects with the wrist stiff • Pain when straightening arms or contracting them against resistance • Associated with desks that are too high
Medial epicondylitis (also known as golfer's elbow—tendon inflammation of the muscles attaching to the medial epicondyle of the elbow [inner elbow])	• Inflammation of the tendon • Tenderness and pain at the medical epicondyle made worse by flexing the arm
Rotator cuff tendinitis (inflammation of the shoulder tendons that rotate the arm inward/outward)	• Pain when reaching behind with arms in "winged" position • Often from keyboards that are too high • The most common shoulder tendon disorder
Carpal tunnel syndrome (compression and neuropathy of the median nerve inside of the carpal tunnel of the wrist)	• Pressure on the nerve causes numbness and tingling in thumb and fingers • Sleep interruption • Caused by excessive wrist and finger movement, like striking computer keys
Thoracic outlet syndrome (compression of the nerves and blood vessels between the neck and shoulder—the neurovascular bundle)	• Weakness, numbness, tingling, swelling, fatigue, or coldness of the arm and hand • May present in pain patterns in the wrist, neck, or shoulder
Guyon's tunnel syndrome (ulnar nerve compression as it passes through a tunnel in the wrist called Guyon's canal)	• Caused by overuse of the wrist, especially in tasks bending the wrist down (flexing) and out (ulnar deviation) or putting constant pressure on the palm

(continued)

TABLE 12-5 *(continued)*

SYMPTOMS AND PHYSICAL SIGNS OF COMMON WORK-RELATED DISORDERS OF THE UPPER LIMB AND NECK

Common Disorders	*Signs and Symptoms*
Vibration syndrome (also known as "white finger" and Raynaud's syndrome involving vasospasms to the hands and fingers causing intermittent blanching)	
Trapezius myositis/spasm (muscle inflammation from repetitive trauma and/or overexertion injury, may be caused by disk bulge or degenerative joint disease)	• Muscle guarding • Limited neck range of motion • Pain
Paraspinals/rhomboid/spasm (muscle inflammation from repetitive trauma and/or overexertion injury, may be caused by disk bulge or degenerative joint disease)	• Muscle guarding • Limited neck range of motion • Pain
Cervical radiculopathy (nerve root irritation by pressure from a bulging disk or by narrowing between vertebrae)	*Bulging Disk:* • Muscle spasm in the neck in the morning • Difficulty swallowing • Limited neck movement *Osteoarthritis:* • Neck and shoulder pain • Radiating pain in the arm • Numbness in an extremity • Muscle weakness

Adapted from lecture by Professor Alan Hedge on Work-Related Musculoskeletal Disorders at Cornell University, August 2005 and Environmental & Occupational Health & Safety Services.

Other tools for assessment include a scale to weigh items lifted or moved in some way and a dynamometer to measure grip strength.

Posture screening is a useful feedback mechanism for clients and, more importantly, a recognized tool to prevent the prolonged positioning in "poor" posture, leading to pain and dysfunction. Postural impairments can be performed by a quick test, the Matthias Posture Test (also known as the Alexander Technique), based on the principle that the mind and body form one continuous unit.[22] The theory contends that habits of poor posture result in many of the everyday aches and pains commonly experienced and are attributed to the imbalances created by the incorrect positioning of the head in relation to the neck and torso. Poor postural alignment results in inefficient or misplaced muscular effort and unnecessary muscle tension, diminishing both the physical health and the mental attitude of an individual.[22] To perform this quick screen, the therapist stands the client with feet and back placed against a wall and flexes their shoulders to 90 degrees, then holds the pose for 30 seconds. If clients have poor muscle control and inefficient postural responses, they begin to exhibit those patterns of poor posture during the 30 second standing trial.[22]

A more conventional postural screening technique, developed by Kendall, involves looking at each segment of the body responsible for posture and teases out the most common faults of each area.[23] Any position contributing to the increase in joint stress is termed *faulty posture* and is thought to cause excessive wearing of the articular surface of the joint. Excessive wearing of the joint results in (1) the production of *osteophytes* (projections of bone occurring at sites of cartilage degeneration near joints), (2) *traction spurs* (abnormal bone growths), (3) soft tissue stretch, and (4) weakening.[23]

TABLE 12-6

WORKPLACE SCREENING FOR MUSCULOSKELETAL RISK

Does your job require you to:

1. Repeatedly bend and twist your wrists?
2. Repeatedly twist your arm?
3. Repeatedly hold your elbows away from your body?
4. Repeatedly use a pinch grip?
5. Repeatedly reach behind your body?
6. Repeatedly reach or lift things above your body?
7. Repeatedly reach or lift items above shoulder-level?
8. Repeatedly use a tool that vibrates?
9. Repeatedly use your hand as a hammer?
10. Repeatedly twist or flex your body?
11. Repeatedly lift objects from below knee-level?
12. Repeatedly work with your neck bent?

How much time is spent in a static position?

How many hours are spent in front of a visual display terminal or computer?

How often does your job require you to perform this task?

Prevention Practice Using Job Analysis and Design

The National Institute for Occupational Safety and Health (NIOSH), the agency established to help assure safe and healthful working conditions for working men and women by providing research, information, education, and training in the field of occupational safety and health, recommends several ways to prevent cumulative trauma disorders and the sequelae from these repetitive motion disorders. The NIOSH outlines the primary mechanisms for secondary prevention of cumulative trauma disorders, including (1) redesigning tools, work stations, and job duties; (2) educating the employee regarding care of joints, proper lifting techniques, and posture; and (3) recommending that employees take frequent and scheduled breaks from static positioning.[24] NIOSH also recommends seven elements of an effective program for evaluating and addressing musculoskeletal concerns in an individual workplace:

1. Looking for signs of a potential musculoskeletal problem in the workplace, such as frequent worker reports of aches and pains or job tasks that require repetitive, forceful exertions
2. Showing management commitment in addressing possible problems and encouraging worker involvement in problem-solving activities
3. Offering training to expand management and worker ability to evaluate potential musculoskeletal problems
4. Gathering data to identify problematic conditions, using injury and illness logs, medical records, and job analyses
5. Identifying effective controls for tasks that pose a risk of musculoskeletal injury and evaluating various approaches to determine their effectiveness in injury prevention
6. Establishing health care management to emphasize the importance of early detection and treatment of musculoskeletal disorders
7. Minimizing risk factors for musculoskeletal disorders when planning new work processes and operations, as it is less costly to build than to redesign or retrofit later

Physical therapists may find it helpful to use a quick questionnaire to determine the likelihood for potential musculoskeletal problems in the workplace. The questionnaire should include the questions listed in Table 12-6.

After evaluating the work site and its potential for musculoskeletal problems, the redesign phase should begin. The redesign stage can be accomplished by recommending that the client's company have a qualified ergonomist or a qualified physical or occupational therapist perform a careful analysis of the risk factors in each job. Both worker input and input by the local union's Health and Safety Committee should be incorporated into this analysis. In addition, worker and union input is critical in developing the best redesign solutions. The physical therapist has available to him or her several ergonomic guidelines on lifting and materials-handling tasks to help them provide ranges of activity alterations at work. These guidelines are based on various biomechanical assumptions and theoretical equations to build a margin of safety for individuals who have to lift at work or perform repeated movements over prolonged periods of time.[25] When recommending activity modifications for clients who work, the clinician should obtain a written description of the physical demands of required job tasks. The nature and duration of limitations will depend on the clinical status of the patient and the physical requirements of the job. Activity modifications must be time-limited, clear to both patient and employer, and reviewed by the clinician on a regular basis. It is also helpful to establish activity goals, in consultation with the client and the employer when applicable. Such goals are particularly important for the small percentage of clients who are still not able to overcome activity intolerance after 1 to 2 months of symptoms.

The literature is rich with suggestions and discussion regarding physical ergonomics of the work area, the workstation, and potential modifications for both. Only recently has there been data supporting the importance of frequent breaks during the work day for employees and, especially, for those employees susceptible to cumulative trauma or repetitive motion disorders. The most significant factor associated with symptoms of CTIs was the length of time workers spent in a static position with unchanging postures (eg, keyboarding, prolonged standing activities).[26] An optimal work-rest schedule of 45 minute shift, 15 minute break is ideal when considering the viscoelastic deformation of the spine and the prevention of secondary changes from faulty posture changes.[26] Rest breaks decrease musculoskeletal soreness and discomfort, decrease levels of eyestrain and visual blurring, and slightly increase the work rate after rest breaks.[26,27] Scheduled breaks were found to be generally more effective than allowing the worker to take breaks on his or her own.[27] Rest breaks should be short and often to avoid fatigue. These are short breaks of perhaps only 5 to 10 seconds taken every 5 to 10 minutes of continuous use.[28] Activity modifications, including rest breaks and job redesign (based on principles of ergonomics) are important options for the clinician treating clients with repetitive motion disorders to reduce the impairment, functional limitations, and potential sequelae.

Prevention Practice by Screening for Psychosocial Factors Leading to Chronic Pain

Physical therapists are adept at examining clients for mechanical injury, faulty posture, and clinical manifestation of pathology but may not be as prepared to recognize the psychosocial factors contributing to these disorders. When a physical therapist performs the examination portion of an evaluation of persons with repetitive motion disorders, back pain from repetitive mechanical stress, or degenerative joint conditions, attention must be paid to psychological and socioeconomic problems in the individual's life. It has been commonly recognized that these nonphysical factors can complicate both assessment and treatment.[29] These nonphysical factors, such as emotional distress or low work satisfaction and depression, can affect an individual's symptoms and response to treatment. The physical therapist should question the client regarding sociodemographic indices, stressors, moderators in work and nonwork settings, psychological symptoms, attitudes about health care, and symptom reporting, as these are potential "extenders" of the client's initial complaints. Objective indices of *work characteristics* (lighting, job essentials, hours in static position, work site description) as well as *subjective work stressors* (such as psychological demands, decision latitude, work and social support, and job satisfaction) should be included in the initial history taking of a client with repetitive motion symptoms or chronic low back pain. The impact of these nonwork stressors, in addition to financial problems and social support, have a huge impact on patient functioning and outcomes and need to be screened.[29]

The Job Demand-Control-Support Model (D-C-S) has served as a research tool for several years to assess the interaction of two main dimensions in the work environment: *psychological demands* and *job control*.[30] Job control, also called decision latitude, includes two components: decision authority and skill discretion. These terms are further defined as *decision authority* (the workers' ability to make decisions on the job) and *skill discretion* (the breadth of skills used by the worker). Physical therapists have a high/high rating in their occupation when looking at decision authority and skill discretion compared with meatpackers or persons on assembly lines. According to the D-C-S model, the highest strain, most work-related injuries, and lowest job satisfaction arises in a work environment when demands are high, control is low, and social support is low.[30] The combination of job demand and job control determines stress ratings, while decision latitude predicted energy ratings on the job. In addition, social support is related to both stress and energy ratings. Stress ratings are significantly related to symptoms of shoulder, neck, and back pain. These findings indicate that perceived job stress, an employee's ability to control the environment by making decisions, and the latitude of those decisions have a direct effect on work-related injuries. These data raise the issue of the impact of job characteristics on workers' health in a specific work environment. The better understanding of the interactions between workers and their work conditions will be significant for reconstruction of the work environment, helping to improve productivity in industry and quality of life for workers.

Depression is by far the most common emotion associated with pain syndromes, particularly back pain. Major depression is thought to be four times greater in people with chronic back pain than in the

TABLE 12-7

PrimeMD Brief Patient Health Questionnaire

Patient Name: ______________________________

Today's Date: ______________________________

This questionnaire is an important part of providing you with the best health care possible. Your answers will help in understanding problems that you may have. Please answer every question to the best of your ability.

Over the last 2 weeks, how often have you been bothered by any of the following problems?	Not at all (1 pt)	Several days (2 pt)	More than half the days (3 pt)	Nearly every day (4 pt)
a. Little interest or pleasure in doing things				
b. Feeling down, depressed, or hopeless				
c. Trouble falling or staying asleep or sleeping too much				
d. Feeling tired or having little energy				
e. Poor appetite or overeating				
f. Feeling bad about yourself or that you are a failure or have let yourself or your family down				
g. Trouble concentrating on things, such as reading the newspaper or watching television				
h. Moving or speaking so slowly that other people could have noticed. Or the opposite—being so fidgety or restless that you have been moving around a lot more than usual				
i. Thoughts that you would be better off dead or of hurting yourself in some way				

Make a referral to a psychologist or other mental health professional for any client scoring greater than or equal to 12 points (at a minimum, 6 or more items of "several days" occurrences or 4 or more items of "more than half the time"). Note: PrimeMD attempts to differentiate diagnoses of Major Depressive Disorder and Other Depressive Disorder from normal bereavement, a history of a Manic Episode (Bipolar Disorder), and a physical disorder, medication, or other drug as the biological cause of the depressive symptoms

Signature: ______________________________

general population.[31] In research studies on depression in chronic low back pain clients seeking treatment at pain clinics, prevalence rates are even higher with 32% to 82% of clients showing some type of depression or depressive problem, with an average of 62%.[31] The rate of major depression increases in a linear fashion with greater pain severity.[32,33] Also, the combination of chronic pain and depression is associated with greater disability than either depression or chronic pain alone.[32] Given these staggering findings, it is imperative that physical therapists screen for depression in their populations with any pain syndrome. In a study examining the accuracy of physical therapists' screening for depressive symptoms in the clients with low back pain, the therapists did not accurately identify symptoms of depression, even symptoms of severe depression.[33] The examiners recommend that physical therapists managing clients with low back pain use the 2-item depression screening test featured in the PrimeMD patient health questionnaire (PHQ), as illustrated in Table 12-7. Administration of this screening test would improve physical therapists' ability to screen for symptoms of depression and would enable referral for appropriate management and potentially lessen the secondary effects from musculoskeletal conditions.

Summary

As experts in management of musculoskeletal conditions, physical therapists need to be aware of the changes in muscular and skeletal systems across the lifespan. This baseline knowledge serves as a foundation for providing optimal preventive care for children, adults, and older adults as they engage in work and leisure activities. Application of ergonomic principles combined with a background in biomechanics, kinesiology, and preventive care offers physical therapists an opportunity to reduce the high incidence of cumulative trauma injuries and back pain in the workplace. Chapter 19 provides additional information about how to manage a prevention practice business that focuses on corporate wellness.

References

1. APTA. *Guide to Physical Therapist Practice.* 2nd ed. Alexandria, Va: American Physical Therapy Association; 2001.
2. Sinclair D, Dangerfield P. *Human Growth After Birth.* 6th ed. New York, NY: Oxford University Press; 1998.
3. Scoliosis Research Society Terminology Committee. A glossary of scoliosis terms. *Spine.* 1976;1:57–58.
4. Brown M, Kern F, Barr J. How do we look? Functional aging within the physical therapy community. *J Geriatric Phys Ther.* 2003;26(2):17–21.
5. Carlson JE, Ostir GV, Black SA, Markides KS, Rudkin L, Goodwin JS. Disability in older adults 2: Physical activity as prevention. *Behavioral Medicine.* 1999;24(4):157–168.
6. Turner CH, Robling AG. Designing exercise regimens to increase bone strength. *Exerc Sports Sci Rev.* 2003;31:45–50.
7. Colcombe S, Kramer AF. Fitness effects on the cognitive function of older adults: a meta-analytic study. *Psychol Sci.* 2003;14(2):125–130.
8. Mazzeo RS, Cavanagh P, Evans WJ, et al. Exercise and physical activity for older adults—American College of Sports Medicine position stand. *Med Sci Sports Exerc.* 1998;30(6):992–1008.
9. Kohrt WM, Snead DB, Slatopolsku E, Birge SJ Jr. Additive effects of weight-bearing exercise and estrogen on bone mineral density in older women. *J Bone Miner Res.* 1995;10:1303–1311.
10. Jones CJ, Rikli RE, Beam WC. A 30-second chair-stand test as a measure of lower body strength in community-residing older adults. *Res Q Exerc Sport.* 1999;70(2),113–119.
11. Spirduso WW, Francis KL, MacRae PG. *Physical Dimensions of Aging.* 2nd ed. Champaign, Ill: Human Kinetics Publishers; 1995.
12. Stevenson JS, Topp R. Effects of moderate and low intensity long-term exercise by older adults. *Res Nurs Health.* 1990;13(4):209–218.
13. Brown M, Sincacore DR, Host HH. The relationship of strength to function in the older adult. *J Gerontol Biol Med Sci.* 1995;50:A55–A59.
14. Iwamoto J, Takeda T, Ichimura S. Effect of exercise training and detraining on bone mineral density in postmenopausal women with osteoporosis. *J Orthoped Sci.* 2001;6,128–132.
15. Turner CH, Robling AG. Designing exercise regimens to increase bone strength. *Exerc Sports Sci Rev.* 2003;31,45–50.
16. Ettinger WH Jr, Burns R, Messier SP, et al. A randomized trial comparing aerobic exercise and resistance exercise with a health education program in older adults with knee osteoarthritis. *J Gerontol Biol Med Sci.* 1997;54: M184–M190.
17. Board of Certification in Professional Ergonomics (BCPE). PO Box 2811, Bellingham, WA 98227-2811.
18. DHHS (NIOSH) Publication No. 83–110. National Institute for Occupational Safety and Health Publications Dissemination 4676 Columbia Parkway Cincinnati, Ohio: 45226 1998. 1-800-35-NIOSH.
19. Erdil M, Dickerson OB. *Cumulative Trauma Disorders—Prevention, Evaluation, Treatment.* New York, NY: Van Nostrand Reinhold; 1997.
20. Kumar S. *Biomechanics in Ergonomics.* London, England: Taylor and Francis; 1999.
21. Cunningham LS, Kelsey JL. Epidemiology of musculoskeletal impairments and associated disability. *Am J Public Health.* 1984;74(6):574–579.
22. Kodish B. *Back Pain Solutions.* Pasadena, Calif: Extensional Publishing; 2001.
23. Kendall F, McCreary E, Provance P, Rodgers M, Roman W. *Muscles Testing and Function with Posture and Pain.* Hagerstown, MD: Lippincott Williams and Wilkins; 2005.
24. DHHS (NIOSH) Publication No. 97–117. National Institute for Occupational Safety and Health Publications Dissemination. Cincinnati, Ohio: NIOSH; 19980.
25. Battachrya A. McGlothlin JD. *Occupational Ergonomics—Theory and Applications.* New York, NY: Marcel Dekker, Inc; 1996.
26. Green N. Breaks and micropauses—a survey of the literature. Internal Research Document for Niche Software Ltd; 1999.
27. Luczak H, Cakir A, Cakir G. Musculoskeletal disorder, visual fatigue and psychological stress of working with display units: current issues and research needs. Work With Display Units 92: *Proceedings of the Third International Scientific Conference on Work with Display Units.* Berlin, Germany: Technische Universitat; 1992:288–289.
28. Mclean L, Tingley M, Scott RN, Rickards J. Computer terminal work and the benefit of micro-breaks. *Appl Ergon.* 2001;32(3):225–237.
29. Stansfeld S, Tarasuk,V, Shannon H, Frand J. Studying psychosocial risk factors in the etiology and prognosis of low back pain 1: choice of variables. 1994.

30. Skov T, Borg V, Orhede E. Psychosocial and physical risk factors for musculoskeletal disorders of the neck, shoulders, and lower back in salespeople. *Occup Environ Med.* 1996;53(5):351–356.

31. Srunin L, Bodin LI. Family consequences of chronic back pain. *Social Sci Med.* 2004;58:1385–1893.

32. Sullivan MJ, Reesor K, Mikail S, Fisher R. The treatment of depression in chronic low back pain: review and recommendations. *Pain.* 1992;52:249.

33. Haggman S, Maher CG, Refshauge KM. Screening for symptoms of depression by physical therapists managing low back pain. *Phys Ther.* 2004;84:1157–1166.

Chapter 13

Prevention Practice for Cardiopulmonary Conditions

Amy Foley, DPT, PT; Gail Regan, PhD, PT; and Catherine Rush Thompson, PhD, MS, PT

"If you can't breathe, you can't function."

~ MARY MASSERY, PT, DPT

Cardiopulmonary pathologies affect millions of Americans. Recent statistics for the United States show that coronary heart disease is the single leading cause of death in America. Coronary artery disease causes *angina* (pains associated with poor heart circulation) and, ultimately, *heart attacks (myocardial infarctions)*. There are 1.2 million new and recurrent coronary attacks per year.[1] Over 13 million people (7.2 million males and 6.0 million females) suffer from angina, myocardial infarctions, or other forms of coronary artery disease. It should be noted that women often experience a more "silent" form of heart disease—one lacking significant angina or discomfort prior to myocardial infarction.[1]

Likewise, pulmonary pathology is nearly as prevalent in America. In 2001, chronic obstructive pulmonary disease (COPD) was the fourth leading cause of death in the United States, resulting in more than 118,000 deaths. More than 90% of these deaths were attributed to smoking.[2] Many cardiopulmonary diseases are preventable, and physical therapy plays a key role in prevention.

Cardiopulmonary conditions may be primary impairments or secondary complications resulting from ineffective preventive strategies for other pathologies. Heart disease, hypertension, hyperlipidemia, arteriosclerosis, coronary artery disease, congestive heart failure, peripheral vascular disease, bronchitis, asthma, and emphysema are all conditions impairing the cardiovascular and pulmonary systems. The physical therapy practice patterns for delivering all levels of primary, secondary, and tertiary care for patients with cardiopulmonary conditions include the following[3]:

- *6A:* Primary prevention/risk reduction for cardiovascular/pulmonary conditions
- *6B:* Impaired aerobic capacity/endurance associated with deconditioning
- *6C:* Impaired ventilation: respiratory exchange, and aerobic capacity/endurance
- *6D:* Impaired aerobic capacity/endurance associated with cardiovascular pump dysfunction or failure
- *6E:* Impaired ventilation and respiration/gas exchange associated with ventilatory pump dysfunction or failure
- *6F:* Impaired ventilation, and respiration/gas exchange associated with respiratory failure
- *6H:* Impaired circulation and anthropometric dimensions associated with lymphatic system disorders

These practice patterns provide patient/client management elements of examination, evaluation, diagnosis, prognosis, and intervention once a cardiopulmonary disease process has been identified. This chapter describes the physical therapist's role in the prevention of some of these disease states and their sequelae.

Changes in the Cardiopulmonary System Across the Lifespan

The cardiopulmonary system begins functioning as early as 4 months in utero and continues to function throughout the lifespan. During fetal development, the heart differentiates and enlarges, then begins beating at approximately 4 months gestational age.[4] Defects in the heart structure, such as atrial or ventricular septal defects, can reduce the efficiency of the heart and can potentially limit function early in life.

Typically, respiratory rate and pulse rates decline as a child matures into adulthood, while blood pressures concomitantly rise. The more forceful *myocardium* (heart muscle) uses more efficient contractions to deliver blood to the body, and finally, the resting heart rate of children over age 10 is comparable to the adult resting heart rate of 60 to 100 beats per minute. Beginning at approximately age 25, aerobic capacity generally begins to decline as one ages, but the rate of decline can be diminished through physical activity.[4] *Maximum ventilatory uptake* (the maximum amount of oxygen the body inhales) usually drops between 5% and 10% per decade between the ages of 20 and 80.[4] Aerobic capacity, as measured by maximal rate of oxygen consumption *(VO_2 max)*, declines with aging; however, the rate may be modulated by exercise training.

Decline in VO_2 max can be attributed to a decrease in maximum heart rate with aging and to decreased muscle mass and decreased muscle demands, requiring less oxygen. The metabolizing tissue that contributes to VO_2 max measurement is almost exclusively muscle tissue and, unless they exercise to preserve muscle mass and strength, older adults experience a gradual loss of both.[5] It appears that improving the lungs' functional capacity and functional reserve are keys to slowing the rate of decline of VO_2 max. Consistent physical activity over the course of one's life has been found to maintain ventilatory oxygen uptake at a higher level than in those who are inactive. In the absence of regular physical activity, there is an increased risk of cardiopulmonary pathology and generalized deconditioning over the lifespan. Additional factors contribute to pathologies of the cardiopulmonary system and should be identified to reduce the risk of disease.

Screening for Cardiopulmonary Conditions

The cardiopulmonary system should be screened through client observation and testing of vital signs. Chapter 5 discusses simple tools for screening an individual for potential pathology and the need for referral. Table 13-1 provides an overview of screening information for common cardiovascular and pulmonary pathologies and positive findings warranting special attention. For example, if an individual has general health problems and is not being seen regularly by a physician, a referral is warranted. If another individual has a chronic medical condition that is stable and under medical care, consultation for a prevention program is appropriate. If an individual is in general good health and has no health complaints, a prevention program should begin immediately through health education and advisement on appropriate physical activity.

A simple and informative way to assess the pulmonary system is the check the respiratory rate. Simply watching the rate of chest expansions or shoulder elevations while an individual is resting provides baseline values. Irregularities in respiratory rates not caused by imposed exercise or activity suggest a problem that may need medical attention. For example, infections, such as pneumonia, commonly present with elevated respiratory rates. In addition, the respiratory system should be screened for common pathologies, such as asthma. Individuals who present with chest pain, shortness of breath, a cough, or wheezing should receive a more comprehensive examination. Chronic smokers have an increased risk of developing lung, throat, and mouth cancers and should be examined more extensively for early detection. Other types of breathing problems may suggest either a respiratory or a cardiovascular problem.

Common Cardiovascular Pathologies

Heart Disease

Heart disease includes a wide variety of cardiac and vascular conditions affecting the entire body. Congenital heart disease is caused by abnormal heart development before birth and is responsible for more deaths in the first year of life than any other birth defects.[4] While there may be genetic factors contributing to congenital heart disease, prevention focuses on maternal health education to reduce risks associated

TABLE 13-1

SCREENING FOR CARDIOPULMONARY CONDITIONS

Screening Information	Resources Needed	Positive Findings
Family History Hypertension Hypotension Heart disease Pulmonary conditions Lifestyle behaviors of family, such as smoking	Screening form	History of congenital, genetic, or family heart or pulmonary conditions. Consider the possibility of second-hand smoke exposure.
Prior History of Individual History of pulmonary illness History of cardiac illness	Screening form	Note any history of congenital, genetic, or prior pulmonary conditions (eg, asthma).
Lifestyle Habits of Individual	Screening form	Note smoking, exercise, and diet information. Detail FITTE (frequency, intensity, types, time, and enjoyment of exercise).
Anthropometrics of Individual Body weight Body height Location of body fat		Check body mass index (BMI) for body composition. Note distribution of body fat, including presence of central obesity.
General Health of Individual Blood pressure Pulse Respiratory rate	Screening form Stethoscope Sphingmomanometer	Note evidence of fatigue, weakness, malaise, fever, or illness. Note measures of blood pressure, pulse, and/or respiration rates outside of age- and gender-matched norms.
Medication/Drugs	Screening form	Note use of any prescribed or over-the-counter medications or supplements.
Nose and Sinuses	Screening form Otoscope	Note nasal or sinus discharge, sinus pain, unusual and frequent colds, and/or changes in smell.
Mouth and Throat	Screening form Otoscope	Note any reports of pain, lesions or sores on the mouth or throat, and altered taste.
Neck	Screening form Palpation	Note pain, limitations in movement, lumps, swelling, tenderness, or discomfort.
Respiratory System	Screening form Auscultation	Note chest pain, shortness of breath, or cough wheezing.
Cardiovascular System	Screening form Auscultation	Note pain with or without exertion, dizziness when standing, and/or problems breathing while sleeping.
Peripheral Vascular System	Screening form Observation Auscultation	Note any coldness, numbness, tingling, or swelling of legs or hands, pain in the legs, discolored hands or feet, and/or varicose veins.

with drug use, alcohol consumption, and prescribed medicines.

Common heart diseases of adulthood include coronary artery disease, congestive heart failure, ischemic heart disease, rheumatic heart disease, and myocardial infarction. Approximately 22 million adults or 1 in 12 people had heart disease in the United States in the year 2000.[6]

According to one estimate from experts with the American Heart Association, the prevalence of heart disease in the United States may double by 2050.[1] Since heart disease is one of the primary preventable causes of death, a thorough screening of the cardiovascular system is essential during physical therapy management. Chest pain near the heart before, during, or after exercise warrants special attention. While diseases such as *pleurisy* (inflamed membranes around the lungs) and indigestion (often causing heartburn) may present with chest pain, this symptom is usually a cardinal sign of heart pathology. Another common symptom of cardiac pathology is dizziness when standing up, potentially due to inadequate venous return to the heart. *Orthostatic hypotension* (a condition associated with dizziness when changing position from lying to upright) may be caused by low blood pressure from other types of pathology as well.

While rheumatic heart disease is best prevented through infection control to reduce the incidence of rheumatic fever, other types of heart disease are more amenable to preventive practice. Unmodifiable factors contributing to this high prevalence rate, such as advanced age and a family history of early heart disease, should be noted along with modifiable risk factors that can be affected by preventive care, as listed in Table 13-2.

Individuals with a personal or family history of heart problems are particularly vulnerable to heart pathology. Heredity plays a major role in determining blood lipid profile and heart rate variability (two major risk factors for coronary artery disease). For Caucasians and African-Americans, lipid levels (high density [HDL] and low density lipoprotein [LDL] levels and triglycerides) are 60% to 80% determined by genetics.[1] Prevention of cardiopulmonary disease involves recognizing and addressing the greatest risk factors. According to a study at McMaster University with over 29,000 participants from 52 countries, cigarette smoking and an abnormal blood lipid profile are the two most important risk factors for myocardial infarction.[7] Other risk factors that contribute to heart disease include high blood pressure, diabetes, abdominal obesity, stress, lack of consumption of fruit and vegetables, and lack of regular exercise. Protective factors, on the other hand, include regular consumption of small amounts of alcohol. According to this study, more than 90% of heart attacks are predictable based on these risk factors. Additional symptoms that may suggest heart disease include problems with breathing when sleeping, fatigue, a racing heart rate, or feeling "winded" after exercise. Individuals complaining of these symptoms should have a more thorough medical examination before initiating a regular exercise program.

Suggested secondary prevention interventions include the following[7]:

- Controlling weight
- Eating a healthy, low saturated fat diet
- Quitting smoking
- Controlling diabetes
- Controlling blood pressure
- Controlling cholesterol
- Controlling homocysteine
- Taking antioxidants
- Considering the benefits and risks of hormone replacement therapy (HRT)
- Taking low-dose aspirin if you are a female. In a study of over 87,000 women, those taking low-dose aspirin were less likely to suffer a first heart attack than those without aspirin.[8] Women over age 50 appeared to benefit most. Aspirin, however, can increase the risk of getting ulcers, kidney disease, liver disease, and a hemorrhagic stroke, so this intervention should be supervised by the client's physician.
- Engaging in physical activity. Physical activity can indirectly decrease LDL levels, known to play a key role in the development of fatty depositions.[1] According to the Centers for Disease Control and Prevention, over 50% of Americans

TABLE 13-2

MODIFIABLE CONTRIBUTORS TO HEART DISEASE

- High blood pressure
- High blood cholesterol
- High LDL cholesterol
- Low HDL cholesterol
- Diabetes. Adults with diabetes have heart disease death rates about 2 to 4 times as high as those of adults without diabetes.
- Obesity
- Overweight
- Smoking
- Physical inactivity. Physical inactivity doubles the risk of heart disease.
- Apple-shaped body—worse than a "pear-shaped" body
- High blood homocysteine
- Atherosclerosis
- High fat diet
- High levels of stress
- Depression

Adapted from American Heart Association. Heart attack and angina statistics. Available at: http://www.americanheart.org/presenter.jhtml?identifier=4591. Accessed February 6, 2006.

do not engage in regular physical activity,[1] so physical therapists can advocate of increased physical activity levels across all populations to help decrease the incidence of cardiovascular disease. When the heart condition is stabilized, the training should continue outside the hospital. Suitable activities are daily walks, jogging, cycling, swimming, aerobics, and dance, depending on the individual's interest and physical condition. Even patients with chronic heart failure benefit from controlled physical training, leading to increased cardiovascular function, load tolerance, and muscular strength.[1]

- Using healthy interventions to manage stress. One study demonstrated that patients with stable ischemic heart disease who engaged in aerobic exercise and stress management training reduced emotional distress and cardiovascular risk more than usual medical care alone. One effective intervention included aerobic exercise training for 35 minutes 3 times per week for 16 weeks plus 1.5-hour stress management training for 16 weeks.[9]
- Reducing hostility. Younger patients with heart disease have a higher prevalence of hostility symptoms that adversely affect their condition.[9] Physical therapists should encourage younger patients who present with these symptoms to seek psychological counseling to reduce these symptoms and other psychological stressors contributing to their unhealthy condition.

HYPERTENSION

Hypertension (defined as a mean systolic blood pressure of 140 mm Hg and a mean diastolic blood pressure of 90 mm Hg or currently taking antihypertensive medication) is prevalent in 50 million Americans (ie, 1 of 5 people in the United States) with an additional 15 million Americans who are undiagnosed.[10] Increased prevalence rates are seen in adults who are overweight.[11] The prevalence for obese adults (body mass index [BMI] 30) is 38.4% for men and 32.2% for women.[11] Compounding factors of obesity and metabolic disorders can put patients with hypertension at increased risk for more serious pathologies, such as coronary artery disease or enlargement of the heart's left ventricle.

Desired exercise includes regular aerobic physical activity, preferably at least 2 to 3 times per week for approximately 1 hour, while carefully keeping a regular heart rate of 70% to 85% of the theoretic age-related maximum rate.[1] According to the American Heart Association, "Physical inactivity is a major risk factor for developing coronary artery disease. It also increases the risk of stroke and such other major risk factors as obesity, high blood pressure, low HDL ("good") cholesterol, and diabetes." The American Heart Association recommends a daily combination of moderate and vigorous physical activity for both children and adults: "Specifically, we recommend a total of 30 minutes of moderate-intensity activities on most days of the week and a minimum of 30 minutes of vigorous physical activity at least 3 to 4 days each week to achieve cardiovascular fitness."[1] In addition, clients should discontinue or at least sharply reduce cigarette smoking, possibly replacing it with pipe smoking. All of these measures combined are effective in reducing tensive values in most patients.

Nonpharmacological measures to control hypertension, especially those who are borderline or mildly hypertensive, include a combination of diet and lifestyle changes. Other measures, such as reduced coffee consumption to a maximum of two cups per day; increased intake of potassium, calcium, or magnesium-rich substances (ie, some types of fruits and legumes and hard mineral water); increased intake of polyunsaturated fats (mainly contained in white meat and sea fish); and a reduced saturated-fat intake (mainly due to all animal-derived products) may also prove beneficial.

Obese patients can benefit from weight loss, and those consuming alcohol can reduce their intake to the recommended 20 to 30 gm per day. A diet that is low sodium (a maximum 5 gm of sodium chloride per day), low calorie, and high fiber (at least 30 gm per day including 50% of soluble and 50% of insoluble fibers) is also recommended. The control of associated diabetes by means of dietary and therapeutic measures represent another related measure required for both male and female hypertensive patients. Discontinuing of any estroprogestinic contraceptive treatments is also required for female patients. ACE-inhibitors and calcium antagonists appear to be the drugs of choice, since they may also positively affect the development of vascular plaques as well as reduce the left ventricular mass, which may influence the outcome for hypertensive patients.[12]

Physical therapists should work closely with their physicians, dietitians, and other health professionals to ensure that optimal prevention includes dietary, behavioral, and medical considerations. Whenever mild pressure increases are not monitored, arterial pressure values are very likely to shift from moderate to considerably high in the relatively short term.

HYPERLIPIDEMIA

Hyperlipidemia is an increase in the blood levels of triglycerides and cholesterol that can lead to cardiovascular disease and other chronic pathologies. An estimated 101 million Americans have cholesterol greater to or equal to 200 mg/dL; in other words, one in three Americans have hyperlipidemia.[13] It has been shown that patients aged 65 to 75 years can benefit from intervention at least as much as younger patients.[17] Despite the clear demonstration that lowering LDL cholesterol improves cardiovascular risk, most adults who are eligible for cholesterol-lowering therapy do not receive it, including over half of those who qualify for drug therapy.[13] Lipid-lowering therapy can prevent cardiovascular mortality and morbidity for patients with known coronary artery disease and type II diabetes.[13] Risk factors for hyperlipidemia include fatty diets, diabetes, hypothyroidism, Cushing's syndrome, kidney failure, certain medications (including birth control pills, estrogen, corticosteroids, certain diuretics, and beta-blockers), and lifestyle factors (including habitual, excessive alcohol use and lack of exercise, leading to obesity). Physical therapists working with individuals diagnosed with hyperlipidemia should encourage their clients to seek pharmacological management of this condition to complement nonpharmacological interventions, including screening for risk factors and providing education on disease and diet.

While eating a healthy diet and following the American Heart Association exercise guidelines for healthy populations can affect hyperlipidemia, one study demonstrated that intense lifestyle interventions are more effective for improving not only blood lipids but also other risk factors and the individual's quality of life. In one study, more intense supervised aerobic exercise as opposed to unsupervised exercise increased the participants' exercise capacity (1.6 to 1.9 METS), reduced body weight by 10%, and reduced LDL by 7.6%.[14] Physical therapists can play a key role in secondary prevention by ensuring that sufficiently aggressive exercise training is coupled with a diet recommended by a registered dietitian and appropriate medical intervention. Not only can clients with hyperlipidemia reduce their cholesterol, they can also increase their exercise capacity, lower their blood pressure, and lose weight, further reducing risk for pathology.

Arteriosclerosis

Arteriosclerosis is used to describe several diseases characterized by the loss of elasticity and thickening of the arterial wall. The arteriosclerotic damage of the arterial endothelium is initiated by risk factors like dyslipidemia, hypertension, diabetes mellitus, and smoking, which account for the majority of vascular morbidity and mortality.[15] Since arteries supply the body with needed nourishment, vascular diseases caused by arteriosclerosis can affect all vital organs and ultimately lead to death. Coronary artery disease is an example of pathology resulting from arteriosclerotic processes affecting the myocardium. In the same manner, all body systems are vulnerable to arteriosclerosis, including the brain and peripheral vascular system. Atherosclerosis, a form of arteriosclerosis, is the most common vascular disease. Atherosclerosis is characterized by the deposition of plaques containing cholesterol and lipids on the innermost layer of the walls of large and medium-sized arteries. The deposition of plaques narrows the vessels, potentially leading to hypertension and impaired blood flow. The same lifestyle changes needed to prevent heart disease and hypertension can be employed to reduce the risk of arteriosclerosis.

Peripheral Vascular Disease

People aged 50 or older who have diabetes, smoke, have high blood pressure, or have high cholesterol levels are at risk for peripheral vascular disease (PVD) or damage to their peripheral vascular system impairing normal blood circulation.[16] PVD is a highly treatable disease in its early stages and can often be detected by the appearance of the extremities. The hands or feet may appear swollen or may be discolored. The individual may complain of coldness, numbness, tingling, or pain. Often individuals will report a family history of vascular problems or will have evidence of varicose veins ("spider veins") prominent on their legs. Bruises and other skin discolorations may also be attributed to peripheral vascular pathology. PVD can be an early warning sign of a potential heart attack, stroke, or aneurysm, so individuals presenting with these clinical manifestations should be examined and followed by a physician.

Most people with PVD can be treated with lifestyle changes, medications, or both. Lifestyle changes are the same listed as modifiable risk factors for heart disease. These lifestyle changes can be augmented by medications to improve vascular flow, antiplatelet drugs to slow blood clotting, and cholesterol-lowering agents (statins).[16] See Table 13-3 for examples of common cardiovascular pathologies and risk factors.

Common Pulmonary Pathologies

Sudden Infant Death Syndrome

Sudden infant death is the sudden, inexplicable death of an infant under the age of one.[17] While the Back to Sleep campaign urging parents to put their infants to sleep on their backs has reduced the

TABLE 13-3

EXAMPLES OF COMMON CARDIOVASCULAR PATHOLOGIES AND RISK FACTORS

Life Span	Pathology	Modifiable Risk Factors	Prevention
Childhood	Congenital heart disease	Maternal health	Health education
Adulthood and older adulthood	Heart disease (including coronary artery disease, congestive heart failure, ischemic heart disease, rheumatic heart disease, and myocardial infarction)	Sedentary lifestyle, smoking, poor diet	Exercise, smoking cessation, diet modification, stress management
	Heart disease (rheumatic heart disease)	Prevent rheumatic fever	Education for infection control
	Hypertension	Sedentary lifestyle, smoking, poor diet	Exercise, smoking cessation, diet modification, stress management
	Hyperlipidemia	Sedentary lifestyle, smoking, poor diet, excessive and habitual alcohol use, certain medications	Exercise, reduce alcohol consumption, diet modification, medical management
	Arteriosclerosis	Hyperlipidemia, hypertension, diabetes mellitus, smoking	Exercise, smoking cessation, diet modification, stress management
	Peripheral vascular disease	Hyperlipidemia, hypertension, diabetes mellitus, smoking	Exercise, smoking cessation, diet modification, stress management
	Heart disease (myocardial infarction, congestive heart failure)	Sedentary lifestyle, smoking, poor diet	Exercise, smoking cessation, diet modification, stress management

incidence of this syndrome, thousands of babies in the United States die from this condition. Risk factors for this condition include the following[17]:

- Babies who sleep on their stomachs
- Babies who have soft bedding in the crib
- Multiple birth babies
- Premature babies
- Babies with a sibling who had sudden infant death syndrome (SIDS)
- Mothers who smoke or use illegal drugs
- Teen mothers
- Short intervals between pregnancies
- Late or no prenatal care
- Situations of poverty

The American Academy of Pediatrics (AAP) provided the following recommendations for preventing SIDS[18]:

- Always put a baby to sleep on its back. Allowing the baby to roll around on its tummy while awake can prevent a flat spot (due to sleeping in one position) from forming on the back of the head.
- Only put babies to sleep in a crib. NEVER allow the baby to sleep in bed with other children or adults, and do NOT put them to sleep on surfaces other than cribs, like a sofa.
- Let babies sleep in the same room (NOT the same bed) as parents. If possible, babies' cribs should be placed in the parents' bedroom to allow for nighttime feeding.
- Avoid soft bedding materials. Babies should be placed on a firm, tight-fitting crib mattress with no comforter. Use a light sheet to cover the baby. Do not use pillows, comforters, or quilts.
- Make sure the room temperature is not too hot. The room temperature should be comfortable

for a lightly clothed adult. A baby should not be hot to the touch.

- Let the baby sleep with a pacifier. Pacifiers at nap time and bedtime can reduce the risk of SIDS. Doctors think that a pacifier might allow the airway to open more, or prevent the baby from falling into a deep sleep. A baby that wakes up more easily may automatically move out of a dangerous position. However, do not force the infant to use a pacifier. Although pacifier use has been associated with dental problems and breast-feeding difficulties, researchers say the potential benefit (decreased SIDS risk) outweighs the risks. The AAP says that one SIDS death could be prevented for every 2,733 babies who suck on a pacifier during sleep.[18]
- Do not use breathing monitors or products marketed as ways to reduce SIDS. In the past, home apnea (breathing) monitors were recommended for families with a history of the condition. However, research found that they had no effect, and the use of home monitors has largely stopped.

ASTHMA

Asthma is a chronic inflammatory pulmonary disorder characterized by reversible obstruction of the airways seen in nearly 7% of the population of the United States, including 12 million adults and 8 million children.[19] Annually, approximately 5,000 deaths are related to asthmatic attacks.[19] Almost all asthma patients can become free of symptoms with proper treatment. Removal of asthma triggers, as described in Chapter 6, can help reduce the incidence of asthma. For adults, workplace irritants need to be determined as well as home-based triggers of asthmatic reactions. Various products are available to help reduce the allergens in the individual's environment; these items include specialized bedding, water filtration, air filtration, and mold control product. The use of bronchodilators and exercise is also recommended.

While breathing exercises may not result in significant reduction of bronchospasms, they contribute to improved quality of life. According to a study in the *Cochrane Database Systematic Review*[20]:

> *Two studies demonstrated significant reductions in rescue bronchodilator use, three studies showed reductions in acute exacerbations, and two single studies showed significant improvements in quality of life measures. Overall, benefits of breathing exercises were found in isolated outcome measures in single studies.*

Swimming is one type of exercise that is beneficial and has been shown to be less asthmogenic than other forms of exercise.[21] Exercise programs, featuring whole-body exercise training and local resistance training, have resulted in significant changes in perceived dyspnea and fatigue, utilization of health care resources, exercise performance, and health-related quality of life.[21]

For children who have asthma, the family should be advised to reduce or eliminate the triggers of asthma symptoms. Educating parents about recognized methods to address asthma triggers may help families use more effective measures. These triggers include airborne allergens; upper respiratory tract infections; smoke and other lung irritants; cold, dry air; intense emotional expressions; endocrine factors (menstrual cycle and thyroid disease); and various types of medications (eg, aspirin and other nonsteroidal anti-inflammatory drugs and beta-blockers).[21]

SLEEP APNEA

Sleep apnea is a common breathing problem that occurs while lying down. Sleep apnea is defined as the cessation of breathing for 10 or more seconds during sleep.[22] Consequences of sleep apnea range from simple annoyance to life threatening. A thorough medical examination is warranted if sleep apnea is suspected.

Early recognition and treatment of sleep apnea is important because it may be associated with irregular heartbeat, high blood pressure, heart attack, and stroke. According to the National Sleep Foundation, nearly 18 million Americans have sleep apnea, 4% being middle-aged men and 2% being middle-aged women.[23] These individuals may complain of excessive daytime sleepiness, problems with their weight, high blood pressure, loud snoring, or possible obstructions in their airways. They may have additional symptoms including depression, irritability, sexual dysfunction, learning problems, and memory difficulties as well as falling asleep while at work, on the phone, or driving because of their excessive sleepiness. Obese patients with sleep apnea are at increased risk of death, so patients with possible sleep apnea, especially those with obesity, should be referred for a more extensive examination of their sleep problems.

Prevention of sleep apnea includes reducing risk factors that commonly cause the problem, including use of alcohol, excess body weight, smoking, and congestion. Recommended prevention measures for sleep apnea also include the following[22]:

- Avoiding the use of sedatives that can relax throat muscles and slow breathing and antihistamines that cause drowsiness. Decongestants can decrease drainage from colds or allergies without increasing sleep apnea.
- Changing sleeping posture to sidelying with pillows between the knees.

- Raising the head of the bed by 6 inches to reduce respiratory efforts.

Chronic Obstructive Pulmonary Disease

COPD, also known as chronic obstructive lung disease and chronic obstructive airway disease, is the fourth leading cause of death and is expected to be the third leading cause of death by 2020.[24] Primarily resulting from smoking, the condition is associated with *emphysema* (damaged lung alveoli or air sacs become enlarged as they lose elasticity for ventilation), *chronic bronchitis* (excess mucus in large airways), and *obstructive bronchitis* (small airway obstruction, inflammation, and fibrosis). The early stages of COPD are asymptomatic, but severe cases can lead to death. In addition to smoking, risk factors for COPD include genetic predisposition, premature birth, deficiency of antioxidants (vitamins A, C, and E) in diet, exposure to vehicle fumes, industrial pollution, and bacterial or viral infection in young children. It is estimated that biomass fuels contribute to 40,000 deaths annually.[25] These same risk factors contribute to lung cancer and emphysema.

Generally, individuals with COPD are not seen until the individual is symptomatic with changes in chest shape to increase lung efficiency (a barrel-shaped chest evolves over time), *dyspnea* or difficulty breathing (also known as shortness of breath [SOB]), and coughing. As the disease progresses, chronic coughing may develop, and the individual may become *cyanotic* (bluish coloring, especially of the skin, lips, and nail beds, as the body copes with lung inefficiency). Physical therapists should alert their clients to see a physician for changes in chronic coughing or a new cough. In addition, individuals should be encouraged to change lifestyle habits incompatible with their health, including smoking and working in areas filled with vehicle fumes or other industrial pollutants.

Patients with COPD frequently exhibit physiologic and psychological impairments, such as dyspnea, peripheral muscle weakness, exercise intolerance, decreased *health-related quality of life (HRQOL)*, and emotional distress. Aerobic exercise, such as walking, should be strongly advocated for improving health and quality of life. In one study, patients with chronic obstructive lung disease, using a bronchodilator in combination with pulmonary rehabilitation, improved treadmill walking endurance and health status. Improved ventilation from *bronchodilation* (opening of the airways) enhanced the individuals' ability to perform ambulation and increase exercise tolerance. Improvements with the bronchodilation medication were sustained for 3 months following pulmonary rehabilitation completion. In the National Emphysema Treatment Trial, individuals engaged in a rehabilitation program increased their scores on the 6-minute walk distance and their quality of life measures.[26]

Pneumonia

Pneumonia (an inflammation or infection of the lung) is commonly caused by lung infection or aspiration of food into the lung and oftentimes develops as a secondary complication in individuals who have restrictive or obstructive lung diseases and difficulties with pulmonary hygiene.[26] Ideally, infectious pneumonia is prevented through proper infection control with individuals infected with pneumonia and with others at risk for infection, such as immunosuppressed and elderly patients. The physical therapist may recommend extra vigilant behaviors to the client with COPD in order to avoid community-acquired pneumoniae. Pneumonia may present as a high fever, shaking chills, and a cough with sputum production or very gradually with a worsening cough, headaches, and muscle aches.

Tuberculosis

Pulmonary tuberculosis (TB) is a contagious bacterial infection caused by inhaling droplets sprayed into the air from a cough or sneeze by an infected person. TB is a preventable disease, even in those who have been exposed to an infected person. Skin testing (PPD) for TB is used in high-risk populations or in individuals who may have been exposed to TB, such as health care workers.[27] Pulmonary impairments associated with TB include localized pulmonary signs, such as coughing up phlegm or blood, wheezing, chest pain, and difficulty breathing, and systemic signs, such as fever, fatigue, excessive sweating at night, and weight loss. See Table 13-4.

As with all infectious conditions, infection control is the most appropriate method of preventing the spread of disease. The Centers for Disease Control and Prevention offers a helpful website listing the infectious diseases that may be transmitted and/or acquired in health care settings (see Appendix C).[28]

Summary

As members of the health care team, physical therapists play a key role in identifying risk factors for persons with cardiopulmonary conditions and disease states. It is incumbent on physical therapists to employ strategies to promote health and wellness and prevent secondary complications from cardiopulmonary conditions through screening that adequately

TABLE 13-4

EXAMPLES OF COMMON PULMONARY PATHOLOGIES AND RISK FACTORS

Life Span	Pathology	Modifiable Risk Factors	Prevention
*Infancy**	Sudden infant death	Positioning prone while sleeping, loose bedding	Back to Sleep program augmented by prone to play
Childhood	Asthma	Environmental triggers, emotional stress, infections	Removal of triggers, stress management, infection control
Adulthood and Older Adulthood	Sleep apnea	Obesity, sleeping on back, antihistamines for colds and allergies	Weight loss, sleeping on side, decongestants for colds and allergies
	Lung cancer	Smoking, occupational exposure	Smoking cessation, protective gear to reduce inhalation of toxins
	Chronic obstructive pulmonary diseases (bronchitis and emphysema)	Smoking	Smoking cessation
	Pneumonia Tuberculosis	Exposure to infection	Infection control

*Adapted from Dewey C, Fleming P, Golding J, ALSPAC Study Team. Does the supine sleeping position have any adverse effects on the child? II. Development in the first 18 months. *Pediatrics.* 1998;101(1):e5. Available at: http://www.pediatrics.org/cgi/content/full/101/1/e5. Accessed October 15, 2005.

assesses cardiovascular and pulmonary risk factors, health education about risk factors and infection control, and promoting healthy lifestyle behaviors, particularly regular physical activity, smoking cessation, and heart-healthy foods.

Physical therapists should use teamwork to optimize secondary prevention strategies enabling individuals with pulmonary pathology to exercise and improve their quality of life. Contact with the physician, pharmacologist, psychologist, social worker, and respiratory therapist may be appropriate when developing optimal secondary prevention for those with COPD and emphysema.

References

1. American Heart Association. Heart attack and angina statistics. Available at: http://www.americanheart.org/presenter.jhtml?identifier=4591. Accessed February 6, 2006.
2. Martin T. About Fitness. Respiratory disease statistics: your guide to smoking cessation. The prevalence of COPD. Available at: http://quitsmoking.about.com/od/tobaccostatistics/a/COPDstatistics.htm. Accessed February 6, 2006.
3. APTA. *Guide to Physical Therapist Practice.* Alexandria, Va: American Physical Therapy Association; 2001.
4. Sinclair D, Dangerfield P. *Human Growth After Birth.* 6th ed. London, England: Oxford Publishers; 1998.
5. Pimentel AE, Gentile CL, Tanaka H, Seals DR, Gates PE. Greater rate of decline in maximal aerobic capacity with age in endurance-trained than in sedentary men. *J Appl Physiol.* 2003;94:2406–2413.
6. Wrong Diagnosis. Prevalence and incidence of heart disease. Available at: http://www.wrongdiagnosis.com/h/heart_disease/prevalence.htm. Accessed February 12, 2006.
7. Anand SS, Yusuf S. Risk factors for cardiovascular disease in Canadians of South Asian and European origin: a pilot study of the Study of Heart Assessment and Risk in Ethnic Groups (SHARE). *Clin Invest Med.* 1997;20(4):204–210.
8. US Department of Health and Human Services. National Institutes of Health, National Heart, Lung, and Blood Institute, SERVICES. NIH Publication No 98–3654. 1998.
9. Blumenthal J, Sherwood A, Babyak M, et al. Effects of exercise and stress management training on markers of cardiovascular risk in patients with ischemic heart disease. *JAMA.* 2005;293:1626–1634.
10. Giles TD, Berk BC, Black HR, et al. Expanding the definition and classification of hypertension. *J Clin Hypertens.* 2005;7(9):505–512.
11. Hedley A, Ogden C, Johnson C, Carroll M, Curtin L, Flegal K. Prevalence of overweight and obesity among US children, adolescents, and adults, 1999–2002. *JAMA.* 2004;291:2847–2850.

12. Censori B, Agostinis C, Partziguian T, Guagliumi G, Bonaldi G, Poloni M. Spontaneous dissection of carotid and coronary arteries. *Neurology.* 2004;63:1122–1123.

13. Merck Manual. Hyperlipidemia. Available at: http://www.merck.com/mrkshared/mmanual/section2/chapter15/15a.jsp. Accessed February 12, 2006.

14. Lalonde L, Gray-Donald K, Lowensteyn I, et al. Comparing the benefits of diet and exercise in the treatment of dyslipidemia. *Prev Med.* 2002;35(1):16–24.

15. Henzen C. Risk factors for arteriosclerosis. *Schweiz Rundsch Med Prax.* 2001;25;90(4):91–95.

16. American Heart Association. Peripheral vascular disease. Available at: http://www.americanheart.org/presenter.jhtml?identifier=4692. Accessed February 12, 2006.

17. Committee on Fetus and Newborn. American Academy of Pediatrics. Apnea, sudden infant death syndrome, and home monitoring. *Pediatrics.* 2003;111(4[Pt 1]):914–917.

18. Task Force on Sudden Infant Death Syndrome. The changing concept of sudden infant death syndrome: diagnostic coding shifts, controversies regarding the sleeping environment, and new variables to consider in reducing risk. *Pediatrics.* 2005;116(5):1245–1255.

19. The Ad Council. Child asthma attack prevention. Available at: http://www.adcouncil.org/issues/Childhood_Asthma. Accessed February 12, 2006.

20. Holloway E, Ram F. Breathing exercises for asthma. *Cochrane Database of Systematic Reviews.* 2005;2:1–2.

21. Spruit M, Troosters T, Trappenburg J, Decramer M, Gosselink R. Exercise training during rehabilitation of patients with COPD: a current perspective. *Patient Educ Couns.* 2004;52:243–248.

22. WebMD. Sleep apnea prevention. Available at: http://www.webmd.com/hw/sleep_disorders/hw49354.asp. Accessed February 6, 2006.

23. National Sleep Foundation. Facts and stats. Available at: http://www.sleepfoundation.org/hottopics/index.php?secid=10&id=226. Accessed February 6, 2006.

24. National Center for Health Statistics. Report of Final Mortality Statistics. 2002.

25. Goddard Institute for Space Studies. Submitted testimony: 5. Alternative scenario: air pollution. 2005. Available at: http://www.giss.nasa.gov/research/features/senate/page7.html. Accessed February 12, 2006.

26. National Lung Health Education Program. Treatment of advanced disease. Available at: http://www.nlhep.org/resources/erly-rec-mng-copd/treatment-6.html. Accessed February 12, 2006.

27. US Centers for Disease Control. Treatment of tuberculosis. *MMWR.* 2003;52.

28. Centers for Disease Control and Prevention. Infectious diseases in health care settings. Available at: http://www.cdc.gov/ncidod/dhqp/id.html. Accessed February 12, 2006.

Chapter 14

Prevention Practice for Neuromuscular Conditions

Paul Hansen, PhD, PT and Catherine Rush Thompson, PhD, MS, PT

"To be able to feel the lightest touch really is a gift."

~ CHRISTOPHER REEVE

Some neuromuscular disorders make life difficult, such as when a person damages an isolated peripheral nerve; other conditions change the very fabric of one's life, such as Alzheimer's disease. Unfortunately, conditions that change neural and muscular function are often life-changing events. Young men who pride themselves on their athletic prowess one day may find themselves dependent in their daily living skills following a motor vehicle accident that severs their spinal cords or causes traumatic brain injury (TBI). Many older adults face the devastating memory losses associated with Alzheimer's disease that profoundly change their quality of life. Primary prevention can reduce the risk of neurological pathologies that can completely alter an individual's lifestyle, while secondary and tertiary prevention helps those afflicted with neurological impairments to live longer and healthier lives while adjusting to the changes chronic conditions induce.

This chapter focuses on the following *Guide to Physical Therapist Practice* patterns[1]:

- *5D:* Impaired motor function and sensory integrity associated with nonprogressive disorders of the central nervous system—acquired in adolescence or adulthood.
- *5E:* Impaired motor function and sensory integrity associated with progressive disorders of the central nervous system.
- *5F:* Impaired peripheral nerve integrity and muscle performance associated with peripheral nerve injury.
- *5H:* Impaired motor function, peripheral nerve integrity, and sensory integrity associated with nonprogressive disorders of the spinal cord.
- *5I:* Impaired arousal, range of motion, and motor control associated with coma, near coma, or vegetative state.

All interventions, including exercise prescription, are individually designed based on the cognitive and physical abilities of the patient that may put the individual at increased risk for injury.

Normal neural physiological function is dependent upon the nervous system being anatomically intact, isolated from the external milieu by the blood-brain barrier and the meninges, stable ionic concentrations and pH, and a constant supply of oxygen and glucose. If damaged, the nervous system has limited ability to repair itself. Trauma and toxins can disrupt neuroanatomy; cardiovascular accidents breach the blood-brain barrier; infections damage the meninges; gastrointestinal dysfunction can alter ion concentrations; cardiac arrest cuts off oxygen; and diabetes alters glucose availability. Most adult neuromuscular disorders fall into several broad etiology categories: cardiovascular impairment, metabolic dysfunction, trauma, primary and secondary neoplasms, toxin or drug exposure, infections, nutritional deficiencies, and genetic anomalies. Some conditions are due to a specific cause, such as traumatic head injury; some conditions arise without any known cause (*idiopathic*); other conditions, such as multiple sclerosis (MS), appear to arise from multiple, interacting factors. Primary prevention is directed toward identifying and reducing these risk factors through screening, education, and promoting healthy lifestyles. Secondary and tertiary prevention practices attempt to reduce sequelae and optimize the person's the quality of life, regardless of neurological impairment.

Stroke

Stroke is the most common and, perhaps, the most preventable neuromuscular dysfunction. Stroke, or brain attack, is defined as a loss of blood flow to the central nervous system.[2] While strokes usually occur in the cerebral hemispheres (a cerebral vascular accident [CVA]), they can occur anywhere in the nervous system, including the brainstem and spinal cord. An ischemic stroke (88% of stroke cases) occurs when a supplying artery is occluded, while a hemorrhagic stroke occurs when the artery ruptures with the extra-arterial blood then displacing brain within the cranial vault.[2] Each year approximately 700,000 people sustain a stroke in the United States, with 500,000 having a first stroke and 200,000 having a recurrent stroke.[3] Stroke risk increases with age, gender (more common in males), and ethnicity (substantially higher in black males and females than in white males and females).[3] The actual prevalence of stroke is probably much higher than these rates suggest as many strokes go unreported and some strokes do not result in observable deficits. "Silent" ischemic strokes occur in 11% of individuals aged 55 to 64 years and 43% of individuals over 85 years.[4] In an ischemic stroke the blood vessel is rapidly occluded by an embolus (often arising from the heart) or, more slowly, by a thrombosis (often arising from atherosclerosis). Due to the similar etiologies and prevention strategies for stroke and heart disease, the American Heart Association merged with the American Stroke Association.

The risk for stroke includes unmodifiable factors, such as the age, ethnicity, gender, and genetic predisposition. Physical therapists can more easily address the modifiable factors that can reduce the incidence of initial strokes and subsequent strokes by identifying risk factors and educating their clients to avoid these risks. For example, *transient ischemic attacks (TIAs)* are strokes that resolve within 24 hours without apparent deficit or functional loss. There is a 10% risk of stroke in the 3 months following a TIA.[4] With such a high stroke risk, a person who experiences a TIA should expediently address and be particularly vigilant in addressing the modifiable stroke risk factors. Modifiable risk factors for stroke include diabetes mellitus, hypertension (a systolic pressure of 160 mm Hg or higher and/or diastolic pressure of 95 mm Hg or higher quadruples stroke risk), smoking (smoking more than 40 cigarettes per day quadruples risk, though cessation can reduce risk to baseline values over 5 years),[5] carotid artery disease, cardiac dysfunction, blood disorders that increase clot formation, high LDL levels and low HDL levels, obesity, excessive alcohol intake (more than one drink per day and binge drinking), illegal drug use (intravenous drug abuse carries a high risk of stroke), and use of oral contraceptives.[5] To help identify these risk factors, the National Heart Association has prepared a community screening program. While such screenings help distribute information on stroke risk, the positive impact of such programs dissipates quickly.[6]

Physical therapists should also caution their clients about signs indicating that a stroke may be occurring as emergent medical treatment can minimize a stroke's damage. The signs of stroke include the following:[3]

- Sudden weakness or numbness of the face, arm, or leg, especially on one side of the body
- Sudden confusion, trouble speaking, or understanding
- Sudden trouble seeing in one or both eyes
- Sudden trouble walking, dizziness, loss of balance, or coordination
- Sudden severe headaches with no known cause

Secondary prevention should address prevention of stroke recurrence and death. Approximately 25% of stroke survivors die within 1-year poststroke.[7] Over 50% of younger stroke survivors (less than 65 years of age) die within 8 years of their stroke, and 14% of people who have a first stroke will have another stroke within 1 year.[7] Thus, the occurrence of a first stroke foretells a potentially bleak future unless aggressive secondary prevention is implemented to prevent mortality or recurrence.

Secondary prevention primarily addresses the factors that increase stroke risk. In contrast, a positive thing people can do to reduce their stroke risk is exercise. Physical activity reduces stroke risk in a dose-dependent manner; the greater the level of physical activity, the greater the reduction in stroke risk.[8] The Washington University at St. Louis Stroke Center website offers a variety of stroke scales and assessment tools that can be used to assess individuals poststroke.[9]

More than 1 million American adults report difficulties with ADLs and IADLs due to a stroke.[9] Three months poststroke, approximately 50% to 70% of stroke survivors regain functional independence, with 15% to 30% dependent and greater than 20% being institutionalized.[9] The most common disabilities apparent poststroke include the following:

- 50% exhibit *hemiparesis* (weakness on one side of the body)
- 35% show depression
- 30% have a gait dysfunction
- 26% require assistance to perform ADLs
- 19% have communication problems

Duncan and her colleagues point out that many measures that quantify stroke severity do not address all areas affected by a stroke, especially the cognitive and fine motor domains.[9] Therefore, stroke's true impact may be significantly underestimated.

Determining a person's secondary prevention needs poststroke requires knowledge of the stroke's vascular etiology, the function of the affected brain region, pre-existing and poststroke comorbidities, and the individual's residual capabilities and remaining debilities.[9] Common problems that occur poststroke include pneumonia, incontinence, urinary tract infections, mental health issues (such as depression, increased social isolation, altered emotional control), and altered communication. Other common impairments include motor impairments affecting vital functions and the performance of ADLs, IADLs, fine motor skills, and walking.[9] These problems may arise due to problems with muscle weakness, fatigue, poor coordination, *hypertonicity* (increased muscle tone), *spasticity* (velocity-dependent, increased resistance to passive muscle stretch), or *dyskinesia* (abnormal movement).[9] These impairments are further confounded by pain, soft tissue or articular *contractures* (abnormal joint movement limitation), sensory dysfunction (such as *anesthesia*—loss of sensation, *hyperesthesia*—increased sensory sensitivity, *dysesthesia*—abnormal, disagreeable sensory feelings, *paraesthesia*—burning or prickling sensations, *hemi-neglect*—lacking awareness of one side of the body, *hemianopsia*—loss of half of the visual field, and *pusher syndrome*—a tendency to push out of postural alignment), altered nonsensory/motor functions (such as fatigue, inattention, and lack of safety awareness), and sexual dysfunction.[9]

Physical therapists need to monitor their clients poststroke to ensure that these problems are addressed. The American Heart Association offers guidelines to prevent a second stroke at their website.[10] Also, the National Stroke Association offers stroke prevention guidelines with information for stroke survivors, caregivers and families, and medical professionals on their website.[11] In addition, exercise programs should be implemented to maintain health and wellness after intensive therapy is no longer appropriate. Table 14-1 illustrates exercise programs that can benefit stroke survivors.[12]

When developing a prevention program for stroke survivors, physical therapists should keep in mind that these individuals are usually physically deconditioned prestroke, are at increased risk for sustaining a second stroke or cardiovascular disease, and are often taking antihypertensive, cardiovascular, and/or anticonvulsant medications. Due to motor paralysis, sensory loss, and/or cognitive impairments, certain exercises may not be possible, and other activities need to be adapted to meet individualized needs.

Spinal Cord Injury

Working to improve the health and wellness of individuals who have a spinal cord injury (SCI) presents unique challenges for the clinician. As with all nervous system injuries, there is no "typical" case; each person who has a SCI has a unique clinical presentation. The spinal cord can be traumatically damaged by direct cutting (eg, cut by a knife), a crush injury (eg, injured in a car accident), or edema or swelling following an acute injury. Traumatic injury often disrupts the bony spinal column, leading to vertebral fracture or articular instability. Nontraumatic spinal cord injuries (SCIs) include disruption of blood flow from an ischemic stroke, tumor encroachment (abnormal growth causing pressure on the spinal cord), and spinal stenosis (spinal canal narrowing).[13]

Cord damage can occur at any spinal level. While the injury may be ascribed to one spinal segment, the damage often extends across multiple segments. If only the lower extremities are involved, the paralysis (loss of muscle strength) is called paraplegia (loss of strength in the legs). Tetraplegia (weakness in all four limbs) refers to loss of function in both upper and lower extremities. The injury is incomplete if any sensory or motor function is preserved below the injury level. The classification scale published by the American Spinal Injury Association (ASIA) incorporates the injury completeness with the level of injury. This scale is used in the clinic and in sport participation, such as the Paralympic Games.[14]

In the United States, there are approximately 11,000 individuals with new SCI each year, split evenly between paraplegia and tetraplegia. Approximately 247,000 people are alive today living with their cord injuries.[13] Most injuries occur between 16 and 30 years of age, with the mode at 19 years, although there is an increasing incidence over the age of 60.[13] The vast

TABLE 14-1

SUMMARY OF EXERCISE PROGRAMMING RECOMMENDATIONS FOR STROKE SURVIVORS

Mode of Exercise	Major Goals	Intensity/Frequency/Duration*
Aerobic: Large-muscle activities (eg, walking, treadmill, stationary cycle, combined arm-leg ergometry, arm ergometry, seated stepper)	• Increase independence in ADLs • Increase walking speed/efficiency • Improve tolerance for prolonged physical activity • Reduce risk of cardiovascular disease	• 40% to 70% peak oxygen uptake; 40% to 70% heart rate reserve; 50% to 80% maximal heart rate; rating of perceived exertion (RPE) 11 to 14 (6 to 20 scale) • 3 to 7 days/week • 20 to 60 min/session (or multiple 10-min sessions)
Strength: Circuit training Weight machines Free weights Isometric exercise	• Increase independence in ADLs	• 1 to 3 sets of 10 to 15 repetitions of 8 to 10 exercises involving the major muscle groups • 2 to 3 days/week
Flexibility: Stretching	• Increase range of motion of involved extremities • Prevent contractures	• 2 to 3 days/week (before or after aerobic or strength training) • Hold each stretch for 10 to 30 seconds
Neuromuscular: Coordination and balance activities	• Improve level of safety during ADLs	• 2 to 3 days/week (consider performing on same day as strength activities)

* Recommended intensity, frequency, and duration of exercise depend on each individual patient's level of fitness. Intermittent training sessions may be indicated during the initial weeks of rehabilitation.

Adapted from Gordon NF, Gulanick M, Costa F, Fletcher G, Franklin BA, Roth EJ, Shephard T. Physical activity and exercise recommendations for stroke survivors: an American Heart Association scientific statement from the Council on Clinical Cardiology, subcommittee on exercise, cardiac rehabilitation, and prevention. *Circulation.* 2004;109(16):2031-2041.

majority of cord injuries are to Caucasian males.[13] Motor vehicle crashes account for over half the SCI cases, followed by falls, acts of violence (primarily gunshot wounds), and sporting activities.[13] Falls are the leading cause of SCI for people 65 and older.[13] Over time, sports injuries have decreased while fall injuries have increased. In sports, two-thirds of the injuries are due to diving accidents, and over 90% of sports injuries result in tetraplegia.[13] In all cases, the presence of alcohol in the blood worsens the damage, possibly due to the ethanol directly contacting the neural tissue due to the injury.

PROGNOSIS FOR INDIVIDUALS WITH SPINAL CORD INJURY RELATED TO SECONDARY COMPLICATIONS

The vast majority (88%) of individuals with SCI are discharged to home.[14] At 1 year postinjury, 32% of those with paraplegia and 26% with tetraplegia are employed.[14] The postinjury employment picture is better among persons with paraplegia than among their tetraplegic counterparts.

In the mid-1900s, individuals with SCI were expected to live only a few years after injury, with death occurring due to *decubitus ulcers* (pressure sores), urinary tract infections, or respiratory infections. Today, individuals with SCI live approximately 85% to 90% of a normal adult life span.[15] In recent years, the leading cause of death in tetraplegia is respiratory complications, while in paraplegia it is heart disease and cancer, thus mirroring the overall change in mortality in the United States population.[16] Individuals with SCI often mirror the medical conditions acquired in aging populations, although these conditions occur at an earlier age. For example, many older adults remain independent in their IADLs and ADLs well into their 70s, while individuals with SCI often see increasing dependence beginning in their mid-40s.[16]

Other long-term changes that occur in individuals with SCI include lower extremity osteoporosis and fractures, substance abuse, autonomic dysreflexia, *neurogenic bowel* (a bowel without voluntary control), nutritional adjustments, and changes in musculoskeletal, cardiorespiratory, endocrine, integumentary, genitourinary, and alimentary systems, as well as psychosocial adjustment and issues related to aging.[17] Pressure sores are a real problem following a SCI with nearly three-quarters of individuals experiencing at least one pressure sore, with yearly treatment costs exceeding $1.2 billion.[17] Several wellness-based approaches have shown the potential for dramatically reducing pressure sore occurrence and severity. For example, in Arkansas, an intervention project assessed if in-home education reduced the incidence and severity of pressure sores.[18] In a 1-year period, participants in the intervention group experienced a 46% decrease in occurrence and a 36% decrease in sore severity, saving over $660,000 in hospitalization expenses.[19]

Major depressive disorder is common among all medical clients (6% to 10%) but is more common after SCI (23% to 30%).[20] Clinical depression may be five times more prevalent than in the general population.[21] Urinary tract infections seem almost inevitable. Fertility problems affect most men with SCI. Pain, contractures, and spasticity are common occurrences. Other problems that affect the long-term health of individuals with SCI include cardiovascular disease, bowel dysfunction, musculoskeletal repetitive trauma, and scoliosis.[21] The presence of these conditions is closely related to these individuals' psychosocial function with resultant social isolation, depression, and substance abuse.

Mobility and perceived health appear to be the consistent predictors of life satisfaction 2 years post-SCI.[22] The following tips may reduce the risk of secondary conditions related to SCI[23]:

- *Diet:* Encourage the individual to eat a well-balanced diet, including protein foods, fresh fruits, and vegetables, to help keep skin, urinary tract, and bowel functions healthy. Water throughout the day benefits the skin, the urinary tract, and bowel functions.
- *Mobility:* Have the individual change position frequently in a wheelchair and in bed to prevent pressure sores. Regular exercise improves cardiovascular and respiratory function, increases bone strength, regulates bodily functions, and may reduce spasticity. Immobilization of the lower limbs may also precipitate venous stasis, blood pooling, and edema due to inactivity of the venous muscle pump. This situation may lead to *deep venous thrombosis* (a clot that forms in a vein, commonly in the lower leg but can occur anywhere in the body) and a *pulmonary embolism* (occlusion of a pulmonary artery from a dislodged thrombus).
- *Smoking:* Smoking constricts blood vessels, restricting blood flow to body tissues. Smoking also negatively affects cardiorespiratory and skin health.
- *Skin Care:* Teach each individual how to regularly examine the skin, paying special attention to bony areas such as heels, tailbone, and shoulder blades. Mirrors are often needed.
- *Regular Medical Care:* Encourage regular physicals to monitor health conditions both related and unrelated to the SCI.
- *Respiratory Hygiene:* For individuals with high-level lesions, encourage exercises, such as coughing, that can clear the lungs. Paralysis of intercostal and abdominal muscles can severely limit pulmonary ventilation and the ability to cough, increasing the probability of developing life-threatening pulmonary problems.

Altered autonomic nervous system function can limit individuals with SCI in their ability to exercise as sympathetic stimulation, which is required to stimulate normal cardiovascular reflex responses. Autonomic nervous system reflexes normally augment blood flow to metabolically active skeletal muscles to provide increased oxygen and fuel substrates, while removing metabolic end-products. When these reflexes are disrupted, the body does not have the normal balance of blood flow to internal organs, skeletal muscles, and vital other tissues. Lesions above the sixth thoracic level (T6) can affect sympathetic nerves innervating the heart and that ensure adequate blood flow during exercise. With a lesion at or above T6, the blood flow can be impaired as well as the ability to sweat while exercising. Blood pressure testing should always accompany exercise testing and exercise training.

For those individuals with tetraplegia affecting all extremities, endurance training may not have the same effects as seen with normal individuals. Arm ergometry supplemented by *functional electrical stimulation* (a device to activate muscles electrically) may help improve cardiopulmonary training for increased endurance.[24]

Chronic urinary tract infections lead to multiple hospitalizations, increased costs, and long-term morbidity regardless of how the bladder is emptied.[23] Secondary complications include *septicemia* (blood poisoning), *calculi* (stone) formation, inflammation, urine reflux, *abscess* (a pus accumulation secondary to infection), and renal failure. Suggestions for preventing urinary tract infections can be found on the Internet.[25,26] Keeping the catheter bag clean and using proper clean techniques for bladder management reduce infection incidence.

In addition, some individuals have problems with bowel elimination since the sensation of rectal fullness and the ability to control the anal sphincter may be absent. Bowel and bladder programs can help reduce concerns associated with bowel and bladder dysfunction. Strategies to prevent bowel disorders center on establishing a predictable elimination pattern. These strategies include a high-fiber diet, increased fluid intake, digital stimulation, use of a rectal suppository, manual removal, and Valsalva maneuvers.[26] Craig Hospital, a well-recognized center for rehabilitation post-SCI, provides information about bowel management at its website.[27]

A wide variety of problems and complications are associated with the neurological and musculoskeletal systems, including pain caused by the lesion itself, *myelopathy* (spinal cord disease), weakness, spasticity, *heterotopic ossification* (new bone formation in the connective tissue or muscle surrounding the major joints), musculoskeletal pain (from tendon, bursa, or joint inflammation), peripheral neuropathy, autonomic dysfunction, joint contracture, degenerative joint disease, and osteoporotic fracture.[17] Pain and impaired function increase with time. The overused shoulder is the most common painful joint. Common conditions include tendonitis, bursitis, and impingement syndrome. Later complications include rotator cuff tears and glenohumeral or acromiohumeral joint degeneration.[17] These conditions can be severely disabling for persons with SCI who depend on their arms for locomotor power and prehensile tasks. Physical therapists need to educate these individuals about overuse prevention and methods to protect their musculoskeletal systems without compromising their ability to function.

Traumatic Brain Injury

TBI results from either intentional or nonintentional trauma to the brain. While a direct traumatic impact causes some brain injury, the major impairments and functional limitations result from vascular hemorrhage and *diffuse axonal injury (DAI)* (tearing of nerves located throughout the brain); the functional deficit is positively correlated with the amount of DAI.[28] Although the injury usually happens in a single event, such as a motor vehicle accident, repetitive microtraumatic neural injury from activities such as boxing or heading the ball in soccer can summate to negatively affect cognitive and motor functions.

Males are almost twice as likely as females to sustain a TBI.[29] African-Americans have the highest death rate from TBI.[29] There are two high-risk ages: ages 15 to 24 years and those over age 75. The younger group is prone to sustain the injury in a motor vehicle accident or in a fall while participating in a high-risk activity.[29] Alcohol or drugs are often involved. The older age group often acquires a brain injury in a slip/fall accident.[29] The risk of sustaining another head injury increases with each subsequent injury. Note that this profile closely resembles that for SCI; in fact, the two injuries too often occur together.

A TBI can be mild, resulting in a brief concussion, or severe, leading to death or a *persistent vegetative state* (a condition characterized by the inability to speak, follow simple commands, or respond in a meaningful way).[30] While each person's presentation is unique, there are general classification schemes for categorizing individuals who have a TBI. The Glasgow coma scale is used in the acute medical setting, while in physical therapy the revised Ranchos Los Amigos Levels of Cognitive Functioning[31] is more common. The "Rancho" scale has 10 levels ranging from severe functional limitations to near-normal function.[31] This scale provides a guide to the individual's general behavior but does not take into account alterations in the individual's function as related to community reintegration.

The most devastating problems following a TBI are the cognitive deficits. Cognitive deficits are further complicated by motor and sensory dysfunction, such as a *hemiparesis* (weakness on one half of the body), *apraxia* (inability planning voluntary movement), and *dystonia* (abnormal muscle tone). The types of complications that arise are dependent upon the severity of the injury, the neural functions involved, the concurrent injuries, and comorbid conditions.

A major concern following a TBI is the person's increased risk of sustaining another TBI. This risk needs to be actively addressed by suggesting use of protective gear when engaged in sports and avoiding high-risk activities. A relatively unique complication of TBI, as well as SCI, is *heterotopic ossification* (the formation of bone in abnormal locations). This condition generally occurs within 1 year of the injury and is most frequently noted in the hip flexor muscles, although it can occur later and in other muscles.[32] Treatment for heterotopic ossification is maintaining as much movement as possible at the joints without further tissue damage. If needed, surgery sometimes is undertaken to remove the heterotopic ossification. In addition to the above risks, the person with a TBI faces a myriad of challenges. Neurological dysfunction includes movement disorders, seizures, headaches, visual deficits, and sleep disorders. Nonneurological problems include pulmonary, metabolic, nutritional, gastrointestinal, musculoskeletal, and dermatologic dysfunction. Behaviorally, the person may exhibit verbal and physical aggression, agitation, learning difficulties, shallow self-awareness, altered sexual functioning, impulsivity, social disinhibition, mood disorders, personality changes, altered emotional control, and depression. Socially, the person with a TBI is at increased risk for suicide, divorce, chronic unemployment, economic strain, and substance abuse.[32]

Parkinson's Disease

Parkinson's disease (PD) and a number of other movement disorders are due to subcortical and brainstem damage that occurs due to various etiologies, including genetic abnormalities, metabolic dysfunction, stroke, environmental toxins, infections, and oxidative stress. PD is described here, as it is the most common movement disorder.

The incidence rate for PD increases with advancing age, with the median onset at 62.4 years. Although PD is a condition that afflicts primarily the elderly, up to 10% of cases begin before the age of 40. Prevalence is approximately 300 per 100,000, although due to the difficulty in diagnosis, as many as 40% of cases may be undiagnosed.[33] Its etiology is unknown, although its incidence increases with advancing age. It may result from the interaction of weak environmental toxins and a genetic predisposition.[33]

PD is the most common neurodegenerative condition. The impairments arise primarily due to damage to the *substantia nigra's* dopanergic neurons. The diagnosis of PD relies on clinical observation, as there are no imaging or laboratory findings specific to PD. Its cardinal signs are (1) *resting or postural tremor* (small movements at rest), (2) *bradykinesia* (slow movement), (3) *rigidity* (increased resistance to the passive movement of a limb), and (4) postural instability. While the tremor is often the most clinically apparent symptom, the bradykinesia, rigidity, and postural instability can be the most disabling.[33] These motor signs may present as micrographia (small handwriting), *masked facies* (a reptilian stare), *stooped shuffling* (simian) gait with decreased arm swing, difficulty arising from a chair, difficulty turning in bed, and *hypophonic* (low volume) speech. Nonmotor symptoms and signs are often apparent before the motor signs. Nonmotor signs may include autonomic dysfunction, slowed gastric and intestinal motility, urinary dysfunction, sexual dysfunction, pain, cognitive changes, speech problems, and swallowing dysfunction.[33] Although more difficult for the clinician to observe, the nonmotor signs may change a person's health and wellness more than the motor signs. Dementia can occur in up to one-third of individuals who have PD. Depression occurs in about half of these individuals and arises from the neurological impairment, rather than as a secondary symptom.[33] Aspiration pneumonia is a major cause of morbidity and mortality in PD. Physical therapists must address these complications and caution these individuals of risks associated with motor and nonmotor impairments that can influence functional abilities.

Medications currently are the best treatment for PD. Progress in pharmacological treatment and PD's progressive nature means that an individual's medications can frequently change. To optimize a person's abilities the medications require continuous monitoring and adjustment by a physician, usually a neurologist.[33] Overmedication can lead to problems with hallucinations, *dyskinesias* (uncontrolled movements), insomnia, nausea, reduced appetite, weight loss, and *dystonia* (abnormal muscle tone).[32]

As PD is a progressive condition, there is increasing interest in discovering ways to slow the progression rate. A most promising avenue is exercise's effect on slowing the progression of Parkinson's disease.[34]

Many of the signs and symptoms of PD may respond to nonpharmacological treatments. Nonpharmacologic and pharmacologic treatments for PD give often transient results, producing an effect only while the person is using or engaged in the treatment. Therefore, adherence to the intervention program should be encouraged. Problems that may be managed with nonpharmacologic interventions include the following[35]:

- Difficulties with motor control, balance, posture, gait, and mobility
- Difficulties with ADLs and IADLs
- Problems with speech and swallowing
- Issues with proper nutrition
- Sleep dysfunction

- Pain
- Constipation
- Sexual dysfunction
- Psychosocial issues, including depression

Physical therapy can address the motor problems in an effort to maintain or increase activity levels, decrease rigidity and bradykinesia, optimize gait, and improve balance and motor coordination. The impact of physical therapy interventions tends to persist only while the person continues with the activity. Features of a physical therapy program may include the following[36]:

- Regular exercise, such as walking, swimming, dancing, and bicycle ergometry
- Stretching
- Strengthening
- Providing mobility aids, as needed
- Training in transfer techniques
- Training in techniques to improve posture and walking
- Fall prevention, including balance activities such as tai chi

Referrals to occupational therapists, dietitians, and speech and language pathologists who specialize in oromotor training and management of swallowing problems are often appropriate. Sexual dysfunction experienced by this population includes erectile dysfunction in men, vaginal dryness in women, loss of libido, and hypersexuality from dopaminergic drugs.[37]

Alzheimer's Disease

Alzheimer's disease, the most common form of dementia, is a degenerative brain disease characterized by a relatively rapid, progressive impairment in memory, judgment, decision-making, performing routine tasks, orientation to time and physical surroundings, and language. Motor dysfunction is not a hallmark of Alzheimer's disease. It is important to differentiate Alzheimer's disease from normal age-related gradual decline in cognitive functions that minimally affect a person's capabilities and other forms of dementia that may be treatable. Alzheimer's disease is diagnosed by excluding other causes for a person's loss of cognitive function; a definitive diagnosis of Alzheimer's disease can only be made through autopsy. Table 14-2 shows the stages of the disease.

The incidence of Alzheimer's disease increases with age. One percent of individuals 65 to 70 years have Alzheimer's disease, while 40% to 50% of those older than 95 years have Alzheimer's, with the mean age of onset at age 80 years.[38] "In the United States, the disease accounts for about $100 billion per year in medical and custodial expenses, with the average patient requiring an expenditure of about $27,000 per year for medical and nursing care. In addition, 80% of caregivers report stress, and about 50% report depression."[39]

At present, there is no known cure for Alzheimer's disease, although there are medications that may slow its progression, including drugs that inhibit the degradation of acetylcholine within synapses.[38] Thus, the primary focus is on palliative care and on the prevention of secondary complications. The involvement of psychologists in providing education, support, and counseling is appropriate. Caring for a person with Alzheimer's disease is extremely demanding on the caregiver, so intervention should address the patient's secondary prevention needs and the caregiver's primary and secondary prevention needs. Respite care and psychosocial support for the caregiver are often necessary. The American Health Assistance Foundation provides information about the Alzheimer's Family Relief Program at its website.[40]

The secondary prevention needs of a person with Alzheimer's disease can be identified by inspection of the problems that are encountered at each stage of the disease. For example, in the early stage of Alzheimer's disease, social isolation is an issue. In a later stage, a person with Alzheimer's disease who is bedridden with incontinence of bowel and bladder has a high risk for integument breakdown.

Epilepsy

Epilepsy is the most common brain disorder. It is characterized by repeated seizures that range from short lapses in attention to severe, frequent convulsions. The seizures can occur several times a day or once every few months. The seizures are due to bouts of excessive electrical activity in the brain. Usually, the brain region involved in the seizure remains the same from one seizure to the next, so an individual's seizure presentation is relatively predictable, although there can be dramatic differences among individuals.

While the cause of the abnormal neural activity is not known, 70% of individuals with epilepsy can be seizure-free with antiepileptic drugs.[41] Most individuals who take antiepileptic drugs are satisfied with the medication's ability to control their seizures, yet antiepileptic drug side effects, including fogginess or lack of clear headedness, sleepiness, and

TABLE 14-2
Stages of Alzheimer's Disease

Early Stage

The individual may be aware of the diagnosis and be able to participate in care decisions. Symptoms may include difficulties with memory and communication. Some individuals remain active while others become passive or withdrawn. Depression and anxiety are common.

Mental abilities	• Mild forgetfulness • Difficulty learning new things and following conversations • Difficulty concentrating or limited attention span • Problems with orientation, such as getting lost or not following directions • Communication difficulties such as word finding	Moods and emotions	• Mood shifts • Depression
		Behaviors	• Passiveness • Withdrawal from usual activities • Restlessness
		Physical abilities	• Mild coordination problems

Middle Stage

Memory continues to deteriorate with forgetting of personal history and loss of recognition of family and friends. The person will need assistance with ADLs. Some people become restless and pace or wander. The person may react to the decline by becoming less involved in activities or endlessly repeating the same action or word.

Mental abilities	• Continued memory problems • Forgetfulness about personal history • Inability to recognize friends and family • Disorientation about time and place	Moods and emotions	• Personality change • Confusion • Anxiety/apprehension • Suspiciousness • Mood shifts • Anger • Sadness/depression • Hostility
Behaviors	• Declining ability to concentrate • Restlessness (pacing, wandering) • Repetition • Delusions • Aggression • Uninhibited behavior • Passiveness	Physical abilities	• Assistance required for daily tasks (eg, dressing, bathing, using the toilet) • Disrupted sleep patterns • Appetite fluctuations • Language difficulties • Visual spatial problems

Late Stage

The individual is unable to remember, communicate, or participate in self care, eventually becoming bedridden with loss of bodily functions such as swallowing and bowel and bladder continence. Care is required 24 hours a day. Death occurs often due to secondary complications, such as pneumonia.

Mental abilities	• Loss of ability to remember, communicate, or function • Inability to process information • Severe speaking difficulties • Severe disorientation about time, place, and people	Physical abilities	• Sleeps longer and more often • Becomes immobile (bed-ridden) • Loses ability to speak • Loses control of bladder and bowels • Has difficulty eating and/or swallowing • Unable to dress or bathe • May lose weight
Behaviors	• Nonverbal methods of communicating (eye contact, crying, groaning)		
Moods and emotions	• Possible withdrawal		

Adapted from Alzheimer's Society of Canada. The progression of Alzheimer's disease. Available at: http://www.alzheimer.ca/english/disease/progression-3stages.htm. Accessed October 15, 2005.

dizziness, can limit an individual's ability to perform daily tasks.[41]

Mistakenly, some clinicians views epilepsy as a condition of children and young adults. In fact, older populations have the greatest prevalence of epilepsy. Often, the older individual's seizure is not of the grand mal type but rather presents as brief gaps in conversation, periods of confusion, blank stares, or unresponsiveness. These may be small, treatable seizures, but too often, they are described as "senior moments" and go untreated. Secondary prevention in this population should focus on injury prevention when the person is seizing. Protection may involve having the person wear a helmet to prevent a head injury or hip protectors to reduce the risk of a fractured hip if a fall were to occur during a seizure. Also important is education for the individual and his or her family on what occurs during a seizure and how to respond to that individual's seizure. Limits on high-risk activities, such as driving, may be necessary.

When not experiencing a seizure, the person with idiopathic epilepsy usually has normal cognitive and motor function. Yet, the knowledge that a seizure may occur can induce the person to self-limit activities with resulting social isolation. Thus, secondary prevention must work toward maintaining or reintegrating the individual into a supportive social network.

Multiple Sclerosis

MS, with a prevalence ranging from 50 to 100/100,000 people, is a pathology that damages the myelin that surrounds axons in the central nervous system, resulting in *sclerosis* (scarring) and neurological dysfunction.[42] The multiple sclerotic areas, also called a plaque, that appear over time, are relatively small, but their impact can summate, so large neural areas can be effected.[42] The plaques can occur anywhere in the nervous system, including in the spinal cord, cerebellum, occipital lobe, and frontal lobe. Where the plaques occur determines the symptoms and signs that a particular person will exhibit.

The cause of MS is unknown; however, environmental and genetic factors appear to interact to cause an autoimmune dysfunction. This condition most commonly affects young adults between the ages of 20 and 40, with women affected twice as often as men, and in individuals with a Northern European genetic history. Common signs and symptoms are listed in Table 14-3.[42] As noted above, the particular symptom cluster a person may experience depends upon where the plaques are located in the nervous system. The clinical manifestations may progress continuously, or *exacerbate* (increase in intensity and frequency), or go into *remission* (reduce in intensity and frequency; this form is referred to as relapsing-remitting MS) depending upon the course of the pathology for any given individual.

Early clinical manifestations of MS include fatigue; uncomfortable sensations in the arms, legs, trunk, or face (eg, tingling, numbness, pain, burning, or itching); and muscle weakness. These physical changes can be accompanied by psychological changes, such as mood swings, euphoria, depression, or apathy. In addition, the individual with MS may have problems with memory, judgment, or attention. Since the demyelination process is unpredictable and may vary in each individual, these subtle changes may not be recognized unless it is a very aggressive pathology. The subtle onset and progression make MS often difficult to diagnose.

Several MS features are unique to the disease; exacerbations, fatigue, and thermal sensitivity. During an exacerbation, it is advised that the individual not engage in strenuous physical activity. The fatigue seen in MS can be very profound. It is described as more of a lassitude rather than being tired. It can come on quickly and be so debilitating that the person can not function for hours or even days after onset. A person with MS is often thermally sensitive, usually to heat but sometimes to cold. To avoid the heat, some people with MS are "strongest" in the morning and then sequester themselves in an air-conditioned room for the rest of the day. While exercise is beneficial for a person with MS, exercise can cause fatigue and increase body temperature. These factors must be closely monitored and controlled when working with individuals who have MS.[44-46]

Often, the person's movements become more erratic, lacking the smooth coordination of muscle activity. This lack of muscular coordination is also evident in speech patterns and hand dexterity. Muscles can become spastic (increased muscle tone), further limiting movement and causing motor dysfunction. While medications are used to manage muscle tone, movement control can pose problems with work and leisure activities. Over time, individuals with MS experience the same problems that many with neurological impairments face: decreased mobility, contracture formation, skin breakdown, urinary tract infections, and pneumonia, compounded by progressive weakness, sensory disturbances, and depression.[42]

According to the *Merck Manual of Medical Diagnosis*[42]:

People with multiple sclerosis can often maintain an active lifestyle, although they may tire easily and may not be able to keep up with a demanding schedule. Regular exercise such as riding a stationary bicycle, walking, swimming, or stretching reduces

TABLE 14-3

IMPAIRMENTS ASSOCIATED WITH MULTIPLE SCLEROSIS

Psychological Impairments	Sensory Impairments	Motor Impairments
• Inappropriate giddiness or elation • Inability to control emotions (eg, laughing or crying without reason) • Mood swings • Subtle or obvious mental impairment • Depression	• Visual disturbances (eg, partial blindness and pain in one eye, double vision, loss of central vision, and blurred or dim vision) • Abnormal sensations (eg, pain, tingling, numbness, itching, and/or burning) • Vertigo or dizziness • Difficulty in reaching orgasm, sexual impotence in men, and lack of sensation in the vagina	• Uncoordinated eye movements • Clumsiness and weakness • Problems with control of bowel movements and urination • Constipation • Difficulty with walking or maintaining balance • Unsteadiness, stiffness, and unusual fatigue • Tremor

Adapted from The MERCK Manuals Online Medical Library. Multiple sclerosis. Available at: http://www.merck.com/mmhe/sec06/ch092/ch092b.html. Accessed October 15, 2005.

spasticity and helps maintain cardiovascular, muscular, and psychologic health. Physical therapy can help with maintaining balance, walking ability, and range of motion as well as reduce spasticity and weakness.

While these individuals tend to fatigue easily, one study demonstrates that resistance training can be effective for improving mobility and function in individuals who are moderately disabled by MS.[45] Another study found that incorporating aerobic exercise was beneficial for both moderately and severely involved individuals. This study further recommends that programs should incorporate balance training and socialization, taking into account time constraints, access, impairment level, personal preferences, motivations, and funding sources influence the prescription for exercise and other components of rehabilitation.[46]

Finally, stress management and time management, as described in Chapter 10, can be helpful in dealing with the chronic fatigue and weakness commonly associated with MS.

Peripheral Neuropathy

Neuropathy refers to a dysfunction in a peripheral nerve. It may be a polyneuropathy (involving multiple nerves), such as *Guillian Barre syndrome* (an acquired immune-mediated inflammatory disorder); or *diabetic peripheral neuropathy* (neuropathy caused by diabetes mellitus); or it may affect only a single nerve or nerve root, such as *carpal tunnel syndrome* (median nerve compression in the wrist's carpal tunnel) or lumbar *radiculopathy* (nerve root damage). There are many causes for neuropathies, including entrapment with compression, inflammation, genetic predisposition, trauma, and metabolic dysfunction. The neuropathy may disrupt a peripheral nerve's sensory, motor, or autonomic nervous system components.

If motor function is disrupted, there will be flaccid paralysis of the muscles innervated by the nerve(s). Secondary prevention must address the resultant articular instability and potential for deformity that the muscular weakness produces. If the phrenic nerve is involved, respiratory support is required emergently to compensate for the paralyzed diaphragm. If the nerves innervating the muscles of chewing or deglutition are involved, alternative means for eating and aspiration prophylaxis need to be implemented. Some motor paralysis can result in very abnormal gait, such as Legg-Perthes neuropathy that weakens the distal musculature of the lower extremities. If sensory function is disrupted, the person may have an *anesthetic* (without feeling) region in the area supplied by the nerve(s), or may experience *paresthesias* (abnormal, often painful sensations). Some lower extremity sensory neuropathies can alter walking, as exhibited by sensory ataxic gait. See Table 14-4 for characteristics of chronic neurological impairment and associated wellness concerns.

Tension Headache

Annually, over 10 million people go to the emergency department because of headache; about 69% of men and 88% of women develop a tension headache sometime during their lives.[47] Tension headache can occur at any age but most commonly begins during

TABLE 14-4

CHARACTERISTICS OF CHRONIC NEUROLOGICAL IMPAIRMENT AND ASSOCIATED WELLNESS CONCERNS

Key Features of the Medical Condition	Associated Wellness Concern
Age of onset • Pediatric or young adult onset (eg, SCI and head injury) • Intermediate onset: (eg, peripheral neuropathies) • Older adult (eg, stroke, Alzheimer's disease, PD)	Address the individual's age-appropriate biological and developmental tasks. Consider changes in body structure that can result from motor dysfunction.
Speed of onset • Rapid (eg, SCI, stroke) • Progressive onset (eg, MS) • Insidious onset (eg, Alzheimer's disease, PD)	Consider if the symptoms are sudden or insidious throughout the screening process. A rapid onset usually results in a clearly delineated injury
Progression • Relatively static (eg, SCI) • Variable course (eg, MS, peripheral neuropathies) • Progressive (eg, PD and Alzheimer's disease)	Consider how the progression of the pathology impacts the person's coping mechanisms and ability to anticipate future needs. Consider how chronic conditions may burden caregivers.
Etiology • Inborn mechanism of injury (eg, arteriovenous malformation, Huntington's chorea) • Interaction with genetics and lifestyle (ie, possibly MS) • Acquired through lifestyle choices (eg, SCI or ischemic stroke)	Consider how lifestyle behaviors can prevent initial injuries and subsequent injuries. Educate these individuals about genetic predisposition to disease when family histories are positive.
Lifestyle behaviors • High risk activities (eg, SCI and TBI) • Long-term lifestyle habits (eg, atherosclerosis leading to stroke)	Educate these individuals about healthy lifestyle choices to reduce the risk of chronic pathology.
Cognitive impairment • No cognitive impairment (eg, peripheral neuropathy) • Cognitive impairment (eg, TBI and Alzheimer's disease)	Consider how a cognitive impairment may impair the person's ability to comprehend and implement the treatment.
Sensory changes • Changes (eg, diabetic peripheral neuropathy) • No change (eg, poliomyelitis)	Provide precautions regarding the risk of self injury.
Perceptual changes • Probable change (eg, right parietal stroke) • Minimal changes (eg, SCI)	Consider that these individuals may have altered perceptions of reality.
Communication changes • Profound changes (eg, brain injury with aphasia) • No changes (eg, SCI with paraparesis)	Consider how difficulty with communication can impact interventions. Offer various options for communication and refer to speech pathology, as appropriate.
Respiratory involvement • Minimal (eg, paraparetic SCI) • Variable (eg, PD) • Significant impairment (eg, tetraparesis)	Consider how impaired respiration predisposes individuals to pneumonia and reduces their exercise tolerance.

adolescence or young adulthood, with the highest frequency among those aged 20 to 50 years.[47] Headache types are described as primary or secondary. Ninety percent of people present with primary headaches, including migraine, tension-type, and cluster headaches. While generally harmless, primary headaches may return periodically. Episodic headaches are characterized by mild-to-moderate nausea, vomiting, or tightening on both temples that is not aggravated by physical activity as well as possible sensitivity to light or sound.

People with chronic tension-type headaches have an average headache frequency of 15 days a month for 6 months or 180 days a year and must also meet the criteria for episodic tension-type headache.[47] In addition, people with chronic tension-type headaches must not have another disorder, as shown by physical and neurological examination.

Given the wide array of headache types and their medical management, it is important to refer individuals with lingering symptoms to a physician. People without a history of headache who are older than 50 years and experience pain in the temporal region (near the temple on the head) should see a doctor to be evaluated for temporal arteritis. In addition, those older than 50 years with new-onset headache should be evaluated for possible malignancy.[47] Studies show that some people with primary headache disorders respond to medications that specifically target and influence serotonin. In a comparison of 12 sessions of frontal electromyographic biofeedback training, 12 sessions of trapezius electromyographic biofeedback training, and 7 sessions of progressive muscle relaxation therapy for tension headaches, significant improvement was noted for 50% of subjects in the frontal biofeedback group, 100% in the trapezius biofeedback group, and 37.5% in the relaxation therapy group. These results suggest that psychophysiological measures, such as biofeedback and relaxation techniques, may prove useful for relief of tension headaches and should be considered viable treatment options.[48]

Psychological Disorders

Common psychological disorders in adulthood include bipolar affective disorder, schizophrenia, and substance abuse. Substance abuse, specifically drug abuse, plagues all ethnic groups and social classes worldwide and is a top priority of the United States Surgeon General, as outlined in the *Healthy People 2010* goals for the nation.[49] *Drug abuse* is defined an intense desire to obtain increasing amounts of a particular substance or substances to the exclusion of all other activities.[50] *Drug dependence* is the body's physical need, or addiction, to a specific agent.[48] Over the long term, this dependence results in physical harm, behavior problems, and association with people who also abuse drugs. Stopping the use of the drug can result in a specific withdrawal syndrome.

Vital sign readings can be increased, decreased, or absent completely. Sleepiness, confusion, and coma are common. Because of this decline in alertness, the drug abuser is at risk for assault or rape, robbery, and accidental death. Skin can be cool and sweaty or hot and dry. Chest pain is possible and can be caused by heart or lung damage from drug abuse.[50] Alcoholic individuals are sometimes difficult to identify since alcohol can influence people very differently. Certain behaviors suggest that someone may have a problem with alcohol, including alcohol on the breath, insomnia, frequent falls, bruises of different ages, blackouts, chronic depression, anxiety, irritability, tardiness or absence at work or school, employment loss, divorce or separation, financial difficulties, frequent intoxicated appearance or behavior, weight loss, or frequent automobile collisions.[50] A physical therapist should consult a physician whenever any of these signs or symptoms is observed or reported during a client screening. Additional details about drug and substance abuse are discussed in Chapter 10.

Summary

Medical conditions affecting the nervous system may be transient or chronic depending upon the etiology, the part of the nervous system affected, and the lifestyle habits of the individual at risk for further injury. Physical therapists play an essential role in identifying risk factors for neurological conditions that can irreversibly alter the lives of those with acute and chronic medical conditions affecting the brain, the spinal cord, and the peripheral nervous system. Through promoting healthy lifestyle habits and identifying risk factors for neuropathology, physical therapists can substantially reduce the costly loss of neurological function for those at greatest risk and decrease the number of sequelae that often accompany debilitating neurological conditions.

References

1. APTA. *Guide to Physical Therapy Practice.* Alexandria, Va: American Physical Therapy Association Press; 2001.
2. Greenberg DA, Aminoff MJ, Simon RP. *Clinical Neurology.* 5th ed. New York, NY: Lange Medical Books/McGraw-Hill; 2002.
3. Department of Health Human Services, Centers for Disease Control and Prevention, National Center for Chronic Disease Prevention and Health Promotion, Division of Adult and Community Health. Stroke fact sheet. Available at: http://www.cdc.gov/cvh/library/fs_stroke.htm. Accessed November 1, 2005.
4. Leary MC, Saver JL. Annual incidence of first silent stroke in the United States: a preliminary estimate. *Cerebrovascular Diseases.* 2003;16:280–285.

5. Johnston SC, Gress DR, Browner WS, Sidney S. Short-term prognosis after emergency department diagnosis of TIA. *JAMA*. 2000;284(22):2901–2906.
6. American Heart Association. Heart disease and stroke statistics: 2005 Update. Dallas, Tex: American Heart Association; 2005. Available at: http://www.americanheart.org/downloadable/heart/1105390918119HDSStats2005Update.pdf. Accessed February 6, 2006.
7. DeLemos CD, Atkinson RP, Croopnick SL, Wentworth DA, Akins PT. How effective are "community" stroke screening programs at improving stroke knowledge and prevention practices? Results of a 3-month follow-up study. *Stroke*. 2003;34(12):e247–e249. Epub November 20, 2003.
8. Patel AT, Duncan PW, Lai SM, Studenski S. The relation between impairments and functional outcomes post-stroke. *Arch Phys Med Rehab*. 2000;81(10):1357–1363.
9. Washington University at St. Louis Stroke Center. Stroke scales and clinical assessment tools. Available at: http://www.strokecenter.org/trials/scales/scales_links.aspx. Accessed February 13, 2006.
10. Stroke Journal Report. New guidelines address how to prevent a second stroke. Available at: http://www.americanheart.org/presenter.jhtml?identifier=3037102. Accessed February 13, 2006.
11. National Stroke Association. Stroke prevention guidelines. Available at: http://info.stroke.org/site/PageServer?pagename=PREVENT. Accessed February 13, 2006.
12. Gordon NF, Gulanick M, Costa F, Fletcher G, Franklin BA, Roth EJ, Shephard T. Physical activity and exercise recommendations for stroke survivors: an American Heart Association scientific statement from the Council on Clinical Cardiology, subcommittee on exercise, cardiac rehabilitation, and prevention. *Circulation*. 2004;109(16):2031-2041.
13. NSCISC. The 2005 annual statistical report for the model spinal cord injury care systems. Available at: http://images.main.uab.edu/spinalcord/pdffiles/facts05.pdf. Accessed February 6, 2006.
14. El Masry WS, Tsubo M, Katoh S, El Miligui YH, Khan A. Validation of the American Spinal Injury Association (ASIA) motor score and the National Acute Spinal Cord Injury Study (NASCIS) motor score. *Spine*. 1996;21(5):614–619.
15. Winkler T. *Spinal Cord Injury and Aging*. 2002. Available at: http://www.emedicine.com/pmr/topic185.htm. Accessed February 6, 2006.
16. Capoor J, Stein AB. Aging with spinal cord injury. *Spinal Cord*. 2005;43(2):96–101.
17. Spinal Cord Injury Program. Washington University School of Medicine. Complications. Available at: http://www.neuro.wustl.edu/sci/complica.htm. Accessed February 6, 2006.
18. Clark F, Rubayi S, Jackson J, et al. The role of daily activities in pressure ulcer development. *Adv Skin Wound Care*. 2001;14(2):52,54.
19. Injury Fact Book 2001–2002. Spinal cord injury. Available at: http://www.cdc.gov/ncipc/fact_book/25_Spinal_Cord_Injury.htm. Accessed February 6, 2006.
20. Groah SL, Stiens SA, Gittler MS, Kirshblum SC, McKinley WO. Preserving wellness and independence of the aging spinal cord injured: a primary care approach for the rehabilitation medicine specialist. *Arch Phys Med Rehab*. 2002;83(3 Suppl 1):S82–S89, S90–S98.
21. Graitcer PL, Maynard FM. *First Colloquium on Preventing Secondary Disabilities Among People with Spinal Cord Injuries*. Atlanta, Ga: US Department of Health and Human Services; 1990. Available at: http://www.cdc.gov/ncbddd/dh/Publications/Conferences/1990PrevSecDisabilitySCI/1990PrevSecDisabSCI.htm#functexpect. Accessed February 6, 2006.
22. Putzke JD, Richards JS, Hicken BL, DeVivo MJ. Predictors of life satisfaction: a spinal cord injury cohort study. *Arch Phys Med Rehabil*. 2002;83(4):555–561.
23. Centers for Disease Control and Prevention. Spinal cord injury (SCI): prevention tips. Available at: http://www.cdc.gov/ncipc/factsheets/sciprevention.htm. Accessed February 6, 2006.
24. Sommer JL, Witkiewicz PM. The therapeutic challenges of dual diagnosis: TBI/SCI. *Brain Injury*. 2004;18(12):1297–1308.
25. Northwest Regional Spinal Cord Injury System (NWRSCIS). Bladder management. Available at: http://depts.washington.edu/rehab/sci/pamp_bladder_manage.html. Accessed February 13, 2006.
26. Spinal Cord Injury Information Network. Effect of cranberry pills to prevent and treat urinary tract infection among persons with spinal cord injury. Available at: http://www.spinalcord.uab.edu/show.asp?durki=59866&site=1021&return=21544. Accessed February 13, 2006.
27. Craig Hospital. Bowel program. Available at: http://www.craighospital.org/SCI/METS/bowel.asp. Accessed February 10, 2006.
28. Centers for Disease Control and Prevention (CDC). Traumatic brain injury—Colorado, Missouri, Oklahoma, and Utah, 1990–1993. *MMWR*. 1997;46(01):8–11.
29. Thurman D, Alverson C, Dunn K, Guerrero J, Sniezek J. Traumatic brain injury in the United States: a public health perspective. *J Head Trauma Rehab*. 1999;14(6):602–615.
30. Merck Manual Online. Trauma of the head. Available at: http://www.merck.com/mrkshared/mmanual/section14/chapter175/175a.jsp. Accessed February 6, 2006.
31. Hagen C, Malkmus D, Durham P. (original scale). *Communication Disorders Service, Rancho Los Amigos Hospital, 1972*. Revised 11/15/74 by Malkmus M, Stenderup K. Available at: http://www.braininjury.com/recovery.html. Accessed February 6, 2006.
32. Practice Guidelines: 2. Rehabilitation for traumatic brain injury. Available at: http://www.ncbi.nlm.nih.gov/books/bv.fcgi?rid=hstat1.chapter.1280. Accessed February 6, 2006.
33. MD Virtual University. Parkinson's disease. Available at: http://www.mdvu.org/library/disease/pd. Accessed February 13, 2006.

34. Tillerson JL, Caudle WM, Reveron ME, Miller GW. Exercise induces behavioral recovery and attenuates neurochemical deficits in rodent models of Parkinson's disease. *Neuroscience.* 2003;119(3):899–911.

35. Butler RN, Davis R, Lewis CB, Nelson ME, Strauss E. Physical fitness: benefits of exercise for the older patient. *Geriatrics.* 1998;53(10):46,49–52,61–62.

36. Canning CG, Alison JA, Allen NE, Groeller H. Parkinson's disease: an investigation of exercise capacity, respiratory function, and gait. *Arch Phys Med Rehabil.* 1997;78(2):199–207.

37. Klos KJ, Bower JH, Josephs KA, Matsumoto JY, Ahlskog JE. Pathological hypersexuality predominantly linked to adjuvant dopamine agonist therapy in Parkinson's disease and multiple system atrophy. *Parkinsonism Relat Disord.* 2005;11(6):381–386.

38. Khachiaturian Z. *Alzheimer's Disease.* Boca Raton, Fla: CRC Press; 1996.

39. Delagarza VW. Pharmacologic treatment of Alzheimer's disease: an update. *Am Fam Phys.* 2003;68(7):1365–1372.

40. American Health Assistance Foundation. Alzheimer's family relief program. Available at: http://www.ahaf.org. Accessed February 13, 2006.

41. Centers for Disease Control and Prevention. Epilepsy: increasing awareness and improving care. Available at: http://www.cdc.gov/programs/chron02.htm. Accessed February 10, 2006.

42. Centers for Disease Control and Prevention. Disability/condition: multiple sclerosis and exercise. Available at: http://www.ncpad.org/disability/fact_sheet.php?sheet=186. Accessed February 10, 2006.

43. The Merck Manual Online. Multiple sclerosis. Available at: http://www.merck.com/mmhe/sec06/ch092/ch092b.html. Accessed February 10, 2006.

44. Gutierrez GM, Chow JW, Tillman MD, McCoy SC, Castellano V, White LJ. Resistance training improves gait kinematics in persons with multiple sclerosis. *Arch Phys Med Rehabil.* 2005;86(9):1824–1829.

45. Schwid SR, Covington M, Segal BM, Goodman AD. Fatigue in multiple sclerosis: current understanding and future directions. *J Rehabil Res Dev.* 2002;39(2):211–224.

46. Rietberg MB, Brooks D, Uitdehaag BMJ, Kwakkel G. Exercise therapy for multiple sclerosis. The Cochrane Database of Systematic Reviews, 3(CD003980.pub2); 2004.

47. Scher AI, Stewart WF, Liberman J, Lipton RB. Prevalence of frequent headache in a population sample. *Headache.* 1998;38(7):497–506.

48. Arena JG, Bruno GM, Hannah SL. A comparison of frontal electromyographic biofeedback training, trapezius electromyographic biofeedback training, and progressive muscle relaxation therapy in the treatment of tension headache. *Headache.* 1995;35(7):411–419.

49. National Institutes of Health and Substance Abuse and Mental Health Services Administration. Healthy People 2010: Substance abuse. Available at: http://www.healthypeople.gov/document/HTML/Volume2/26Substance.htm.. Accessed February 13, 2006.

50. Medline. Drug abuse and dependence. Medical Encyclopedia. Available at: http://www.nlm.nih.gov/medlineplus/ency/article/001522.htm. Accessed February 13, 2006.

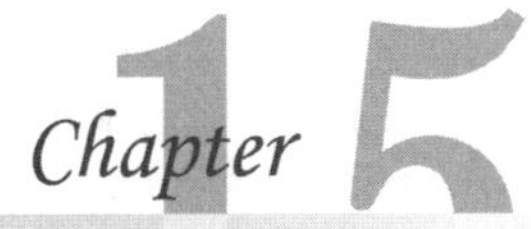

Secondary Prevention for Integumentary Disorders

Amy Foley, DPT, PT and Catherine Rush Thompson, PhD, MS, PT

"There are over 1 million new cases of skin cancer diagnosed in the US each year, outnumbering all other cancers combined."

~ NATIONAL COUNCIL ON SKIN CANCER PREVENTION

Lifespan Changes in the Integumentary System

The integumentary system contains the largest organ of the body, the skin. This system also includes subcutaneous tissues (responsible for storing energy and absorbing trauma), the nails, the hair, and the structures immediately under the superficial skin layer (dermis). The most important function of the integumentary system is protection. In addition to serving as a barrier against infection and injury, the skin helps to regulate body temperature, removes waste products from the body, protects internal structures (to some extent) from ultraviolet (UV) radiation, and produces vitamin D, an essential nutrient for maintaining normal blood levels of calcium and phosphorus needed to form and maintain strong bones. When the skin is compromised from overexposure to radiation, infectious agents, toxins, allergens, insect bites, and other types of injurious agents, the entire body becomes vulnerable. Maintaining skin integrity is essential for health and wellness. Simply observing someone's skin provides some clues about the overall health of that person.

A healthy full-term baby is born with extra fat and increased skin elasticity. With babies having proportionately greater skin surface than adults, they are especially prone to losing heat. As soon as the infant becomes more active, some of this "baby fat" is lost. Changes in the skin become more apparent during puberty when hormones influence sexual changes in hair and fat distribution and, in some cases, increased secretion from sebaceous glands. With aging and exposure to UV radiation, toxins, and other damaging agents, the skin tends to lose its elasticity, its vascularity, its thickness, its strength, and its thermoregulation properties. In older adults, the overall function of the skin is compromised with the graying of hair and the physiological changes underlying changes in physical appearance, including tissue dehydration and impaired wound healing. Primary practice includes health education about maintaining skin hydration as well as avoiding the various risk factors leading to premature aging and pathology.

Integumentary Pathology

One of the primary physical therapy practice patterns, as outlined in the *Guide to Physical Therapist Practice*,[1] is the integumentary system, since the skin is commonly affected by other pathologies, such as amputation, congestive heart failure, diabetes, malnutrition, neuromuscular dysfunction, obesity, peripheral nerve involvement, spinal cord dysfunction, and vascular disease. Any clients with impairments limiting levels of activity, reducing sensation, or causing edema, inflammation, pain, or ischemia are at increased risk for integumentary problems and should be monitored carefully by the physical therapist. Primary prevention of integumentary problems secondary to these common pathologies is an important role of physical therapists with management guided by *Practice Pattern 7A:* Primary prevention/ risk reduction for integumentary conditions.[1]

Patients with existing skin pathologies, such as superficial burns, cellulitis, and dermatitis, are managed using *Practice Pattern 7B:* Impaired integumentary integrity associated with superficial skin involvement. These conditions also include many of the skin pathologies commonly seen in the adult, discussed in Chapter 7. More serious integumentary conditions such as severe burns (partial- or full-thickness), pressure ulcers, serious skin infections, and skin cancers are addressed in the following practice patterns[1]:

7C: Impaired integumentary integrity associated with partial-thickness involvement and scar formation

7D: Impaired integumentary integrity associated with full-thickness skin involvement and burn formation

7E: Impaired integumentary integrity associated with skin involvement extending into fascia, muscle, or bone and scar formation

Physical therapists are fortunate in their practices to have the time to complete a comprehensive and thorough examination of their clients. A comprehensive examination and assessment of the patient includes identification of secondary complications related to chronic pathology, such as loss of integumentary integrity. Suspected risk to integumentary integrity should lead the physical therapist to three vital areas of skin care education: risk reduction for skin cancers, avoidance of pressure sores or wound development, and medication side effects with integumentary manifestations. In addition, physical therapists can help clients prevent losses of skin elasticity and range of motion by encouraging passive and active movement, a healthy diet (including adequate hydration), and protection from irritants and infections affecting the skin's integrity.

As integumentary conditions become more severe, the client becomes more vulnerable to complications resulting from exposure of underlying tissue. Physical therapists can play a key role in primary, secondary, and tertiary preventive care of clients presenting with integumentary risk factors and clinical manifestations of dermatological pathology.

Skin Cancer

One growing concern is the risk of skin cancer. The incidence of skin cancer is greater than the incidence of breast, lung, prostate, colorectal, and kidney cancers combined. In the United States, about 1.3 million new cases of skin cancer are diagnosed each year.[2] Individuals at the highest risk include children, those with increased outdoor time, those with decreased clothing worn outdoors, and those in areas were there is a decrease in atmospheric ozone levels. The American Academy of Dermatology has developed a quick screen for skin cancer. The ABCDE rule[3] of skin cancer helps to identify any abnormal skin lesions that are suspect and includes the following:

- "A" represents *asymmetry* in the lesions (ie, one half of the lesions is unlike other half).
- "B" represents *borders* that are irregular or poorly circumscribed.
- "C" represents *color* variation in the lesions (melanomas tend to have color variations that include tan, brown, black, white, red, and blue).
- "D" represents *diameter* greater than 6 mm (the size of a pencil eraser) since cancerous skin lesions tend to grow.
- "E" represents *elevation* since normal skin lesions tend to be flat and raised lesions may represent abnormal growth.

As part of a routine screening of all patients, the physical therapist should include questions incorporating the ABCDE rule. The ABCDE characteristics should be noted by physical therapists every time they examine a patient's skin, looking for moles that are irregularly shaped, have varied colors, are asymmetric, are greater than the size of a pencil eraser, or have grown or changed since your client's last visit.

The American Cancer Society recommends a thorough skin exam every 3 years between the ages of 20 and 40, every year age 40 or older, and monthly skin self-exams, most easily performed after a bath or shower.[4] A thorough screening demands that the entire surface of the body be palpated and inspected in good light. The onset and duration of each symptom should be recorded, together with a description of the lesion and any subsequent changes. Any suspected skin lesions should be reported to the physician immediately. Primary prevention includes educating individuals about monthly checks as well as the need to use a full-length mirror and brightly lit room to examine the entire body, including the scalp, inside the mouth, between the toes, and the bottoms of the feet. Individuals at an increased risk for melanoma are those with fair complexions; excessive exposure to UV radiation from the sun or tanning booths; occupational exposure to coal, tar, pitch, creosote, arsenic compounds, and radium; or human immunodeficiency virus (HIV). Preventive practice to reduce melanoma risk includes wearing effective protective sunscreens (containing para-aminobenzoic acid), avoiding sunlight as much as possible, and performing regular skin checks.[5] Individuals should be advised to report any skin changes, such as any sore or mark on the skin with changes in size, height, color, or shape, to their physician. In addition, any area on the skin that becomes itchy or painful and bleeds or ulcerates is also suspect.[5]

Examination of skin for suspicious lesions is considered primary prevention, especially when the person is at risk for skin cancer. For individuals with a previous history of skin cancer or with clinical evidence of precursor lesions (eg, dysplastic nevi and certain congenital nevi), skin examination should be performed regularly during physical therapy visits.[5] Most skin cancers develop mainly on areas of skin exposed to direct sunlight, including the scalp, face, lips, ears, neck, chest, arms and hands, and on the legs in women. They can also develop on unexposed areas, such as the palms, the spaces between toes, and the genital area. A cancerous skin lesion can appear suddenly, or it can develop slowly.

Secondary prevention includes reducing risk factors that can cause a recurrence of malignant skin lesions, including sun protection, self examination, and early diagnosis of potential malignant melanoma, basal cell carcinoma, and squamous cell carcinoma—common forms of skin cancer.

Basal cell or squamous cell carcinomas, the most common of skin cancers,[4] are likely to present in one of the following ways: as an open sore that bleeds, oozes, or crusts and is present for more than 3 weeks; as an irritated red patch that may itch or hurt; as a growth with a rolled border and central indentation; as a shiny bump or nodule; or as a scarlike area. Additional warning signs for malignant melanoma include sudden or continuous enlargement of a lesion; surface changes such as bleeding, crusting, erosion, oozing, scaling, or ulceration; changes in the surrounding skin such as redness, swelling, or satellite pigmentation; changes in sensation such as itching, tenderness, or pain; changes in consistency such as softening or friability; and the development of a new pigmented lesion, particularly in clients older than 40 years of age.[4] Physical therapists suspecting skin cancer should contact the physician immediately.

Pressure Sores

Physical therapists are vital members of health care teams when treating clients at risk for skin breakdown, including clients with periods of immobility, prolonged pressure on bony prominences, poor nutrition, incontinence of bowel and/or bladder, lowered mental alertness, history of pressure sore or open wound, or lack of sensation. Healthy People 2010 defines "persons at risk" as persons with a disability.[6] In this case, disability is defined as having either an activity limitation, a need for assistance in ADLs or IADLs, or a self-perception of having a disability. In 1994, 54 million people in the United States, or roughly 21% of the population, had some level of disability based on these criteria.[7] Although rates of disability are relatively stable or falling slightly for people aged 45 years and older, rates are on the rise among the younger population. One of the Healthy People 2010 initiatives for health care providers is identifying individuals at risk for pressure ulcers and ensuring the initiation of preventive measures to decrease their incidence.[6] Physical therapists are part of this initiative through their involvement in the initial assessment and in providing ongoing interventions for clients at significant risk for loss of integumentary integrity due to disability.

The National Pressure Ulcer Advisory Panel (NPUAP) recommends that a pressure ulcer risk assessment be performed on a patient's admission to a health care facility and on an ongoing basis as patients' conditions change.[8] This assessment should include follow-up by the physical therapist at home or as an outpatient, especially if the client has any disability. In 1996, the American Medical Directors Association (AMDA), a professional association of medical directors and physicians practicing in the long-term care continuum, developed clinical practice guidelines on pressure ulcers, highlighting the following additional responsibilities of the health care team in the prevention of pressure sores[9]:

1. Identify and manage underlying medical risk factors including disease states, nutritional compromise, skin disorders, and drugs that affect skin, such as corticosteroids
2. Identify and treat modifiable causes of decreased alertness, incontinence, and immobility
3. Identify and manage acute changes in condition that may increase the risk of skin breakdown, such as delirium
4. Identify subacute changes that increase risk, such as weight loss or progression of dementia

5. Clarify overall condition, prognosis, and realistic goals, if appropriate to the resident's situation.

The Agency for Health Care Policy and Research (AHCPR; now the Agency for Healthcare Research and Quality) recommended the Braden Scale and the Norton Scale as appropriate tools for assessing a patient's risk for pressure ulcers.[10] The primary objective of these scales is to predict pressure sore occurrence of clients in inpatient and outpatient settings. Since the scores are determined by direct observation, health care providers can individualize interventions needed for clients with pressure ulcers and those who are at risk. The Braden Scale, presented in Table 15-1, is a risk assessment incorporating six subscales: (1) sensory perception, (2) skin moisture, (3) activity, (4) mobility, (5) nutritional status, and (6) friction and shear factors. Each subscale is delineated by a status level with a weighted value, ranging from 1 to 4. For example, in the category of activity, a score of 1 is assigned to a patient who is bedfast, and a score of 4 indicates an individual who walks frequently. Total scores, ranging from 6 to 23, are based on subscale scores and determine an individual's level of risk for developing pressure ulcers. Predictive validity has been established for scores of 16 or less. Reported sensitivity for the tool ranges from 83% to 100%, and specificity ranges from 64% to 90%.[10]

Very often, the older adult patient, seen by the physical therapist for an unrelated condition, will present with a unique risk for skin breakdown. These clients are commonly seen in long-term care facilities but can as easily be seen in acute care environments. Berlowitz, Morris, and Brandis[11,12] collected clinical information on large numbers of nursing home residents researching the development and assessment of pressure sores. Using the Minimum Data Set from 1997, they developed a risk-adjustment model for pressure ulcer development, a tool that could be used to assess the quality of nursing home care. The study involved 14,607 nursing home residents without blistered skin and tissue damage or larger pressure ulcer on an initial assessment (stage 2). Pressure ulcer status was determined 90 days later, and the researchers identified potential predictors of pressure ulcer development. A total of 17 resident characteristics were associated with pressure ulcer development, including dependence in mobility and transferring (eg, from bed to wheelchair), diabetes mellitus, peripheral vascular disease, urinary incontinence, lower body mass index, and end-stage disease. The researchers developed the risk-adjustment model based on these characteristics and validated it in 13,457 nursing home residents. They used patients' risk of developing pressure ulcers to calculate expected rates of pressure ulcer development for 108 nursing homes; expected rates ranged from 1.1% to 3.2%, and observed rates ranged from 0% to 12.1%, demonstrating the model's effectiveness.[11,12]

Attention should also be given to the potential complications associated with pressure ulcers once they have occurred. Complications such as *endocarditis* (heart infection), *heterotopic bone formation* (bone formation in soft tissue), maggot infestation, *osteomyelitis* (bone infection), *bacteremia* (blood infection), *fistulas* (abnormal openings between organs), *septic arthritis* (infection of inflamed joints), develomement of sinus tracts or abscess, and systemic complications of topical treatment, such as iodine toxicity and hearing loss after topical neomycin and systemic gentamicin, are not uncommon and can result from poor hygiene and exposure to infectious agents.[13] Physical therapists should be cognizant of the potential secondary complication of pressure sores in their patients, measures to prevent these from occurring, and finally, appropriate care of pressure sores once integumentary integrity is compromised.

Health Education for Skin Care

Individuals, particularly those with frail skin or those with type I or type II diabetes, should be educated about keeping nails trimmed, avoiding scratching the skin, and bathing in nonfragranced warm water, rather than hot water. The Lower Extremity Amputation Prevention (LEAP) organization advocates routine and frequent screening of skin for risk factors associated with diabetes. These include prominence of metatarsal heads, dry skin, callus formation, unable to perceive 10 g force (5.07 Simmes-Weinstein filament), and finally, decreased thermal and vibration sensation, which tends to dry the skin.[14] Also, avoidance of allergens and skin irritants such as fabric softeners, perfumed soaps, and household cleansers should be emphasized. For those engaged in aquatic activities, bathing is essential following swimming for removing drying pool chemicals. Protection from the sun can be achieved by avoiding peak sunshine (10:00 am to 4:00 pm) and limiting unnecessary sun exposure through protective clothing and maintained sunscreen. Over-the-counter topical ointments (such as topical steroids) can be used to manage minor skin irritations and to reduce skin infections when there is skin injury; however, any client presenting with chronic skin inflammation, pruritus, or suspicious skin lesions should be more thoroughly examined by a dermatologist.

TABLE 15-1

BRADEN SCALE

Braden Scale for Predicting Pressure Sore Risk

Patient's Name: Evaluator's Name: Date of Assessment:

Sensory Perception Ability to respond meaningfully to pressure-related discomfort	1. Completely limited: Unresponsive (does not moan, flinch, or grasp) to painful stimuli, due to diminished level of consciousness or sedation OR Limited ability to feel pain over most of body surface.	2. Very limited: Responds only to painful stimuli. Cannot communicate discomfort except by moaning or restlessness, OR Has a sensory impairment which limits the ability to feel pain or discomfort over half of body.	3. Slightly limited: Responds to verbal commands, but cannot always communicate discomfort or need to be turned, OR Has some sensory impairment which limits ability to feel pain or discomfort in one or two extremities.	4. No impairment: Responds to verbal commands. Has no sensory deficit that would limit ability to feel or voice pain or discomfort.
Moisture Degree to which skin is exposed to moisture	1. Constantly moist: Skin is kept moist almost constantly by perspiration, urine, etc. Dampness is detected every time patient is moved or turned.	2. Moist: Skin is often but not always moist. Linen must be changed at least once a shift.	3. Occasionally moist: Skin is occasionally moist, requiring an extra linen change approximately once a day.	4. Rarely moist: Skin is usually dry; linen requires changing only at routine intervals.
Activity Degree of physical activity	1. Bedfast: Confined to bed.	2. Chairfast: Ability to walk severely limited or non-existent. Cannot bear own weight and/or must be assisted into chair or wheelchair.	3. Walks occasionally: Walks occasionally during the day but for very short distances, with or without assistance. Spends majority of each shift in bed or chair.	4. Walks frequently: Walks outside the room at least twice a day and inside room at least once every two hours during waking hours.
Mobility Ability to change and control body position	1. Completely immobile: Does not make even slight changes in body or extremity position without assistance.	2. Very limited: Makes occasional slight changes in body or extremity position, but unable to make frequent or significant changes independently.	3. Slightly limited: Makes frequent though slight changes in body extremity position independently.	4. No limitations: Makes major and frequent changes in position without assistance.
Nutrition Usual food intake pattern	1. Very poor: Never eats a complete meal. Rarely eats more than one-third of any food offered. Eats two servings or less of protein (meat or dairy products) per day. Takes fluids poorly. Does not take a liquid dietary supplement, OR Is NPO[1] and/or maintained on clear liquids or IV[2] for more than 5 days.	2. Probably inadequate: Rarely eats a complete meal and generally eats only about half of any food offered. Protein intake includes only three servings of meat or dairy products per day. Occasionally will take a dietary supplement, OR Receives less than optimum amount of liquid diet or tube feeding.	3. Adequate: Eats over half of most meals. Eats a total of four servings of protein (meat, dairy products) each day. Occasionally will refuse a meal, but will usually take a supplement if offered, OR Is on a tube feeding or TPN[3] regimen, which probably meets most nutritional needs.	4. Excellent: Eats most of every meal. Never refuses a meal. Usually eats a total of four or more servings of meat and dairy products. Occasionally eats between meals. Does not require supplementation.
Friction and Shear	1. Problem: Requires moderate to maximum assistance in moving. Complete lifting without sliding against sheets is impossible. Frequently slides down in bed or chair, requiring frequent repositioning with maximum assistance. Spasticity, contractures, or agitation leads to almost constant friction.	2. Potential problem: Moves feebly or requires minimum assistance. During a move, skin probably slides to some extent against sheets, chair, restraints, or other devices. Maintains relatively good position in chair or bed most of the time, but occasionally slides down.	3. No apparent problem: Moves in bed and in chair independently and has sufficient muscle strength to lift up completely during move. Maintains good position in bed or chair at all times.	

ADOPTED 1997

TOTAL SCORE:

Common Integumentary Side Effects of Medications

The majority of clients in physical therapy likely receive some form of adjunctive or primary pharmacological care to assist in the management of their acute or chronic medical conditions. The most common medications encountered in the management of many acute conditions include analgesics, anti-inflammatory agents, and muscle relaxants. Physical therapists should be aware of adverse drug reactions associated with these medications. Adverse drug events are the leading cause of medical injury in hospitalized clients in the United States.[15] The number of persons affected is roughly four times the total number killed in automobile accidents every year. Adverse drug events account for an estimated one-fifth of the total 1 million hospitalized clients who are injured each year. Analgesics and antibiotics cause the majority of allergic reactions.[16]

In general, cutaneous drug reactions are the most common adverse responses to drugs, though not the only adverse reaction. *Urticaria* (itchy, swollen, red bumps or patches on the skin) is the most common reaction; however, there are many different types of drug reactions, and some are life threatening.

Aspirin and *nonsteroidal anti-inflammatory drugs (NSAIDs)* can cause *angioedema* (swelling beneath the skin) and urticaria. The prevalence of aspirin-induced angioedema and urticaria is about 5% in the general population but only about 1.5% in clients with aspirin-induced asthma.[17] Use of aspirin over time effectively prevents aspirin-induced bronchospasm, but very little data support its effectiveness for reducing urticaria or angioedema. Instead, affected clients should be given analgesics with minimal cyclooxygenase inhibition. NSAIDs can cause common cutaneous reactions, such as *pruritus* (itching), *morbilliform rash* (rash appearing like measles), urticaria, and photosensitivity. Urticaria is most frequent in salicylate-sensitive patients. Other skin reactions are unusual, although *purpura* (bruiselike coloration) and *cutaneous vasculitis* (an allergic inflammatory reaction of vessels) have been attributed to NSAIDs.[18]

Acetaminophen was once thought to be a safe alternative to aspirin, and NSAIDs were thought safe for clients with aspirin sensitivity. However, more recent data suggest that high doses of acetaminophen inhibit cyclooxygenase and can exacerbate asthma in aspirin-sensitive patients. Settipane and associates[18] studied cross-sensitivity to acetaminophen doses up to 1,500 mg in asthmatic clients with aspirin sensitivity. The probability of acetaminophen tolerance could be predicted by the degree of aspirin sensitivity. Aspirin-desensitized clients were able to tolerate acetaminophen at higher doses. The study also suggests that high doses of acetaminophen (more than 1,000 mg) may cause sufficient cyclooxygenase inhibition to induce bronchospasm.

Skeletal muscle relaxants are commonly prescribed to relieve the stiffness, pain, and discomfort caused by strains, sprains, or other injury to muscles treated in physical therapy. The common cutaneous reactions to this drug classification are large hivelike swellings on the face (eyelids, mouth, lips, and/or tongue), itching, and redness. Additional cutaneous reactions include tenderness, swelling over a blood vessel, pinpoint red spots on the skin, sores/ulcers/white spots on the lips or in the mouth, and unusual bruising or bleeding.[19] All of these reactions should be reported to the patient's physician.

Summary

The advent of direct access has increased physical therapists' responsibility to closely screen clients for a variety of medical conditions, to differentially diagnose those needing specialized care, to appropriately refer clients to other therapists and health care professionals, and to recognize secondary complication of chronic conditions and their medical management. Screening the integumentary system for potential burns, rashes, lesions, or growths and monitoring the skin when it becomes vulnerable with chronic pathology are important roles for physical therapists. Health education to prevent skin cancer and to prevent secondary complications from pathology should be practiced with all clients.

References

1. APTA. *Guide to Physical Therapist Practice.* 2nd ed. American Physical Therapy Association; 2001.
2. American Cancer Society. Facts on skin cancer. 1599 Clifton Rd, NE, Atlanta, Ga 30329-4251. (800)ACS-2345. Available at: http://www.cancer.org.
3. The Skin Cancer Foundation. The ABCDEs of moles & melanomas; dysplastic nevi and malignant melanoma: a patient's guide; skin cancer: if you can spot it, you can stop it. New York, NY: The Skin Cancer Foundation. Available at: http://www.skincancer.org.
4. American Cancer Society. Prevention and early detection of malignant melanoma. Atlanta, Ga: Available at: http://www.cancer.org.
5. American Academy of Family Physicians. Skin cancer: saving your skin from sun damage. Kansas City, Mo. Available at: http://www.aafp.org.

6. US Department of Health and Human Services. Healthy People 2010. Available at: http://www.health.gov. Accessed October 29, 2002.
7. Zanca JM, Brienza DM, Berlowitz D, et al. Pressure ulcer research funding in America: creation and analysis of an online database. *Adv Skin Wound Care.* 2003;16(4);190–197.
8. AHCPR. Publication No. 95-0652: Clinical guidelines number 15: pressure ulcers. December 1994. Available at: http:www.ahcpr.gov/news/pubcat/c_clin.htm.
9. American Medical Directors Association. *Clinical Practice Guidelines on Pressure Ulcers.* Columbia, Md: American Medical Directors Association; 1996.
10. Prevention Plus, LLC. Braden scale. Available at: http://www.bradenscale.com.
11. Berlowitz DR, Brandeis GH, Morris JN, et al. Deriving a risk-adjustment model for pressure ulcer development using the minimum data set. *J Am Geriatr Society.* 2001;49:866–871.
12. Berlowitz DR, Brandeis GH, Anderson JJ, et al. Evaluation of a risk-adjustment model for pressure ulcer development using the minimum data set. *J Am Geriatr Society.* 2001;49:872–876.
13. MacLean DS. Preventing and managing pressure sores. *Caring for the Ages.* 2003;4(3):34–37
14. National Hansen's Disease Programs (NHDP). Lower extremity amputation prevention program. Available at: http://bphc.hrsa.gov/leap. Accessed February 6, 2006.
15. Bates DW, Cullen DJ, Laird N, et al. Incidence of adverse drug events and potential adverse drug events: implications for prevention. ADE Prevention Study Group. *JAMA.*1995;274(1):29–34.
16. Stevenson DD. Diagnosis, prevention, and treatment of adverse reactions to aspirin and nonsteroidal anti-inflammatory drugs. *J Allergy Clin Immunol.* 1984;74(4[Pt 2]):617–622.
17. Roujeau JC. Clinical aspects of skin reactions to NSAIDs. *Scand J Rheumatol.* 1987;65(Suppl):131–134.
18. Settipane RA, Schrank PJ, Simon RA, et al. Prevalence of cross-sensitivity with acetaminophen in aspirin-sensitive asthmatic subjects. *J Allergy Clin Immunol.* 1995;96(4):480–485.
19. MedlinePlus. Drugs, S=supplements, and herbal information. Available at: http://www.nlm.nih.gov/medlineplus/druginformation.html.

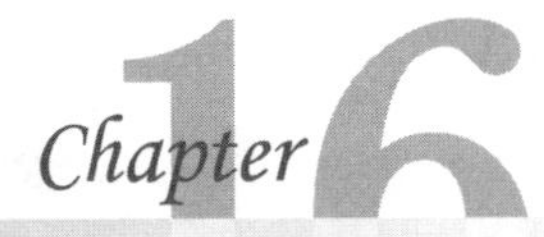

Prevention Practice for Individuals With Developmental Disabilities

Catherine Rush Thompson, PhD, MS, PT

"Due to medical advances people with developmental disabilities are living longer lives. Additionally, there is a large emerging population of 'baby boomers' with developmental disabilities who are experiencing aging issues much earlier than the general population."

~TONY LODUCA, ST. COLETTA

Definitions of Developmental Disabilities

Developmental disability is defined as follows[1]:

A cognitive, emotional, or physical impairment, especially one related to abnormal sensory or motor development, appearing in infancy or childhood and involving a failure or delay in progressing through the normal developmental stages of childhood.

This first definition focuses on the onset of impairments during childhood that alter normal child development. Another definition describes individuals with developmental disabilities as follows[2]:

Persons with *a severe and chronic disability that is attributable to a mental or physical impairment or a combination of mental and physical impairments, is manifested before the person attains age 22, is likely to continue indefinitely, results in substantial functional limitations in three or more of the following areas of major life activity (self-care, receptive and expressive language, learning, mobility, self-direction, capacity for independent living, economic self-sufficiency), reflects the person's need for a combination and sequence of special, interdisciplinary, or generic care, treatment, or other services, which are lifelong or extended duration and individually planned and coordinated.*

This second definition provides more information about the functional limitations evident in one's life activities and the need for continual services across the life span. Another third definition is less specific about the functional limitations, yet provides illustrations of diagnoses that are considered developmental disabilities[1]:

A mental or physical disability, such as cerebral palsy or mental retardation, arising before adulthood and usually lasting throughout life.

While developmental disabilities are considered one category of individuals with disabilities, the range of physical impairments, functional limitations, and disabilities is too great to discuss as one population. Medical diagnoses often included in the category of developmental disabilities include, but are not limited to, those listed in Table 16-1.

From the viewpoint of physical therapy, the majority of these conditions are classified in one of two preferred practice patterns as described in the *Guide to Physical Therapist Practice*[3]:

- *5B* Impaired neuromotor development
- *5C* Impaired motor and sensory integrity associated with nonprogressive disorders of the central nervous system—congenital origin or acquired in infancy or childhood

TABLE 16-1

COMMON DEVELOPMENTAL DISABILITIES

Diagnosis	*Cause(s)*	*Impairment(s)*	*Management*
Autism spectrum disorders	The cause(s) of autism is unknown. Genetic, environmental, immunologic, and metabolic factors could influence the development of the disorder.	Variable Often have communication problems and/or sensorimotor impairments	Refer to speech pathologist for communication needs Provide sensorimotor activities and refer to occupational therapy
Cerebral palsy	Congenital problems, pathology, or trauma resulting in brain damage can lead to cerebral palsy.	Variable Often motor impairments May have cognitive impairments	Provide developmental activities as appropriate for age, skill, and cognition
Mental retardation (including Down syndrome)	The most common preventable cause of mental retardation is the consumption of alcohol during pregnancy, resulting in Fetal Alcohol Syndrome.	Often have motor delays and cognitive delays that present at an early age	Provide developmental activities as appropriate for age, skill, and cognition Medical and educational team intervention covers the spectrum of developmental needs
Hearing impairment	Ear infections, such as otitis media are most common. Genetic problems, congenital problems, and illness or injury after birth may cause impaired hearing.	May have speech, language, and cognitive delays	Provide developmental activities as appropriate for age, skill, and cognition Refer to an audiologist for hearing tests Refer to a speech pathologist for communication skills, as needed
Visual impairment	Congenital problems, pathology, or trauma can result in brain damage causing visual impairment.	May have cognitive and motor delays	Provide developmental activities as appropriate for age, skill, and cognition
Attention deficit hyperactivity disorder (ADHD)	Heredity is the most common cause.	May have difficulties with attending to a task	Provide developmental activities as appropriate for age, skill, and cognition
Epilepsy	Congenital problems, pathology, or trauma can result in brain damage causing cerebral palsy.	May have difficulties with attending to a class and may be at risk for injury	Provide developmental activities as appropriate for age, skill, and cognition
Spina bifida	Unknown cause. Possible environmental and genetic factors	May have cognitive and motor delays, depending upon the level of the lesion(s) and other comorbities	Provide developmental activities as appropriate for age, skill, and cognition

The global outcomes for these children, youth, and adults with developmental disabilities include the following[3]:

- Mitigating or reducing the impact of the condition as much as possible through education about the pathology and awareness of likely complications
- Limiting impairments, especially those contributing to reduced postural control, limited mobility, health-related fitness, and wellness
- Reducing functional limitations through *habilitation* (developing sufficient ability to perform functional activities), *compensation* (using alternative methods to accomplish a task), or *adaptation* (providing assistive devices, etc, as appropriate)
- Reducing health risks and preventing complications associated with the pathology (using secondary prevention measures, such as protecting the skin, preventing musculoskeletal limitations, and reducing exposure to infections)
- Promoting health, fitness, and wellness
- Providing appropriate resources
- Ensuring family and child satisfaction

When providing health, fitness, and wellness resources to individuals with developmental disabilities, the physical therapist must be cognizant of the medical diagnosis and the physical therapy diagnosis, as well as the various physical and psychosocial environments each individual will encounter across the lifespan. This chapter discusses the most common types of developmental disabilities and provides suggestions for preventive practice to enhance health, fitness, and wellness, building on the roles of the physical therapist discussed in previous chapters.

Misconceptions About Individuals With Disabilities

The authors of Healthy People 2010[4] list four main misconceptions about individuals with disabilities that interfere with implementation of this national agenda. These misconceptions are (1) all individuals with disabilities are in poor health, (2) the focus of public health should only be on preventing disabling conditions, (3) a standard definition of "disability" or "people with disabilities" is not needed, and (4) the environment does not play a role in the disabling process. The first step in promoting health is eliminating these four misconceptions.

Misconception #1: Disability Equals Poor Health

It is inaccurate to say that all individuals with disabilities are in poor health. Often, these individuals are at an increased risk of illness, but with proper care, they can be as healthy as individuals without disabilities, depending on their medical diagnoses. The same health education and prevention/protection strategies offered to the general public should be offered to all individuals with disabilities. Physical therapists need to be advocates ensuring multiple health and fitness options for all populations served and should tailor health education and protection/prevention strategies to the unique needs of individuals with developmental disabilities.

Misconception #2: Disability Is the Focus

To eliminate another misconception, the focus of public health should be on health, fitness, and wellness for all individuals rather than disability prevention. For individuals with disabilities, appropriate accommodations should be made to ensure equal access to health promotion.

Misconception #3: What Is "Disability?"

One of the greatest barriers to achieving equitable care is the variance in definitions for the term "disability." There needs to be a universal definition of disability encompassing the educational, medical, legal, social, and economic issues that can be addressed through teamwork and advocacy.

Misconception #4: Environment Is Not Important

Not surprisingly, the environment plays a key role in the disabling process. The "environment," however, includes not only the physical environment but also the psychosocial environment created by the attitudes people share about individuals with disabilities. While it is possible to remove many physical, legal, and civic barriers through time and effort, it takes more time, effort, and vigilance to change peoples' attitudes about disabilities. Negative attitudes can profoundly affect health, wellness, and perspectives of life for those with developmental disabilities. People with disabilities encounter many different forms of attitudinal barriers, including pity, intolerance, impatience, ignorance, and those generated by stereotypes projected through the media. Physical therapists must first assess their own attitudes toward individuals with disabilities to ensure a positive psychosocial environment for their clients. Once they explore their own prejudices or attitudes, then they can help others, including family members, educators, and others, deal more effectively with individuals who are developmentally disabled. Physical therapists can help change the psychosocial environment by educating others about how to interact effectively with people with disabilities, including the use of "people first" language. For example, a child with Down syndrome should not be referred to as a "Down syndrome child."

Assessing Health, Fitness, and Wellness

Many of the screening tools and tests discussed earlier in this book can be used for determining the special needs of a client with developmental disabilities. The range of possible screening and examination tools is listed in the *Guide to Physical Therapist Practice*.[3] These tests and measures should be conducted in the appropriate physical environments to ensure the individuals' safety and full attention. While standardized testing may be valuable for metabolic fitness measures, more creative criterion-referenced tests that examine the individuals' functions can yield valuable information for creating customized health, fitness, and wellness programs.

After completing the examination, with all necessary history and current information, the physical therapist can determine the special needs of the individual seeking resources for health, fitness, and wellness. It is important to examine both the structure and function of each individual to determine if any habitual behaviors have resulted in problems with body structure. Examining each individual's physical fitness provides a baseline for individualized exercise prescription.

Metabolic Fitness

Metabolic fitness, as described in Chapter 3, involves tests of bodily functions at rest, including vital signs and blood tests. Often, individuals with developmental disabilities have stable vital signs and negative blood tests; nevertheless, determining healthy baseline measures enables the physical therapist to either progress to health-related fitness activities or to consult with other health care professionals, as needed, to ensure the individual's health at rest. Individuals with developmental disabilities should have a preparticipation screening conducted by a physician to reveal medical issues that need to be addressed in an exercise program.

Health-Related Fitness

Individuals with disabilities are at a higher risk than the general population for (1) developing medical problems due to limited activity, (2) developing psychosocial problems, and (3) having reduced life spans. Benefits of exercise extend beyond physical fitness to include physical wellness, social wellness, psychological wellness, and emotional wellness, as described in Chapter 1. Overall, the healthy individual develops *salutogenesis* (a complete physical, mental, and social well-being) and not merely the absence of disease. Allowing individuals with disabilities to choose their own options for health promotion is conducive to long-term involvement in healthy activities. Those with developmental disabilities may need specialized adaptations for their activities and to their environments to fitness activities for flexibility, posture, muscular strength, muscular endurance, cardiorespiratory fitness, and body composition.

Flexibility

The majority of children with developmental disabilities have abnormal sensory or motor development contributing to abnormal growth patterns of the body. Children who do not begin walking by the age of 2 may not experience the normal stresses of weight bearing to develop fully. Children with developmental disabilities must be encouraged to bear weight in appropriate positions to promote bone growth without developing musculoskeletal deformities. Children who are at risk for delayed motor development and reduced growth include those with *cerebral palsy* (most commonly those with spastic quadriparesis limiting voluntary movement of the head, neck, trunk, and limbs), *spina bifida* (especially those with spinal cord lesions that compromise muscle strength and muscle balance), and *Down syndrome* (a condition often affecting both physical and cognitive development). In many children with developmental disabilities, delays in motor development result in range of motion limitations that can endure for a lifetime. Providing flexibility exercises, either active exercise performed by the individual or assisted/passive range of motion exercise, is essential for health-related fitness for this population. The physical therapist can monitor range of motion of all "at risk" joints to ensure that growth spurts and functional habits do not affect the individual's flexibility.

Posture

Postural Control

Postural control provides the base of support for the performance of motor skills, such as walking, feeding, and handwriting. Smooth transitions from one posture to another require the fine muscle adjustments of larger muscle groups evidenced with postural control. Postural control provides the individual with *anti-gravity stability* in postures, *automatic reactions with unexpected perturbations*, and postural adjustments when reaching for objects or preparing to catch a ball (ie, *anticipatory postural control*).[5] Many children with developmental disabilities have difficulty with controlling their bodies in sitting and standing postures. For example, individuals with cerebral palsy who have *spastic quadriparesis* (involving reduced motor control of the entire body) often have problems with feeding, swallowing, and speech secondary to poor control of the head, neck, trunk, mouth, and jaw. Working with these children on holding the correct postural alignment in sitting or working in other developmental postures helps to provide a more stable base for muscles to function effectively.

Therapeutic Positioning

When individuals lack postural control in sitting, they are often positioned in prone (on the stomach), supine (on the back), or lying on one side by their caretakers. A number of studies have associated the prone sleeping position in infants with an increased risk of sudden infant death syndrome (SIDS), so pediatricians and nurseries have encouraged parents to position children in other positions, such as supine, as part of the Back to Sleep campaign.[6] In many parts of the country, this Back to Sleep campaign is successful based on the significantly increased proportion of infants sleeping supine and the reduced incidence of SIDS. While reducing SIDS by positioning children supine is important, this change in positioning coincides with an increase in infant cranial deformity with supine sleeping position.[7] "Abnormalities of the occipital cranial suture in infancy can cause significant posterior cranial asymmetry, malposition of the ears, distortion of the cranial base, deformation of the forehead, and facial asymmetry."[7] These cranial abnormalities can be prevented by frequent changes of position and the use of alternate positions, such as sidelying. The role of physical therapists is to clarify that prone positioning *for play* is not a risk factor for SIDS and that it is desirable for infants to spend supervised wakeful time in the prone position, especially for children with developmental disabilities and poor postural control.

For those individuals who do not develop independent sitting, the physical therapist must prescribe therapeutic positioning to support the child, youth, or adult for antigravity activities, such as sitting. The seated postural control measure (SPCM) can be used for seating assessment, offering 22 seating postural alignment items and 12 functional movement items, each scored on a four-point criterion referenced scale.[8] *Adaptive seating devices (ASDs)* are commonly used in the treatment of individuals with developmental disabilities. In one longitudinal study, 19 individuals with multiple handicaps and developmental disabilities (aged 1 to 6 years) were evaluated through direct observation and parent/guardian assessment pre- and postpositioning for 6 months. Activities observed included head control, controlled sitting posture, visual tracking, reach, and grasp. Over the 6 months of intervention, sitting posture, head control, and grasp improved significantly, and parents were freed from handling their children and allowed to engage in other activities with the children and around the home.[6]

Children with Down syndrome need guidance in proper sitting and transitional movements to and from sitting because they tend to have excessive hip external rotation and hip abduction, excessive hip mobility in sitting and transitions to and from sitting, and a wide-based gait. For these children, physical therapy intervention should focus on developing strength in hip muscles, providing support (such as a stretch garment that restricts hip abduction and external rotation), and incorporating body rotation in transitional movement from prone to supine and from sitting to all fours.[9]

Children with spastic cerebral palsy have a tendency to adduct and internally rotate their hips if they are not seated with proper support. In looking at bilateral hand skills, the recommended posture for improving fine motor function is sitting with hip abduction with a straddling device to optimize postural stability by increasing the child's base of support.

MUSCULAR STRENGTH AND ENDURANCE

Muscle strength is essential for controlling the body. Simply encouraging normal motor development provides opportunities to strengthen muscles through daily activities. Older individuals with developmental disabilities can benefit from more directed exercises for general body strengthening, using the principles of progression, overload, and specificity described in Chapter 4. For many individuals, fitness training can be accomplished through standard exercise; however, for individuals with increased muscle tone, movement is more challenging, and spasticity management must be addressed along with efforts to strengthen muscles. While some have thought that maximal efforts to contract muscles could increase spasticity, research suggests otherwise.[10] Using prolonged stretching exercises (including serial casting and positioning in a prone stander), antispasmodic medications (using botulinum toxin A or baclofen), coactivation of antagonistic muscles, and electrical stimulation have been used to reduce spasticity, aiding the development of greater muscle strength and endurance.[10] Studies have consistently shown that children engaged in muscle strengthening have improved motor function.[10,11]

Individuals with low tone also benefit from muscle strengthening activities. Adults with Down syndrome demonstrated significant gains in muscle strength, muscle endurance, and cardiovascular endurance, in addition to slight but significant reduction in body weight, after engaging in a 12-week exercise program (3 days a week for 45 minutes per session) consisting of cardiovascular and strengthening exercises. "Greater effort must be made to promote increases in physical activity participation among persons with Down syndrome and developmental disabilities in order to reduce the potential health risks associated with low fitness and sedentary behavior."[12] Simply engaging in more antigravity activity can increase muscle strength and endurance. In one study comparing the muscle activation of individuals with normal versus delayed motor development, results indicated that children with slower motor development had greater muscle activity in their legs.[12]

Equipment for strengthening can be inexpensive and low risk. Resistive bands are lightweight resistive materials that can be easily adjusted in length and resistance by folding the band, increasing or reducing the slack, or placing them around the extremities to work both arms and legs simultaneously. One precaution is some children are allergic to the materials used to fabricate these bands. It is best to use latex-free materials.

Improving Cardiorespiratory Fitness

Cardiorepiratory endurance is another key component of fitness training. The running and jumping subtests of the Gross Motor Function Measure are helpful in determining a child's level of anaerobic fitness of the legs; however, it is not a suitable tool for determining aerobic capacity of the body or the anaerobic capacity of the arms.[13] Another method of measuring cardiorespiratory endurance is the arm ergometer. In a study using arm ergometry and comparing the oxygen consumption (VO_2), heart rate (HR), and physical working capacity (PWC) of able-bodied individuals and those with cerebral palsy, individuals with cerebral palsy had comparable measures in all except in PWC or the ability to perform maximal work at equal intensities and durations.[13,14] In practice, aerobic work capacity (VO_2 max) is the capacity most often considered. Children and adolescents with cerebral palsy have lower maximal oxygen consumption (VO_2 max) and subnormal values for peak anaerobic power and muscular endurance of the upper and lower limbs when compared with their able-bodied peers.[15]

Gait abnormalities in children with cerebral palsy have been shown to increase sub-maximal walking energy expenditure almost three-fold when compared with healthy children. One study examining the energy costs of gait concluded the following[16]:

> *A certain level of muscle co-contraction is necessary for achieving joint stability during locomotion, particularly at the ankle and knee. There appears, however, to be a co-contraction threshold beyond which there are associated elevated metabolic costs during locomotion in children with cerebral palsy (CP).*

In studies using wheelchair ergometry, measures of maximum oxygen uptake (VO_2 max) can be used as a helpful tool for evaluating the cardiorespiratory fitness of individuals who are nonambulatory.[15] When considering an individual's physiologic demands for increasing cardiorespiratory fitness, it is important to note that these demands are increased for individuals with neurologic and orthopedic disabilities.[15] Furthermore, individuals with intellectual disabilities need supervised treadmill training programs to provide needed cardiorespiratory exercises for endurance and prevention of heart-related diseases.[15]

Continuous exercise, such as walking, cycling, or swimming at slower speeds, is generally less demanding both mentally and physically than interval exercise (exercise with rest breaks). Continuous exercise is effective for cardiovascular fitness and is less likely to produce injury. Interval exercise enables the individual to work at higher intensities for shorter periods, pushing the individual's performance to higher levels for competition.

Body Composition

Individuals who tend to be more sedentary are likely to become overweight. Physical activity is known to have a positive influence on body composition, decreasing body fat and increasing muscle mass. One study examining the effectiveness of a 45-minute exercise program for individuals with Down syndrome found that those with regular activity (consisting of cardiovascular and strength activities) reduced body weight and potential health risks associated with sedentary behavior.[17] In a similar study examining the effects of a 9-month sports program for children with spastic cerebral palsy, researchers found that children with higher intensity programming (4 sessions versus 2 sessions per week) had relatively reduced fat mass and increased peak aerobic power (VO_2 max).[18] These studies suggest that children with abnormal muscle tone, sensorimotor impairments, and cognitive impairments can benefit from cardiovascular and strength training, provided they have no conditions precluding such activities.

Promoting Health for Individuals With Developmental Disabilities

Individuals with disabilities are at a higher risk of developing both physical and psychosocial problems due to limited physical activity. These problems include obesity, hypertension, circulatory problems, reduced muscle strength, reduced flexibility, osteoporosis, scoliosis, skin breakdown, reduced endurance, social isolation, and depression. Proper exercise in an inclusive setting reduces the risk of disease and promotes both physical and mental wellness. Exercise prescription principles for persons with developmental disability should be designed to enhance physical fitness, promote health by reducing the risk for chronic disease, and ensure safety during exercise participation. The focus of the exercise prescription should

TABLE 16-2

IMPROVEMENTS ASSOCIATED WITH PARTICIPATION IN SPECIAL OLYMPICS

Decreased	Increased
• Weight	• Overall fitness and strength
• Body fat	• Aerobic capacity
• Stereotypic, self-stimulatory behaviors	• Athletic achievement
• Inappropriate vocalizations	• Cardiovascular fitness
• Off-task behaviors	• Appropriate or correct academic responding
• Aggression	• On-task behavior at work or school
• Hyperactivity	• Task completion at work or school
	• Self-esteem
	• Social competence
	• Peer relationships

Adapted from Dykens E, Rosner B, Butterbaugh G. Exercise and sports in children and adolescents with developmental disabilities. *Sports Psychiatry.* 1998;7(4):757–768.

be on individual interests, health needs, and each individual's clinical status. Oftentimes the exercise mode, intensity, frequency, and duration are modified according to the individual's clinical condition.

Sometimes caretakers are hesitant to initiate physical fitness programs for fear they might exacerbate any conditions these individuals might have. Encouraging athletic performance through adaptive physical education and Special Olympics can increase engagement in regular activity. Participation in sports is important for the physical and emotional health of all individuals. Sports can improve strength, endurance, and cardiopulmonary fitness while providing companionship, a sense of achievement, and heightened self-esteem.[19] Improved physical and psychosocial functioning are found in studies of both children and adults with mental retardation, as well as in research on athletes enrolled in Special Olympics International, the largest recreational sport program in the world for persons with developmental disabilities (Table 16-2).[20] Physical therapists should educate families about the need for a preparticipation screening by a physician, appropriate athletic options, specialized equipment, and risks associated with specific sports.

Barriers to Health Promotion Opportunities

A disparity exists between what individuals with developmental disabilities seek for fitness and health promotion options and what is available for their use. As stated previously, health problems associated with the limited activity level of this population include obesity, hypertension, circulatory problems, reduced muscle strength, reduced flexibility, osteoporosis, scoliosis, skin breakdown, reduced endurance, social isolation, and depression. Proper exercise in an inclusive setting promotes both physical and mental wellness. Participation in community activities, specifically community-based fitness opportunities, depends on the restrictions, barriers, and facilitators influencing a given environment or social situation. Adaptations of activities, assistive devices/technology, and specialized training often enable individuals with impairments to function in daily activities (mobility, communication, personal care, domestic activities, simple movements, learning, and appropriate behavior). If accommodations are made to meet the individual's needs (modifying or reducing functional limitations for exercise), social restrictions, physical barriers, and facilitators could enhance an individual's participation in fitness activities. Lack of time, money, staffing, transportation, knowledge about specific disabilities, and motivation, as well as negative attitudes are barriers that could limit participation in community-based activities. Identification of these barriers provides a mechanism for matching resources to areas of need.

Resources to Enhance Participation in Health Promotion and Fitness Opportunities

Experts in special adaptations for individuals with physical impairments include physical therapists, occupational therapists, and recreational therapists, and these people can serve as facilitators, addressing concerns and removing barriers to inclusive health promotion opportunities. Lack of self-motivation to exercise is one of the most confounding factors to overcome. Extrinsic motivators for participation in health promotion activities include the following:

- Offering t-shirts as clients reach specific goals
- Creating charts listing progress toward fitness goals (eg, walking across the state)
- Writing news stories featuring active clients in facility's newsletter
- Providing awards or special recognition to clients (eg, "Client of the Month")
- Providing coupons/tickets for local activities or events to clients meeting fitness goals
- Emphasizing socialization as part of fitness programs (create exercise groups)
- Developing a bulletin board that lists activities and regular participants

Local libraries (public, college and university, medical centers and hospitals) and Internet searches provide an array of fitness information for those with special needs. Using the website http://www.google.com, a search for the terms "fitness developmental disabilities" matched 257,000 records of information. Using the term "fitness" alone matched 99,100,000. Interestingly, less than 5 years ago the same search for the terms "fitness developmental disability" revealed only seven matches, the majority of which related to books about physical disabilities. Clearly, there is adequate information to learn about fitness options for individuals with developmental disabilities.

Public law mandates the removal of physical barriers to public facilities, making them accessible to individuals of all ability levels. Educating the private sector about an untapped consumer base of individuals with disabilities could encourage private sector facilities to become more accessible to individuals with impairments.

Many of the negative stereotypes and inappropriate behaviors that restrict socializing can be reduced by regular participation in structured activities. Rather than isolate individuals with developmental disabilities from the community at large, efforts should be made to encourage continuous interaction in leisure activities.

Additional Considerations for Health Promotion Programs

1. *Medical release form:* An annual medical release form listing the client's health problems and special needs (including medications and side effects) should be signed by a physician. A list of recommended activities and special care techniques would also prove useful. A new release form should be signed whenever the individual's health condition changes.
2. *Availability of medical staff for clients with significant health needs:* In addition to providing helpful information for specific clients, medical staff can help to maintain records of body height and weight, as well as maintain records of heart rate and blood pressure at rest and during exercise.
3. *Posted information to encourage self-directed fitness monitoring:* Exercise areas should be equipped with charts and illustrations identifying target heart rates for fitness and how to measure them, muscles of the body, proper body mechanics, proper use of all equipment, and normal height/weight charts.
4. *Community integration:* The best way to accomplish social integration is to schedule activities open to the entire community, develop relationships with other facilities in the community that offer additional amenities, share expertise about health fitness, and wellness, and encourage sports.
5. *Elimination of barriers:* The physical therapist should try to identify barriers to regular exercise and develop resources for ongoing health promotion.
6. *Use available resources:* Many camps offer specialized health and fitness programs for children and adults with developmental disabilities. Checking with local park departments, recreational facilities, special education programs, and health agencies can help identify these programs.

Quality of Life Indicators

According to a survey examining the quality of life (QOL) of individuals with developmental disabilities,[21] people with higher QOL scores were associated with the following characteristics:

1. Living in community settings
2. Having verbal skills
3. Having higher functional abilities
4. Not seeing a psychiatrist or taking psychotropic medications
5. Not having complex medical needs

For nonverbal individuals, higher QOL[22] was associated with the following:

TABLE 16-3

KEY CATEGORIES FOR IMPROVED QUALITY OF LIFE FOR INDIVIDUALS WITH DEVELOPMENTAL DISABILITIES

Being	Belonging	Becoming
Being healthy: 1. Looking after physical health 2. Eating a balanced diet 3. Hygiene and body care	Belonging in a place: 1. Having a place of residence 2. Having space for privacy 3. Living in a neighborhood	Becoming more independent: 1. Learning at work, school, or program 2. Learning how to take care of the home 3. Taking responsibility for self and others
Being in control of thoughts and feelings: 1. Demonstrating self-control 2. Having a clear self-concept 3. Feeling free of anxiety	Belonging to social circles: 1. Having a spouse or special person 2. Having a connection with family 3. Having friends	Becoming healthy, fit, and well: 1. Visiting and socializing 2. Engaging in leisure activities/hobbies 3. Participating in fitness activities
Being aware of beliefs and values: 1. Understanding right and wrong 2. Attaching meaning to life 3. Celebrating life	Belonging to the community: 1. Having access to meaningful work 2. Having access to community places 3. Having access to education	Becoming capable of handling changes in life: 1. Learning more about oneself and the world 2. Attaining new independent living skills 3. Adjusting to life changes

Adapted from Ontario Adult Autism: Research and Support Network. Quality of life indicators. Available at: http://www.ont-autism.uoguelph.ca/STRATEGIES4.shtml. Accessed February 3, 2006.

1. Having some type of occupational activity
2. Having community-based recreational and leisure-time opportunities
3. Having decision-making opportunities
4. Increasing levels of independence for continued development
5. Receiving practical and emotional support from others
6. Not having marked behavior problems

The role of physical therapists is to provide support in whatever areas of life positively affect QOL for individuals with disabilities. "To improve QOL for individuals or groups of individuals, services need to consider all areas of a person's life, and to focus on environments that can enhance life—at the policy level (laws and broad principles) and in culture (values, attitudes and behavior of others) as well as the service level (specific supports)." Physical therapists can help their clients with developmental disabilities by connecting these individuals with social support systems in the community, increasing acceptance by the general public (including advocating for policies and laws discouraging disparities in health care and discrimination in access to health, fitness, and wellness opportunities), and supporting efforts to increase financial resources that ensure a reasonable standard of living for adults with developmental disabilities. Key categories for improved QOL for individuals with developmental disabilities are listed in Table 16-3. When developing a program for individuals with developmental disabilities, it is important to consider that high quality support services exist for people with disabilities.[21] These are described as follows:

- Designed with input of all involved individuals, including those with disabilities
- Considered acceptable by people without disabilities
- Integrated into the community
- Individualized and relevant to each person's needs
- Changed, as needed, to meet the needs of the dynamic individual
- Adequately funded
- Designed to maximum independence

- Developed with respect for the dignity and privacy of individuals

Wellness

Good health is crucial for all individuals, particularly those with developmental disabilities. Every effort should be made to enable persons with developmental disabilities opportunities to access fitness and health promotion opportunities. While impairments and functional limitations can be modified on an individualized basis, participation in community-based fitness programs requires a concerted effort by individuals with developmental disabilities, parents, professionals, and local organizations to provide their varying perspectives and to identify the restrictions and barriers to inclusion. Once these limitations are identified, resources in the community (information, professionals, community organizations, etc) can serve as facilitators to enhance community opportunities for health promotion and fitness.

Summary

Health-related needs of individuals with disabilities are very broad in scope, yet physical therapists have the knowledge to help these individuals, their families, and their caretakers provide optimal health, fitness, and wellness opportunities for all. The prevalence of childhood disability is on the rise, yet life expectancies are improving, and it is not uncommon for children even with severe disabilities to live well into adulthood. The paradigm shift to focus on health and function rather than impairment and disability fits well with the national initiative to promote health for all. The management of individuals with disabilities from childhood throughout adulthood demands continual monitoring and adaptation to deal with disability-related problems. Just as individuals without disabilities must transition into healthy lifestyle habits, individuals with developmental disabilities must be counseled about their perceptions and values, social networks, a sense of personal control, and a readiness to change attitude toward changing lifestyles.

Preventive measures for the management of this population are essential for the individual, for the community, and for society. Optimal management involves teamwork and coordination of services between medical, health, and social agencies for measures such as health education, nutrition, psychological and family support, and funding sources for adaptive equipment and health-related services.

References

1. *The American Heritage Stedman's Medical Dictionary.* New York, NY: Houghton Mifflin Company; 2005.
2. US Department of Health and Human Services. Administration for children and families. Developmental Disabilities Assistance and Bill of Rights Act of 2000, Public Law 106-402. Available at: http://www.acf.hhs.gov/programs/add/ddact/DDACT2.html. Accessed February 3, 2006.
3. APTA. *Guide to Physical Therapist Practice.* 2nd ed. Alexandria, Va: American Physical Therapy Association; 2001.
4. Disability and secondary conditions. Healthy People 2010. Available at: http://www.healthypeople.gov/Document/HTML/Volume1/06Disability.htm. Accessed February 3, 2006.
5. Duff SV, Charles J. Enhancing prehension in infants and children: fostering neuromotor strategies. *Phy Occup Ther Pediatr.* 2004;24(1/2):129–172.
6. Lydic JS, Steele C. Assessment of the quality of sitting and gait patterns in children with Down's syndrome. *Phys Ther.* 1979;59(12):1489–1494.
7. Persing J, James H, Swanson J, Kattwinkel J. Prevention and management of positional skull deformities in infants. American Academy of Pediatrics Committee on practice and ambulatory medicine, section on plastic surgery and section on neurological surgery. *Pediatrics.* 2003;112(1[Pt 1]):199–202.
8. ATOMS. Seated Postural Control Measure (SPCM) [for children]. Available at: http://www3.uwm.edu/CHS/r2d2/atoms/idata/detail-idata.cfm?idata_id=30. Accessed February 3, 2006.
9. Fife SE, Roxborough LA, Armstrong RW, Harris SR, Gregson JL, Field D. Development of a clinical measure of postural control for assessment of adaptive seating in children with neuromotor disabilities. *Phys Ther.* 1991;71(12):981–993.
10. Almeida GL, Campbell SK, Girolami GL, Penn RD, Corcos DM. Multidimensional assessment of motor function in a child with cerebral palsy following intrathecal administration of baclofen. *Phys Ther.* 1997;77(7):751–764.
11. Fowler EG, Ho TW, Nwigwe AI, Dorey FJ. The effect of quadriceps femoris muscle strengthening exercises on spasticity in children with cerebral palsy. *Phys Ther.* 2001;81(6):1215–1223.
12. Pittetti K, Rimmer J, Fernall B. Physical fitness and adults with mental retardation. *Sports Med.* 1993;16(1):23–56.
13. Parker DF, Carriere L, Hebestreit H, Salsberg A, Bar-Or O. Muscle performance and gross motor function of children with spastic cerebral palsy. *Develop Med Child Neurol.* 1993;35(1):17–23.
14. Wei S, Su-Juan W, Yuan-Gui L, Hong Y, Xiu-Juan X, Xiao-Mei S. Reliability and validity of the GMFM-66 in 0- to 3-year-old children with cerebral palsy. *Am J Phys Med Rehabil.* 2006;85(2):141–147.

15. Tobimatsu Y, Nakamura R, Kusano S, Iwasaki Y. Cardiorespiratory endurance in people with cerebral palsy measured using an arm ergometer. *Arch Phys Med Rehabil.* 1998;79(8):991–993.

16. Waters RL, Mulroy S. The energy expenditure of normal and pathologic gait. *Gait and Posture.* 1999;9(3):207–231.

17. Lotan M, Isakov E, Kessel S, Merrick J. Physical fitness and functional ability of children with intellectual disability: effects of a short-term daily treadmill intervention. *Scientific World Journal.* 2004;4:449–457.

18. Van den Berg-Emons RJ, Van Baak MA, Speth L, Saris WH. Physical training of school children with spastic cerebral palsy: effects on daily activity, fat mass and fitness. *Int J Rehabil Res.* 1998;21(2):179–194.

19. Durstine JL, Painter P, Franklin BA, Morgan D, Pitetti KH, Roberts SO. Physical activity for the chronically ill and disabled. *Sports Med.* 2001;31(8):627.

20. Special Olympics. Available at: http://www.specialolympics.org/Special+Olympics+Public+Website/default.htm. Accessed February 3, 2006.

21. Ontario Adult Autism Research and Support Network. Quality of life indicators. Available at: http://www.ont-autism.uoguelph.ca/STRATEGIES4.shtml. Accessed February 3, 2006.

Chapter 17

ADVOCACY FOR PREVENTIVE CARE

Catherine Rush Thompson, PhD, MS, PT

"He who has health has hope; and he who has hope has everything."

~ARABIAN PROVERB

Definition of Advocacy

As physical therapists, we can influence outcomes for others and our profession; this is advocacy.[1] Advocacy can directly affect the lives of millions through public policy and resource allocation throughout governmental, economic, and social systems. Advocacy requires evaluating a current reality, determining the critical issues that have been ignored or overlooked, and bringing to light a new vision that incorporates the needs of those who are disenfranchised.[2] The key to advocacy is using this vision to bring about social justice. While some individuals have the knowledge, the will, and the strength to single-handedly make dynamic changes in institutions and social structures, others may require teamwork and organization to influence the attitudes of those unfamiliar with important needs of others and to enact changes to accomplish their overreaching visions.[2] As health care providers, we should be asking "what if?" and transforming what is into what should be. Advocacy for others protects human rights, whether they are social, political, or economic, and promotes human dignity.[2]

Even self-advocacy, a skill that should be practiced by health professionals and clients alike, can remove barriers to quality health care and improve the lives of others. Advocacy gives those without power some hope of realizing that their needs are being recognized. Physical therapists can be powerful advocates for the health care needs of their clients and the greater community as well as promoters of self-advocacy among their clients.

Key Health Care Issues

Advocacy can be generally understood as empowerment of consumers who may be denied access to services. It can also be thought of enabling health care providers to best meet the needs of intended consumers of health care services. In many respects advocacy is the activity of one individual to act in the interests of another to help that individual gain a certain degree of power to pursue those interests.

As physical therapists, it is important to identify significant health issues, to recognize the populations at greatest risk for health problems, and to determine what cost-effective sources of support can be offered for those specific populations. Some communities, such as a university setting, may need to focus health promotion efforts on the needs of younger adults. For example, health issues for young adults on college campuses may include the following:

- Infectious diseases, including sexually transmitted disease
- Obesity
- Substance abuse
- Lack of access to health care
- Depression
- Rape

Older adults have different risk profiles and need advocacy that addresses issues of greater importance to their population, such as risk for falls, access to health care, affordable health promotion resources, and funding for special health needs.

The Healthy People 2010 initiative provides a wealth of information about these key health issues facing various populations and statistics about populations at the greatest risks for problems, as well as current data on the incidence and prevalence of health problems. These data can be obtained on the Healthy People 2010 website.

There are various ways to advocate for health care issues. Table 17-1 lists several options for the individual who desires to contact policy makers about health care issues.

TABLE 17-1

TIPS FOR INDIVIDUAL ADVOCATES

- Documentation: Keep notes on facts and opinions in one place, either on a computer or in an organized notebook.
- Phone calls: Write the date, time, name and title, and telephone number of the person you spoke with in the documentation records. Prepare written questions on a sheet of paper in advance and allow space for answers to each question.
- Letter Writing: After the phone call, sit down and write a short letter reiterating what transpired during the phone call.
- Meetings: If a meeting is scheduled at a time you are unable to attend, ask for it to be postponed and propose an alternative time. Inform all parties if you know you are going to be late to the meeting.
- Anecdotes: Use anecdotes or examples to make a point and to give added dimension to an issue. Anecdotes are particularly useful when meeting face-to-face meetings with an elected representative, when testifying at a public hearing or public meeting, or when writing a Letter To The Editor of a newspaper. People remember anecdotes.

Adapted from American Physical Therapy Association. Available at: http://www.apta.org. Accessed October 15, 2005.

The Legislative Process

One of the best ways to affect public policy is to get new legislation introduced; however, only members of Congress can introduce legislation. Legislation includes bills, joint resolutions, concurrent resolutions, and simple resolutions. The official legislative process begins when a bill or resolution is numbered; a House bill is labeled HR and a Senate bill is labeled S. The initial step in the legislative process is the referral of the legislation to committee, generally to standing committees in the Senate or House of Representatives. Once the bill has reached committee, it is reviewed carefully by the committee or a subcommittee to determine its chances for passage. Oftentimes, bills referred to subcommittees include a review of testimony (in person or in writing) in support or against the legislation. At this point, physical therapists can affect the opinions of committee members by writing or providing testimony about a specific bill. After subcommittee hearings, the legislation is modified, as needed, to move forward or the bill "dies." The full committee can vote to support recommendations or make additional amendments after reviewing the subcommittee's report on the bill. The full committee then votes on recommendations to the House or Senate.[1]

After the committee votes to have a bill reported, staff prepare a written report on the bill in preparation for presentation to the chamber where it originated. The written report provides information about the intent, the scope, and the impact of the pending legislation as well as the views of those who do not support the bill. When the bill comes up for debate, time is allotted to discuss the strengths and benefits of the bill and the members vote to pass or defeat the bill. If the bill passes, it is referred to the other chamber for the same action. At this point, the legislation may continue to be altered until an agreement is reached between legislators or the bill "dies." If agreement is reached, a conference report summarizing the final bill must be approved by both the House and Senate. Finally, after this approval, it is sent to the President for approval. If approved, the bill is signed and becomes law. The president can take no action for 10 days, and it automatically becomes law. If the President opposes the bill, the bill may be vetoed. If there is no action after Congress has adjourned its second session, the legislation dies. Congress may override the President's veto; this requires two-thirds of members who are present for a quorum. To be successful, most bills must have broad, preferably bipartisan support.[1]

Physical therapists need to contact their legislators about legislation affecting preventive care and the physical therapy profession. While professional lobbyists work with the American Physical Therapy Association (APTA) to advocate for physical therapy issues, many clients and their families are unfamiliar with the legislative process and need advocates for their health care causes.

Contacting Policy Makers

Physical therapists can play a key role in advocating for all health-related issues but are uniquely qualified to advocate for their clients and their families, populations at risk for injury or disease, and individuals in their local community in need of preventive care. Advocacy can be carried out directly with legislators or may be achieved by contacting others to serve as advocates for desired policy changes. Direct advocacy often involves e-mails, telephone calls, or personal contacts with legislators at the national, regional, state, or local level.

E-MAILS OR LETTERS

If e-mails or letters are used, it is useful to have a form that summarizes the key issues. All letters or e-mails should be typed or legibly written with correct grammar and spelling. If the letter is mailed, include the recipient's name and address on both envelope and letter.

Ideally, letters or e-mails should include the following components[1]:

- *Correct Legislative Address and Salutation*

  The Honorable ________________

  US Senate

  Washington, DC 20510

  Dear Senator _________:

  OR

  The Honorable ________________

  US House of Representatives

  Washington, DC 20510

  Dear Representative ________________:
- *Statement of the issue:* Use your own words; avoid form letters. A brief, specific, and focused statement about why the issue is important to you and the legislator's constituents.
- *Acknowledgment of the legislator's position:* References to the legislator's background and voting record on this or similar issues.
- *Restating the issue/anticipation of continued support:* Factual details about the issue/legislation with links to more detailed information about the issue. Enclose applicable editorials or position papers, as appropriate.
- *Identity:* Details about yourself—including your address (constituent), professional credentials, and association with professional, social service, or other organizations.
- *Thanks:* Expression of gratitude for the legislator's time and consideration. Ask the policy maker for a response.
- *Closing:* Closing "Sincerely."

It is also helpful to provide a courtesy copy of the letter or e-mail to organizations supporting the same issues. See Table 17-2 for a sample letter.

TELEPHONE CONTACTS

Telephone contacts with national Senators or Representatives can be initiated by calling the United States Capitol Switchboard at 202-224-3121 and asking for the designated Senator or Representative.[1]

The following suggestions can streamline telephone contacts with legislators[7]:

- *Identify yourself:* State your name, the organization that you represent, and where you live.
- *State your position:* For example, say, "I am calling to support/oppose HB _______/SB _______." Focus on only one or two points with anecdotal evidence to support your facts. Keep the message succinct and clear. Ask about the legislator's position on the issue. Be prepared to supply additional information about the issue, as needed.
- *Do not assume that your legislator is already an expert on the issue:* Be prepared to educate him or her, using local or personal examples in your explanation.

Be aware that telephone calls to the legislators' offices are often taken by a staff member. Ask to speak to the legislator or to the aide who handles health care or preventive care issues. If that individual is not available, leave a message. Note the name and title of the person with whom you spoke and ask that the legislator send you a written response. It is important to be courteous, thanking the person who took the phone call. It is appreciated when an individual's time and effort is recognized.

Personal Contacts

Physical therapists can also meet directly with those in power to effectively advocate for others. The simple steps for meeting with political or health care policy-makers involve preparation and planning. The following are suggestions for planning a meeting with politicians or other policy-makers:

TABLE 17-2

SAMPLE LETTER ASKING FOR SUPPORT FOR HEALTH PROMOTION FUNDING

DATE

YOUR NAME with credentials
YOUR ADDRESS
YOUR CITY, STATE, AND ZIP

Correct Legislative Address
The Honorable John Doe
Missouri House of Representatives
State Office Building
Room Number
Jefferson City, MO 65101

Salutation
Dear Representative Doe:
Statement of Purpose

I am writing to ask you to support health education to reduce childhood obesity in Missouri. This funding, especially for rural Missouri areas like Concordia (hometown of the Representative), is crucial to the health and well-being of Missouri children who are at risk for obesity or who are obese.

Acknowledgment of the Legislator's Position

I recognize your support of health education, especially preventive health care for children.

Restating the Issue/Anticipation of Continued Support

Obesity is considered the number one health risk for children in the United States today, and it is now reaching epidemic proportions. The number of children who are overweight has doubled in the last 20 to 30 years. Funds that are allocated by the Legislature through the Missouri Department of Health help to fill this need by providing both incentives and opportunities for learning strategies and lifestyle habits that reduce obesity.

Identity

As a member of the Northwest District Physical Therapy Association and a member of the Missouri Healthy People 2010 Advisory Board, I regularly have the opportunity to visit with recipients of state funding throughout the region. Also, as a practicing physical therapist dedicated to improving the health, fitness, and wellness of your constituents, I greatly appreciate the opportunity to offer programs designed to reduce childhood obesity. I sincerely appreciate your efforts to help maintain strong funding for health promotion.

Thanks

Thank you for your dedication to this important health care issue as well as your time and consideration.

Closing
Sincerely,
YOUR NAME with credentials

- Make an appointment.
- State your specific purpose.
- Always introduce yourself. If you are with other representatives, select a primary spokesperson.
- Limit discussion to only one or two topics.
- Provide illustrations of the impact of policy change.
- Relate any adverse impact.
- Be flexible and avoid being argumentative.
- Be prepared for questions.
- Offer assistance or further information.
- Provide an accurate, up-to-date fact sheet.
- Thank the person for his/her time and consideration.
- Report to your organization.
- Call or write with answers or information requested.
- Follow up with a note later.

Table 17-3 provides a sample follow-up letter that can be sent following a meeting with policy-makers

TABLE 17-3

SAMPLE THANK-YOU LETTER

DATE

YOUR NAME with credentials
YOUR ADDRESS
YOUR CITY, STATE AND ZIP

Correct Legislative Address
The Honorable Joe Smith
Missouri House of Representatives
State Office Building
Room Number
Jefferson City, MO 65101

Salutation
Dear Representative Smith:
Statement of Purpose

The Northwest District Physical Therapy Association would like to thank you personally for your support in funding health education through the Missouri State Legislature and the State Health Department. Because of a recent grant of $2,000, our organization was able to educate 2,500 obese children about exercise and fitness-related activities as well as healthy eating habits to promote health and wellness.

Acknowledgment of the Legislator's Position

I recognize your support of health education, especially preventive health care for children.

Restating the Issue/Anticipation of Continued Support

This activity would have been difficult, if not impossible, without this small grant support. Hundreds of volunteer hours supported program and will continue their efforts to improve the health, fitness, and wellness of children who are obese or at risk of becoming obese.

Identity

As a practicing physical therapist and a member of the Northwest District Physical Therapy Association, I am dedicated to the health and wellness of children in Missouri.

Thanks

Once again, thank you for your time and energy in supporting this worthy program.

Closing
Sincerely,
YOUR NAME with credentials

who have addressed a health care issue by providing funding for preventive care.

It is helpful to become acquainted with legislators to learn about their personal interests and goals, especially if they focus on community health and wellness. The best times to meet legislators are during a campaign, at fund-raising events, and at town meetings. Most state legislative offices maintain web sites.

The APTA's website for advocacy provides links to state legislative sites and tracks current legislation of interest to physical therapists and their patients.[1] This website also provides a local media guide including national media organizations, newspapers, columnists, magazines, television stations, and radio stations for editorials, articles, and transcripts of discussions related to relevant health care issues.

INDIRECT ADVOCACY

Physical therapists can indirectly affect public policy by becoming actively involved in the American Physical Therapy Association (APTA) or other issue-related organizations. The APTA develops policy statements that guide lobbying efforts to impact national legislation. For more information about policy statements about health and wellness issues, look at the APTA web site. Also, search the Internet for

TABLE 17-4

LEGISLATIVE DO'S AND DON'TS

Do	Don't
• Be polite. • Avoid medical jargon. • Be factual and concise, giving examples when appropriate. • Know the pros and cons of the issue. • Personalize your communication. • Be a patient advocate. • Meet with your local legislators when possible, hopefully, before an issue comes up. • Be a good listener. • Learn the legislative process. • Always answer legislators' questions or requests for more information accurately and promptly. Be truthful if you don't know the answer. • Be willing to testify on issues that are important to you and your patients.	• Threaten or make demands. • Be dictatorial, especially if you don't have a thorough knowledge of the issue. • Use form letters. • Come across as self-serving. • Be impatient. The legislative process can be time-consuming.

organizations seeking support for similar issues. Developing a strong coalition can help move issues into the forefront.

In addition, physical therapists should help empower their clients and families to self-advocate. The United Cerebral Palsy Association has long supported families advocating for individuals with disabilities. One parent with a son who has cerebral palsy stresses how critical it is for parents and family members to not only push the system to maximize access to services for their own children or relatives, but also to speak out as a public advocate for all people with disabilities. "Don't be afraid to raise a little hell because, after all, you are your child's best advocate," says the mother of three who, besides caring for a family, also has a career with the Institute on Disabilities at Temple University.[3] This mother's experience led her to offer the following information to families of children with disabilities:

- "Most importantly, parents and family members are a child's best advocates.
- Get involved in coalitions, parent associations, and support groups.
- Go to public hearings.
- Attend rallies and participate in legislative visit days.
- Get to know the staff in local offices of your Congressional delegation.
- Build on small victories and positions of strength.
- Respond to requests from government agencies for public comment on policy changes.
- Search disability Web sites; you will be surprised at what you can learn.
- Be patient and be prepared to hang in there for the long haul.
- And above all, never give up!"[3]

In addition to supporting clients and families in their advocacy efforts, physical therapists must share their educated opinions about health care issues in addition to addressing legislative issues affecting the practice of physical therapy.

As advocates, physical therapists must be diplomatic and must take a broad view of the multiple factors involved in determining health care policy. Table 17-4 helpful legislative "do's and don'ts."[4]

Polite and meaningful dialogue provides policy makers with needed information to make sound decisions. As advocates, physical therapists should convince their policy makers of the importance addressing key issues for the benefits of their constituents and society in general.

Advocacy at the National Level

Physical therapists can align themselves with national organizations to gain support for preventive care issues. Many organizations advocate for public health and preventive care, including the American Physical Therapy Association, the American Public Health Association (APHA), the American Academy of Pediatrics, and the American Academy of Family Physicians, as well as numerous other professional and national organizations.[5]

The APHA is the oldest and largest organization of public health professionals in the world, representing more than 50,000 members from over 50 occupations of public health.[5] APHA is concerned with a broad set of issues affecting personal and environmental health, including federal and state funding for health programs, pollution control, programs and policies related to chronic and infectious diseases, a smoke-free society, and professional education in public health. The APHA has a website listing the congressional record of support for health issues[5] as well as fact sheets for major health issues, including ergonomics, health disparities, mental health parity, obesity, the patient's Bill of Rights, and others. It's website[5] also links to other organizations offering health information, including aging, children's health, diabetes, cancer, autoimmune diseases, chronic conditions and disorders, health policy and advocacy, and related topics.

The APHA website states the following[5]:

> The APHA has *significant concerns about the ongoing changes in the organization and financing of medical care and health services and the impact of these changes on public health. Specific issues of concern include denials of necessary care, under-funding of public health and prevention services, lack of accountability, loss of choice of health care provider, inadequate access to care (especially specialists), lack of comparable and consumer-friendly information and data about health plans, and abuses in marketing. In addition, APHA is troubled by research findings that raise questions about the effectiveness of managed care organizations in meeting health care needs associated with prevention and with managing chronic conditions.*

These issues need to be addressed through advocacy by physical therapists, other health care providers, patients, and families receiving care, as well as policy-makers.

Working to create a grassroots network for important preventive care issues, as suggested by the APHA, requires time and effort, but affords advocates much needed support for the passage of legislation that benefits community members with unmet health care needs. Contacting the APHA, APTA special interest groups, health organizations who support health promotion, and other groups affected by health care issues can further develop the needed network for influencing public policy at a national level.

Advocacy at the State Level

Physical therapists can have a major impact on health care by addressing policy makers at the state level. If the legislation is a health care bill, it will fare better with support from the state's physical therapy association, health department, specialty medical organizations, and interested consumer groups. Enlisting support may be as easy as making a phone call or sending an e-mail to an organization's president or a university program. Meeting with a group's board of directors to make a brief presentation can help advocate for a specific issue. Some state legislatures have study committees and task force meetings between legislative sessions. The work these groups do often results in legislative recommendations for the upcoming session. Physical therapists can ask their organization(s) if they can serve on these advisory boards as proponents for preventive care. As advisors, physical therapists can educate policy-makers about the cost benefits and societal benefits of health promotion and prevention practice.

Advocacy at the Local Level

Many state allocations for health care are dispersed to local health departments for the dissemination of health-related educational materials as well as the development and management of health-related programs. Preventive care should be designed to meet the specific needs of a given community. Physical therapists should work in concert with their local health departments to ensure that comprehensive preventive care, including fitness programs, can be accessed by all populations in need.

When attempting to work in partnership with local health departments, it is essential to acknowledge the department's overall mission as well as the scope of services available. Generally, the mission of the local health department is to promote, preserve, and protect the health of citizens in the particular locality. Programs meeting local health care needs often include communicable disease control programs, community partnerships and chronic disease programs, health education and health communication programs, environmental health programs, maternal, and child and family health programs. While health departments attempt to meet the needs of their local community, many citizens are not receiving adequate services. Physical therapists should help address issues of accessibility and affordability through advocacy at national, state, and local levels. Additionally, physical therapists should collaborate with local health departments to provide health information and strategies for improving health, fitness, and wellness. Physical therapists are uniquely qualified to address preventive care issues for all segments of the population, especially in the areas of fitness and lifestyle behaviors.

Keys to successful advocacy at the local level include (1) clearly identifying the health issue, (2) describing the impact of the health concern on individual and the community—both positive and negative consequences, and (3) providing cost-effective solutions to the health problem. Offering financial data allows policy-makers to consider whether health promotion options are cost-effective. For example, the following fact could been used to secure financing for education about children's preventive care: "Every $1 spent on child safety seats saves $32.10."[6,7] Encouraging the purchase of child safety seats as a preventive measure can help reduce the overall costs of injuries acquired in motor vehicle accidents. A small investment in educating the public about child safety seats is a cost-effective measure for ensuring child safety and reducing expenses for health care. Thorough research about an issue, including financial data, can provide the needed information to make a particular issue a priority for legislators at the local, state, and national levels.

Advocacy for World Health

More physical therapists are becoming involved in international causes, providing health care services to third world countries and advocating for improved health care. The World Health Organization (WHO), established in 1948, is the United Nations specialized agency for health designed to help all peoples reach the highest possible level of health. Health is defined in the WHO's Constitution as "a state of complete physical, mental and social well-being and not merely the absence of disease or infirmity."[8] The WHO Mega Country Health Promotion Network was developed to significantly impact world health by forming a partnership among the most populous countries. Since 2000, 11 countries, which constitute over 60% of the world's population, have joined in this international effort to promote health. Countries involved in the WHO Network include Bangladesh, Brazil, China, India, Indonesia, Japan, Mexico, Nigeria, Pakistan, the Russian federation, and the United States of America.[8] Working together, Mega countries can speak in a unified voice for global health promotion and move the agenda forward.

The mission of the WHO network is as follows[8]:

To strengthen global and national health promotion capacity to enhance the health of the Mega country populations and support the health of the world's population. Besides tackling important cross-cutting transnational health issues together, Mega countries will continue to address their own national health priorities to build stronger health promotion infrastructures within each country.

The WHO Network has five goals:

- To improve the information base for health promotion by sharing successful health promotion policies and programs, and related surveys and evaluations.
- To develop health promotion strategies in four areas:
    1. *Healthy Lifestyle:* Priority health issues including tobacco use, nutrition, and physical activity.
    2. *Healthy Life Course:* Priority populations including women, children, adolescents, and the aging population.
    3. *Supportive Environments:* Priority health issues including good sanitation, malaria and insect vector control, and safe water.
    4. *Supportive Settings:* Priority settings including schools, cities, workplaces, and communities.
- Mobilize resources from existing, redistributed, and nontraditional sources to increase the status of health as a priority.
- Increase intersectoral collaboration across governmental and non-governmental agencies, and across the public and private sectors, to improve health.
- Address issues of scale that Mega countries share in common, such as reorienting/redistributing resources in large bureaucracies, building capacity with national partners, reaching large populations through the media, and using technology to provide distance education and training.[8]

One of the main objectives of the WHO Network is to improve each nation's capacity for health promotion and to increase awareness, recognition, and advocacy of health promotion among decision-makers and the general public. Physical therapists should work in collaboration with other national organizations to advocate on an international level for health promotion strategies for a healthy lifestyle, healthy life course, supportive environments, and supporting settings, as outlined above. For more information about the WHO Mega Country Health Promotion Network, write to the Department of NCD Prevention & Health Promotion at the World Health Organization, Avenue Appia 20, 1211 Geneva 27 Switzerland.

International facts acknowledged by the WHO Network include the following[8]:

- By 2020, over 70% of premature deaths among adults will be due largely to behaviors initiated during childhood and youth.
- Today, leading causes of death, disease, and disability (eg, CVD, cancer, depression, unintentional and intentional injuries, pulmonary disease, and HIV/AIDS) are significantly influenced by six interrelated categories of behavior: (1) tobacco use, (2) alcohol/substance use, (3) sexual behavior that causes unintended pregnancy and disease, (4) behavior that results in injury, (5) inadequate dietary patterns, and (6) inadequate physical activity. Behavioral patterns/lifestyles are fostered by a range of interrelated environmental conditions, both social and physical, throughout the life course.
- In both developed and developing countries, there is a clear social gradient: those better off have lower morbidity rates and higher life expectancy, those lower on the social ladder have higher morbidity rates and lower life expectancy. The social environment, particularly social determinants of health (such as social cohesion or exclusion), have a significant impact on health and disease.

The mission and goals of the WHO Network parallel the national Healthy People 2010 initiative to reduce the disparities in access to health care for all individuals. Physical therapists can play a key role in international advocacy as proponents of physical activity and healthy lifestyles. Preliminary data from a WHO study on risk factors suggest that inactivity, or sedentary lifestyle, is one of the ten leading global causes of death and disability.

The WHO Network offers a compelling vision of health care needs around the world:

> *More than two million deaths each year are attributable to physical inactivity. In countries around the world between 60% and 85% of adults are simply not active enough to benefit their health. Sedentary lifestyles increase all causes of mortality, double the risk of cardiovascular diseases, diabetes, and obesity, and substantially increase the risks of colon cancer, high blood pressure, osteoporosis, depression and anxiety.*[8]
>
> *In the rapidly growing cities of the developing world, crowding, poverty, crime, traffic, poor air quality, a lack of parks, sidewalks, sports and recreation facilities, and other safe areas make physical activity a difficult choice. For example, in San Paulo, Brazil, 70% of the population is inactive. Even in rural areas of developing countries, sedentary pastimes such as watching television are increasingly popular. In addition to other lifestyle changes, the consequences are growing levels of obesity, diabetes, and cardiovascular diseases. Low- and middle-income countries suffer the greatest impact from these and other non-communicable diseases—77% of the total number of deaths caused by noncommunicable diseases occur in developing countries. These diseases are on the rise. They will have an increasingly severe effect on health care systems, resources, and economies in countries around the world. Many countries that are already struggling to manage the impact of infectious diseases and other development challenges will be forced to spend their meager resources dealing with non-communicable diseases.*[8]

Physical therapists can connect with the international community through various means, but probably the Internet is the easiest route. Advocacy for health education as well as removal of barriers to physical activity can benefit all communities. The WHO website lists information about various countries, including health indicators, health risks, resources/health expenditures, health system organization and regulation (including key legislation), disease prevalence, human resources (doctors, nurses and other health professionals), and media centers. In addition, national contact information is provided for physical therapists seeking additional information about international advocacy for health promotion.

The World Federation of Public Health Associations (WFPHA) is defined as follows[9]:

> *An international, nongovernmental organization bringing health workers throughout the world together for professional exchange, collaboration, and action. Its members, currently numbering 70, are multidisciplinary national and regional public health societies whose own memberships include nurses, sanitarians, administrators, physicians, health educators, pharmacists, anthropologists, researchers, and many other persons interested in public health. Founded in 1967, WFPHA is the only world-wide professional society representing and serving the broad field of public health, as distinct from single disciplines or occupations. WFPHA enjoys official relations status with the World Health Organization and maintains close ties with UNICEF and other international organizations.*

WFPHA's mission is as follows[9]:

> *To promote personal and community health throughout the world by supporting the establishment and development of societies of public health; facilitating the exchange of information, experience, and research; and advocating for policies, programs, and practices that improve public health.*

The goals of WFPHA are as follows:

- To foster the public health profession through the establishment and development of public health associations in all countries where they do not now exist and to strengthen existing associations.

- To promote health worldwide by facilitating collaborative efforts and partnerships among member groups.
- To improve public health practice by exchanging information through publications, meetings, country study tours, and conferences.
- To advance public health policy by providing a medium through which nongovernmental public health organizations can work effectively with national and international health agencies.

More information about joining this organization can be found on its website.

Advocacy for Older Adults

The older adult segment of our population is growing rapidly, and policy-makers seek to implement policies that prevent or delay the onset of disabilities in this population for as long as possible. It is in the public's best interest to help older individuals remain independent and economically active as long as possible. Physical therapists need to advocate for optimal environments that enable older adults to function independently and maintain a good quality of life. Barriers to physical activity and healthy living include limited access to public transportation and physical barriers to health care facilities. Policy makers must be encouraged to implement "age-friendly" environments for optimal health promotion.

In the Closing Session of the American Geriatric Society in 2004, Jessie C. Gruman, PhD, discussed "Health Promotion for Older Adults: Nice or Necessary?" In her presentation, Dr. Gruman discussed the paradox of our current society[10]:

In the past century, Americans—through better nutrition, better medical care, and better social policy—have experienced a 56% increase in life expectancy, from 49 years to 77 years, and have earned the means to enjoy it. Overall, older Americans have the lowest poverty rate of any age group. But they also spend far more of the nation's health care dollars per capita than any other group. Almost 30% of Medicare spending is on those who are in the last year of their lives. So, one "moral values" question we have been asking is how to even things out so that health promotion can reduce unnecessary pain and suffering and thus decrease the need for acute and post-acute medical intervention. This raises another, much tougher question: How much energy are we, in this time of mind-numbing deficits, going to devote to promoting health and preventing disability in older people, when the benefits may be minimal, hard-won or short-lived? The answers to this last question will be powerfully influenced by the three A's—ageism, affordability, and accommodation.

The barriers to health promotion in older populations include not only physical barriers, but also psychological barriers that limit options. Ageism or prejudice against older adults affects the amount of research conducted to fully explore options for healthy aging. Affordability of health promotion options is oftentimes beyond the means of many older adults—a gym membership can cost over $600 a year; personal trainers charge $40 an hour; good shoes cost $100 a year; and a home treadmill can cost between $700 and $1,700. Dr. Gruman continues as follows[10]:

But while the economic barriers are formidable, so, too, are the agglomeration of frustrating annoyances faced by older people who just want to get around like they used to do, if only a bit slower and safer. For example, if you do have good shoes and good knees, what use are they to your health if your neighborhood is poorly lit with high crime and broken sidewalks inviting you to fall?

She later concludes her presentation[10]:

I wish I could foretell a different, more expansive, enthusiastic future for health promotion, but I think that the sage poet, Mick Jagger, nails what I believe should be the new theme song for advocates of health promotion for older adults, "You can't always get what you want—but if you try sometimes, you just might find you get what you need."

Physical therapists must be willing to remove barriers that older adults face when trying to access health promotion education and activities, as difficult as this may be. These challenges are not unique to older adults in the United States. Other countries face similar issues as people age and health care costs soar. The Vienna International Plan of Action on Aging, endorsed by the United Nations General Assembly, serves as the first "international instrument on aging, guiding thinking and the formulation of policies and programs on aging."[11] The plan aims to "strengthen the capacities of governments and civil society to deal effectively with the aging of populations and to address the developmental potential and dependency needs of older persons."[11]

The International plan states the following[11]:

Aging is a life-long process and should be recognized as such. Preparation of the entire population for the later stages of life should be an integral part of social policies and encompass physical, psychological, cultural, religious, spiritual, economic, health and other factors.

For example, the International Plan contains recommendations for health and nutrition for older adults around the world. Additional information about the Vienna International Plan of Action on Aging can be found on the Internet.[11]

Summary

Physical therapists must serve as advocates for access to health care services and products. As knowledgeable health care providers, physical therapists must advocate for children, families, individuals with special needs, older adults, and communities that could benefit from any aspect of preventive practice. Advocacy must penetrate the barriers of ageism, racism, and other discriminatory practices that limit access to health protection, health promotion, and prevention of illness and injury. As health care professionals, physical therapists must be leaders in promoting health care and ensuring that barriers to achieving the overarching goals of Healthy People 2010 are removed. In addition, advocacy must extend beyond national borders to international communities with similar health care challenges. Through organized efforts and actions, such as networking and advocacy, physical therapists can restore hope to people in need.

References

1. American Physical Therapy Association. Advocacy. Available at: http://www.apta.org/Advocacy. Accessed January 18, 2006.
2. Brain Injury Association. Advocacy skills. Available at: http://www.headinjury.com/advocacy.htm. Accessed January 18, 2006.
3. United Cerebral Palsy. Advocacy tools: individual and family advocacy. Available at: http://www.ucp.org/ucp_generaldoc.cfm/1/8/6602/6602-6628/3163. Accessed January 18, 2006.
4. Haggerty P. The most effective do's an don'ts of successful legislative grass roots citizen advocacy. Available at: http://www.jcep.org/reports/donts.htm. Accessed February 3, 2006.
5. American Public Health Association. About APHA. Available at: http://www.apha.org/about. Accessed February 3, 2006.
6. Partnership for Prevention. Prevention: the key to improving the health status of America's children. Washington, DC: July 1997.
7. Children's Safety Network. *Childhood Injury: Cost & Prevention Facts.* Landover, Md: Children's Safety Network: Economics and Insurance Resource Center; 1996.
8. World Health Organization. About WHO. Available at: http://www.who.int/about/en. Accessed February 3, 2006.
9. American Public Health Association. APHA and global health. Available at: http://www.apha.org/wfpha/global_health.htm. Accessed February 3, 2006.
10. Health promotion for older adults: nice or necessary? Remarks by Jessie C. Gruman, PhD. Closing session of the American Geriatric Society confronting ageism and economics in promoting elder health. November 23, 2004. Available at: http://64.233.187.104/search?q=cache:5aMdPAeiXvUJ:www.cfah.org/pdfs/Aging_presentation.pdf+advocating+older+adults+health+promotion&hl=en. Accessed February 3, 2006.
11. The Vienna International Plan of Action on Aging. Available at: http://www.un.org/esa/socdev/ageing/ageipaa.htm. Accessed February 3, 2006.

Chapter 18

Marketing Health and Wellness

Steven G. Lesh, PhD, MPA, PT, SCS, ATC and Catherine Rush Thompson, PhD, MS, PT

"The buyer needs a hundred eyes; the seller, but one."

~ITALIAN PROVERB

With increasing direct access, physical therapists can market their skills to a broad spectrum of clients. Health promotion appeals to healthy individuals, those with disabilities, corporate entities interested in a healthy workforce, and those seeking opportunities to prevent injury. Physical therapists must convince the general population that they have a unique and desirable product or service—providing customized health education and exercise for health, fitness, and wellness.

Definition of Marketing

Marketing is defined as follows[1]:

The process of planning and executing the conception, pricing, promotion, and distribution of ideas, goods, services, organizations, and events to create and maintain relationships that will satisfy individual and organizational objectives.

Marketing professionals preach that if you are not advertising and moving forward, other companies are passing you by. Marketing can be offered through mass media, newsprint, television commercials, and even pop-up ads on a computer screen. Marketing should ideally provide valuable information that is appreciated by its target audience. Above all, the health care practitioner should remember two essential aspects of marketing: (1) knowing the target audience, and (2) building positive relationships with the consumer.

Target Market

Classic marketing is founded at the intersection of the target market and the strategies designed to meet customer expectations. Before any marketing plans can be put into action or before any revenues from converted patrons can be counted, a careful understanding and appreciation of the target audience must be conducted.[2]

A target market is "the group or people toward whom [a] firm decides to direct its marketing efforts, and ultimately its goods and services."[3] As a physical therapist designing a health promotion and wellness program, it is important to ask the following questions:

- Who purchases the product?
- When do they purchase the product?
- Why do they purchase the product?
- Whom is the product intended for?
- Are there any alternatives to purchasing this product?

TABLE 18-1

SAMPLE "MARKET RESEARCH" QUESTIONS

Planning Process

- How does your organization participate in planning processes?
- What kinds of organizations have approached you to be a part of an advisory committee? How do you choose which ones you will join?
- If you were inviting others (members of the target audience) to attend a work group meeting for this project, what would you say to get them to come? What would you avoid saying?
- What was your impression of the state's planning process for health care? What worthwhile came out of it?

Design and Production

- What makes a plan useful? What kinds of plans are not useful?
- If you need detailed information about a topic, do you prefer to have it included at the back of a publication, in a separate publication, or on a web site?
- Which of these formats is easy to use (present two or more visual formats)?
- What do you think the people who wrote this page want you to do?

Marketing

- Where do you get ideas for your work or community activities?
- What kinds of published recommendations and plans have you seen from other state agencies?
- What impression do you have of government planning efforts?
- When you receive plans from other agencies, what do you do?
- If you were in charge of marketing the state's health plan to others (members of the target audience), what would you do?
- What do you read?
- How do you like to get information about emerging objectives in public health?

Adapted from Healthy People 2010. State Healthy People 2010 tool library. Available at: http://www.phf.org/HPtools/state.htm. Accessed October 15, 2005.

Understanding the answers to these questions will help focus the marketing plan. Marketing health promotion, however, can be directed to a diverse target market, spanning all ages and levels of functional abilities.

Groups with varying needs present different challenges and demands. Diversity in the population needs to be appreciated and addressed through a marketing plan with multiple strategies to reach all elements of the target market. Projections of the US Census Bureau show that the Hispanic population will soon be the largest minority group in the United States.[4] If a wellness organization produces a marketing campaign designed to prevent birth defects through regular prenatal care, will it reach all of the target market if it fails to produce Spanish language versions of the plan?

Marketing campaigns must be formulated using input from multiple sources. *Surveys* (a method of gathering information in writing or in person from a sample of individuals) are commonly utilized tools, followed closely by focus groups. *Focus groups* are live samples of members from the desired target market organized to give opinions and reactions to products or a marketing campaign. *Opinion polls* are surveys of opinion using sampling and are designed to represent the opinions of a population by asking a small number of people a series of questions and then extrapolating the answers to the larger group. Table 18-1 lists sample market research questions that the wellness professional can use in developing a cost-effective campaign.

Building a Positive Relationship

The second essential aspect of marketing is building a positive relationship with the target audience.

A positive relationship can be developed if targeted consumers perceive the health, fitness, and wellness services and products to be reliable. Additionally, reduced costs in terms of production time and procurement of services and/or products also enhance the relationship between the provider and consumer. Physical therapists must build positive relationships with their consumers by providing the best possible services designed to meet the unique needs of their constituents. When developing services for target populations, physical therapists should take into account the need to build a positive relationship based on reliable, cost-effective, and easily procured services and products.

The Increasing Role of Physical Therapists in Health Promotion

Employment of physical therapists is expected to grow faster than the average for all occupations through 2008, and the demand for physical therapists should continue to rise as a result of (1) increased number of individuals with disabilities, (2) baby-boomers entering prime age for heart attacks and strokes, (3) advanced technologies to save larger proportion of babies with birth defects, and (4) increased interest in health promotion.[5-7]

It is important to help people think about the costs and potential benefits of health promotion activities. According to health promotion research of people with disabilities, these individuals "face substantial barriers and they fear the costs of participating in health promotion activities will be high. Moreover, if medical providers have said that their condition will not improve, they may expect few benefits from health promotion. Any conversation about health promotion activities must take such expectations into account."[6] Physical therapists must provide information to remove potential barriers that limit participation in preventive care.

Physical therapists need to embrace the challenges of providing health, fitness, and wellness options to all populations in need of preventive care. If physical therapists cannot adequately market their skills and knowledge, less qualified individuals may corner the market on preventive practice and comprehensive health care. A basic knowledge of key marketing concepts can help the entrepreneurial therapist develop a strong business that serves the health needs of targeted populations in the community. Physical therapists have a responsibility to increase public awareness of physical therapy services as the provider of choice for health promotion and prevention of injury promotion.

Marketing Mix: The Four P's

Product, Pricing, Placement, and *Promotion,* the four P's, are the essential domains of the classic marketing model.[8] Marketing plans are developed and implemented within each of these four domains to foster the business-to-customer relationship.

PRODUCT

Product includes the goods and services provided by an organization to meet the needs and expectations of the consumer.[8] The product includes the entire spectrum of goods to services available to meet consumers' needs. Products comprise a wide array of potential goods and services in varying combinations. *Goods* are tangible objects that can be physically used or consumed by the customer, whereas *services* are intangible tasks that are inseparable from the service provider who satisfies the consumer's needs.[8] The key to determining where a product lies on the goods-to-service spectrum is the value derived from the product by the consumer. With any product, there is an associated product life cycle. The life cycle of a product reflects the growth and utilization of the product over time. Early, when the product is introduced, early adopters will rush to use the new product because the mainstream has not yet been enticed to purchase the product. As the mainstream begins to utilize the product, a growth phase is seen in which the number of sales increase as well as the number of consumers making purchases. Eventually, the cycle will see a maturation in which the product becomes very stable in terms of sales and new consumers. Once a product has matured, it can continue unchanged for many years, or can slide into a decline. Industry sales and profits notably decline in this final phase of the product life cycle.[8]

Many strategies can be used to manage the product during its life cycle. Increasing the frequency of use is a common strategy. New customers are not needed, but rather initiating strategies that encourage existing customers to purchase the product more frequently. A second strategy is to find avenues to increase the number of new users to buy the existing product. This strategy is classically implemented to educate and convert potential customers into frequent users of the product. Finding new or alternate uses for an existing product can also be a strategy. A physical therapy clinic with an existing exercise gymnasium may elect to establish "open" gym hours for previous clients and patients in order to exercise for general health rather than the rehabilitation of specific conditions. When all other strategies fail, repackaging the same product with a new appearance and new marketing campaign is possible.

Pricing

Pricing is the exchange value for a good or service.[8] Determining pricing in the health and wellness sector is sometimes determined based on competitors and sometimes based on predeterminates, such as insurance company payments or government regulations. Pricing can be difficult to establish and is often a dynamic entity. The primary issue to consider when establishing a price is that it helps to determine profitability for the organization. In the simplest of terms, collected revenues from the goods and services must exceed the costs of selling the same goods and services. Other considerations include the perception of the product with the attached price tag. Products with higher-than-average price tags impart an image of prestige and possibly greater quality. Conversely, products with lower than average prices may reflect a value purchase, or at times, a below-quality product. When developing a pricing strategy for a health and wellness organization, the price of the product should be comparable to local competition without being significantly higher or lower for a comparable product offering. A method of increasing pricing and profitability is to package or bundle product offerings giving the appearance of great value, but also an increased generation of revenue.[8]

Placement

Placement or distribution is the aspect of the marketing mix that is concerned with how, when and where the product is placed before the target market.[8] Inherent within the domain of distribution and placement are the key factors of the distribution channels and the logistics to make the plan a reality. The distribution channels or supply chain consist of the entire spectrum of events and activities that take the finished good or service from production to the end user of the product. These distribution processes and the inherent efficiencies within the chain can include factors like inventory, materials handling, packaging, ordering, shipping, and warehousing. The logistics of the placement include activities for the coordination and the flow of information.

Promotion

Promotion is the final formal aspect of the marketing mix and accounts for the "...informing, persuading and influencing of the consumer's purchase decision."[9] The promotional elements are all of the strategies and plans that are enacted to create an environment in which the consumer will purchase the product. The key element of promotion is the marketing communication that appears to the potential buyer from a variety of media (eg, television, print, Internet).[10] For a promotional strategy to be effective, the consumers must be made aware of the product and how the product can meet their needs. If a client is not aware of the product or service, the chances of making a purchase are very low.

Packaging

Packaging, while not mutually exclusive to warrant its own domain apart from the classic four P's, is something to consider and respect as part of an established or developing marketing campaign (ie, the fifth P). Product packaging is an important part of the perception of the goods and services. Packaging can mean the simple appearance of the insert sleeve in the latest computer disc program, but it is also the state and condition of the location in which services are provided. A fitness gymnasium that has old and antiquated equipment may not be an appealing sell to a potential client. A common saying relates that there is only one opportunity to make a first impression. Another element to consider in the health and wellness sector is the visual appearance of healthy people from people with various afflictions or even varying age groups or genders. Many health clubs are finding the need to establish gender specific hours in the exercise rooms such that men and women are segregated. Likewise, if the target population is a healthy young adult market, overlapping hours in a swimming pool with an arthritic exercise group or with elementary age children during a physical education field trip may not provide the best packaging of the service.

Health Care Marketing: The SCAP Model

Marketing in the health care world has taken the shape of public relations campaigns, organizational awareness, staff recruitment and retention, direct insurance marketing, and patient satisfaction efforts.[10] In recent years, there has been a more aggressive effort of health care organizations to work to get the health and wellness product directly in front of the client. The marketing domain and target market concepts are sound foundations on which a marketing plan in the health and wellness sector can be built.

The four P's have been redesigned into the SCAP model to more appropriately reflect marketing mix of the goods and services within the health care field: Service, Consideration, Access, and Promotion.[11]

- *Services* are identified and promoted that are designed to meet the health and wellness needs of the target market.
- *Consideration* is the value for the service. In the health care world direct, cash-based reimbursements are not directed to the organization from the consumer of the service. Deductibles, copayments, and coinsurances are the language of payments coupled with allowables and preferred networks from the insurance company perspective. Frequently, the consumer does not fully appreciate the full amount of payment to the provider.
- *Access* is the ease of obtaining the service from the provider. When and how often can the service be accessed is a consideration in the marketing mix and, in part, responsible for the decision whether or not to utilize the service by the client.
- *Promotion* of the health and wellness service is the component, much like as in the four P's model, that makes the target market aware of the existence of the service. The promotion is part informational and awareness, and in part suggestive of which goods and services to use.

Integrated Marketing

Integrated marketing is an expansion on the classic model of marketing founded on the premise that the individual consumer has unique wants and needs coupled with a driving effort to produce a consistent marketing message for the consumer. In today's communication generation, the marketer possesses a wide variety of mediums to reach potential consumers (eg, television, Internet, newsprint, radio, e-mail). With all of the varying opportunities to advertise to the public, great potential also exists for disjointed and inconsistent messages being delivered. Integrated marketing is the push to present a consistent message to the individual consumer. The four foundational elements of integrated marketing include the following:

- Nurturing personal relationships with the customer
- Utilizing current information technology to encourage interactivity and rapid communication
- Fostering mission marketing or a shared organizational vision
- Distributing a consistent message

Nurturing personal relationships was mentioned in the opening of this chapter as one of the most important things for an organization to remember and pursue. Integrated marketing relies on the ability of the organization to connect and make the individual customer feel special. Today's generation of consumers is used to personalization, customization, and immediate gratification. Attempts at personalization are critical to pursue and are necessary to master if success is the ultimate goal. Information is now global and nearly instantaneous. Understanding the target market and how those consumers access information is critical to where, how, and when an organization will dispense its marketing budget. The best use of funds may be directed at print ads or radio spots, but likewise, Internet banner ads and e-mail newsletters may provide greater access. Print ads can mention a web link (URL) to information about fitness, health, wellness, hours of operation, biographies of employees, costs, and even the potential to register or pay fees online.

Fostering mission marketing or supporting a shared organizational vision are valuable elements of the integrated marketing approach. The mission of the organization should be easily understood by the consumer through the marketing and actions of the organization.

Distributing message consistency is the final piece of the integrated marketing approach. After personalization efforts have been fostered through rapid communication exchange technologies and the mission of the organizations is set and shared through all levels, the message that is distributed should be consistent and to the point. A feeling of familiarity is a major selling point for consumers. When a consumer recognizes a familiar and trusted logo or trade name, even if the product is unfamiliar, the consumer is likely to purchase the familiar company as opposed to an unfamiliar company. The consistency of the message should be easily recognized through uniform themes, color schemes, and logos.

Marketing Strategies for Health and Wellness Centers and Organizations

BUDGET

Before the marketing strategies are presented, budget should be discussed. A budget should be developed that matches the goals and objectives of both the marketing plan and the mission of the organization. Many health care organizations develop their marketing budget through a process of what is left over after all other bills have been paid. While this may be the reality, it is not good business sense. Some experts believe that an organization should spend as much on a marketing plan as its chief competitors, while others believe it is not best to follow. The health care industry, hospitals, insurance companies, and drug corporations have implemented enterprising marketing campaigns that are directed to the individual consumer.

For adequate budgeting, an annual percentage of gross revenues should be allocated to marketing. Setting the percentage may be a process of trial and error, and may range drastically depending on business objectives. A business-to-business organization may allot as little as 1% of revenues whereas a company looking to introduce a new product on the market may dedicate as much as 50% of initial target revenues to penetrate the market. For instance, a wellness center has projected annual revenues of $200,000 and allocates 10% annually for marketing.

If resources are not dedicated to marketing, it is difficult to attract new customers and keep existing customers. If the wellness organization does not work to keep the target audience aware of its services and products, a competing organization will work to make its goods and services readily available to the other organization's customers. See Table 18-2 for a list of innovative and cost-effective marketing strategies for health promotion.

Good Will

Good will is a term used in marketing and corporate valuation that reflects the positive attitude and feelings in the community about the product.[11] The perception of a product or corporate good will by the public and potential target market centers on the status, participation, and earned respect within the community. Some organizations establish good will by contributing and donating goods and services to sectors of need within the community. Others establish good will by providing valued quality products, while others still establish good will by simply being long-standing members and contributors to the community. Establishing good will, however, can become an invaluable asset when developing a marketing plan. Products, companies, and wellness causes can build marketing plans on established good will by providing special services to underserved populations and sharing their pro bono efforts through public relations.

Logo and Slogan Products

Logo and slogan products provide many great opportunities for a consistent message and image.[12] An organization can develop an attractive logo that supports the mission and promotes the organizational objectives as part of an integrated marketing plan. Color themes, logos, and slogans should be used consistently across all marketing venues and plans forwarded by the organization. Logos and color schemes can be developed internally using various graphic imaging software programs and the marketing staff, or can be outsourced to local graphics design companies or even via Internet-based companies. For example, logos can be added to polo shirts worn by staff members to present a professional and consistent appearance. Promotional supply companies provide a wide array of creative and professional marketing items. With all of the possible promotional product opportunities to deplete a marketing budget, wise and careful analysis of the anticipated product distribution and expected conversion rate should be considered.

Newsletters

Newsletters, either in the form of a printed circulation that is mailed to current or prospective consumers, or an electronic-based newsletter circulated via the Internet or e-mail, can provide marketing and consumer information elements about the wellness organization.[12] This communication tool can be published weekly, monthly, quarterly, semi-annually, or annually. Newsletters can contain public health information or specific company information. Biographies about employees or healthy eating tips could be regularly included. Updates on product information and services could comprise a regular newsletter installment. Adhering to an integrated marketing approach, at the minimum, the newsletter should contain familiar product or trade names, logos, colors and company contact information. Retail businesses can solicit e-mail addresses from consumers to compile a distribution list for the periodic newsletter.

Websites

Websites have become a staple of information about organizations providing goods and services to the public. Website design and hosting can be done internally if the skills are possessed within the organization, or can be outsourced to companies that provide a professional service to meet the individual needs of the organization. Websites should adhere to a few simple principles[13]:

- Have an easily identifiable URL
- Have all information accessible in less than 3 mouse clicks
- Have complete company contact information for potential customers or current clients who desire to reach the company

TABLE 18-2

MARKETING STRATEGIES FOR HEALTH PROMOTION

The following marketing strategies may be used to increase the awareness of health and wellness programs:

- *Newsprint advertisement:* Newspapers and magazines with large circulations reaching hundreds of thousands of people will charge premium rates for full page ads near the front. However, a small 2" x 2" ad on the final page of the periodical will not cost as much. Circulations will vary depending on the day of the week the newspaper is published. More people are accessing newspapers via dedicated websites, so this option should be taken into account. The key is to make the most effective use of advertising dollars based upon anticipated conversion rates.
- *Television and radio spots:* It costs money to get an advertising spot on the air and the cost is dependent on the duration of time that the spot consumes. When considering television and radio spots, a careful target market analysis should be performed knowing which medium the target market frequently listens to or watches. One efficient way to do explore these media is to ask existing customers their preferences. It is worthwhile to take advantage of the expertise of the radio and television stations about development and production of the advertising spot.
- *Scholarships:* A wellness organization could sponsor a scholarship establishing criteria for receipt of the award, and then present the award at the local ceremony. Publicity would come in terms of recognition at both the ceremony and in the associated program and, possibly, as a public interest story in a local newspapers.
- *Sports team and event sponsorships:* Purchasing banner ads that adorn a community recreation center, school, or college, and printing ads in programs for special events provides exposure and good will to a wide array of potential customers.
- *Billboards:* While billboard are limited in the scope of detailed information they can provide, they can attract attention and provide key information about the organization (eg, how to contact the organization through an Internet address, URL, or a phone number).
- *Membership Discounts:* Offering periodic discounts, incentives, or events for valued clients show them that they are appreciated. Personalized communication (eg, handwritten notes) and cash discounts on products or regular services are additional options for demonstrating appreciation of valued clients. It is more cost effective to keep a valued customer than it is to recruit a new one.
- *Public interest stories and services:* Newspaper columns addressing health and wellness issues and products create public interest and are cost effective. The drawback of this type of marketing is that it cannot be counted on for consistent distribution, as these types of news-based stories are often used as space fillers.
- *Word-of-mouth advertising:* This type of advertising is closely related to good will as people are often more comfortable using goods and services that trusted friends and family also use. One major drawback of word-of-mouth marketing is the potential for negative comments from disgruntled or unsatisfied customers. Conventional wisdom states that it only takes comments from one unhappy customer to offset the positive comments of ten happy customers. The trends are common that unhappy people will tell more people about their negative experience than happy people will tell of their positive experience. At the very least, a regular program of thanking customers and informing them that their positive comments about their experience are much appreciated. Give clients a discount or referral bonus for every customer that they encourage to utilize the product. This type of strategy is highly effective and does not consume a significant part of the marketing budget.
- *Outreach services and health fairs:* There is a wide array of plausible options for outreach services at schools, shopping centers, grocery stores, etc. Health fairs, in particular, have the potential of reaching a large audience in a very small amount of time at a relatively low cost. If there is no organized health fair in the immediate region of the health and wellness organization, then this is a wonderful opportunity to organize and sponsor such an event.
- *Product association:* Physical therapists can work to associate their products (health education, prescription for physical activity, and stress management) with healthy living and stress reduction.
- *Free promotional items and free services:* The term "free" catches eye of the consumer, but will only be effective if the lure of the free item or service converts potential consumers into regular clients. The success of promotional give-away items (eg, paper cups, pens, etc) and services should be ultimately measured in a cost-effectiveness analysis, taking into consideration the actual conversion rate for new customers.

The URL (Uniform Resource Locator) is more commonly known as the web address for the website. It is the string of characters that appears in the navigation bar of the web browser. Typically, the URL begins with "http://" or "ftp://" and may end in a variety of combinations including .com, .org, .biz, .net, .tv, or .gov. This domain name should be easily recognizable, should be easily remembered, and should not take a great deal of effort to key in to a web browser. Note that organizations with similar domain names make identification with any company difficult. In addition, cybersquatters (people who buy domain names corresponding to a famous brand name or trademark in hopes of reselling the domain for a significant profit) may complicate selection of domains. Domain names are secured by paying an annual registration fee to a domain registration company (see Appendix C).[12]

Navigation of a website should be such that information is easily available with only a few points and clicks. A navigation bar should contain corporate information and contact information at the very least. A web page compiled of frequently asked questions (FAQs) can be of great assistance to the web surfer. Complexity of website technology can make for a website that is slow to download or does not easily run on all web browsers. While broadband use is growing, many people still access the Internet via more traditional dial-up connections that do not load complicated or graphic laden websites as easily. It is tempting to use many of the creative tools and software that are at the disposal of website designers, but a site that is too complex for the average user may serve as a source of frustration and reflect negatively on the organization. While developing content for the website, note key criteria listed in Table 18-3 used to evaluate the effectiveness of a health-related website.[14]

TABLE 18-3

WEBSITE EVALUATION

- The purpose of the site is clearly stated or may be clearly inferred.
- All aspects of the subject are covered adequately.
- The information is accurate.
- Sources are clearly documented.
- The site is sponsored by or is associated with a respectable institution or organization.
- For sites created by an individual, author's/editor's credentials (educational background, professional affiliations, certifications, past writings, experience) are clearly stated.
- Contact information (e-mail, address, and/or phone number) for the author/editor or webmaster is included.
- The date of publication is clearly posted.
- The type of audience the author is addressing is evident (academic, youth, minority, general, etc).
- The level of detail is appropriate for the audience.
- The reading level is appropriate for the audience.
- Technical terms are appropriate for the audience.
- Graphics add to the usefulness of the site.
- Site is consistent with other business logos and information.
- Internal links add to the usefulness of the site.
- Information can be retrieved in a timely manner.
- The site is organized in a logical manner, facilitating the location of information.
- Any software necessary to use the page has links to download software from the Internet.

Adapted from Leslie Teach. Health-related web site evaluation form. 1998. Available at: http://www.sph.emory.edu/WELLNESS/instrument.html. Accessed February 2, 2006.

SEARCH ENGINES

Search engines are Internet-based tools that are designed to produce responses or "hits" to keyword queries entered by the computer user.[12] If the wellness organization has a web presence and relies on access to the web from search engines, it may be in its best interest to work with the major search engine providers to ensure that the products and services appear readily at or near the top of the list with associated key words. Search engine marketing (SEM) appearance is assumed by most organizations, and only a minority of companies dedicate marketing funds to take full advantage of the potential revenue streams from this source. Detailed strategies to take advantage of this ever-growing and ever-changing technology are beyond the scope of this chapter, but interested organizations can find many dedicated reference books and sources on the Internet itself for this strategy. Many popular search engines will have locations to submit a company's URL (see Appendix C for examples); however, it can be time consuming to enter a URL for every commercial search engine, and keep in mind that this appearance as a hit is not always guaranteed, nor is it always free of charge.

BANNER ADVERTISEMENTS

A banner advertisement is a web-based advertisement in which a website sells or hosts space on its page to other companies or organizations in the form of a banner or a sidebar.[12] The banner advertisement appears as a would-be billboard either on the top or bottom of the web page. Smaller sidebar advertisements are usually embedded along the periphery of the web page. The user is able to click on the advertisement, which will take him or her to a second page with more information, or preferably to the direct web page of the advertiser. Soliciting banner or sidebar advertisement space on a host web page should be determined by the documented history of hits or number of times the web page is viewed by potential consumers. A critical factor related to the number of hits is the conversion rate, or simply put, the number of actual consumers that are converted from the number of hits observed. If a website claims to have 10,000 hits per month, but only fifteen new customers can be attributed from the advertisement on the website, the monthly conversion rate is 0.15% (15/10,000). Costs of doing this type of advertising are directly related to the size of the advertisement, the location (top of the page is premium), and the anticipated conversion rate. Some hosting companies will charge per actual number of hits generated per month.

SPAM, SPIM, AND POP-UP ADVERTISEMENTS

SPAM, SPIM, and pop-up advertisements are generally undesirable means to support the marketing objectives of a wellness organization. SPAM is unsolicited e-mail advertisements and SPIM is the instant messaging counterpart of SPAM.[15] Pop-up advertisements are the immediate presence of unsolicited windows that open when a website is accessed promoting some product. The key to these marketing elements is that they are unsolicited and are frequently viewed in a negative light by the recipient. Many software companies today are selling products that prevent or block these types of direct communications efforts. Either of these avenues has potentially serious repercussions on the image and good will of an organization and, therefore, should be used judiciously.

Summary

Marketing is the collective processes of establishing a buyer-seller relationship that meets the needs and expectations of both parties. The classic model of marketing includes the four P's or Product, Pricing, Placement (Distribution), and Promotion. Identifying the target market and using current rapid communications technologies to build individual relationships with the potential consumer are key attributes to any well-constructed marketing plan. Health and wellness marketing, while very close to conventional marketing elements, is probably better reflected in the acronym of SCAP: Service, Consideration, Access, and Promotion. An integrated marketing approach is one that fosters a consistency of message and focuses on the needs of the individual. Many strategies ranging from promotional items, to logo based products, websites, print advertisements, and TV/radio spots can be used by the physical therapist to promote health, fitness, and wellness.

References

1. Miller College of Business. Ball State University. Marketing. Available at: http://www.bsu.edu/marketing. Accessed February 2, 2006.
2. Boone LE, Kurtz DL. *Contemporary Marketing 2005*. Mason, Ohio: Thomson Southwestern. 2005.
3. Longest BB, Rakich JS, Darr K. *Managing Health Services Organizations and Systems*. 4th ed. Baltimore, Md: Health Professions Press; 2000.
4. Lesh SG. Integrated marketing for the new millennium. *Bus Educ Technol J*. 2000;2(2):35–37.
5. State Healthy People 2010 Tool Library. Available at: http://www.phf.org/HPtools/state.htm. Accessed February 2, 2006.
6. Rimmer JH. Health promotion for people with disabilities: the emerging paradigm shift from disability prevention to prevention of secondary conditions. *Phys Ther*. 1999;79:495–502.
7. JobBankUSA. Physical therapists. Available at: http://www.jobbankusa.com/ohb/ohb080.html. Accessed February 2, 2006.
8. US Small Business Administration. Strategizing with the four P's. Available at: http://www.sba.gov/starting_business/marketing/fourps.html. Accessed February 2, 2006.
9. Janal DS. *Online Marketing Handbook: How to Promote, Advertise, and Sell Your Product and Services on the Internet*. New York, NY: Wiley and Sons; 1998.
10. Kostrova O. *How to Promote Your Business with a Limited Marketing Budget*. Virginia: Power HomeBiz Guides. 2003. Available at: http://www.powerhomebiz.com/vol113/budget.htm
11. Longest B, Rakich J, Darr K. *Managing Health Services Organizations & Systems*. 4th ed. Baltimore, Md: Health Professionals Press; 2000.
12. Lesh SG, Konin J, DePalma B. Paths to Profits. *Training & Conditioning*. 2002;12(8):20–24.
13. Lesh SG. Innovative technological communication trends in allied health: Instant messaging now appearing on the radar screen. Tampa, Fla: ASAHP Annual Conference "Opportunities for Collaboration" Platform Presentation; October 21, 2004.
14. Rollins School of Public Health. Health-related web site evaluation form. Available at: http://www.sph.emory.edu/WELLNESS/instrument.html. Accessed February 2, 2006.
15. Bruemmer PJ. *Establishing a Search Engine Marketing Budget*. Los Angeles, Calif: Marketing Professionals; 2002.

Chapter 19

Managing a Prevention Practice: A Business Model

Shawn T. Blakeley, PT, CWI, CEES and Catherine Rush Thompson, PhD, MS, PT

"The first goal of Healthy People 2010 is to help individuals of all ages increase life expectancy and improve their quality of life. The second goal of Healthy People 2010 is to eliminate health disparities among different segments of the population."

~ OFFICE OF DISEASE PREVENTION AND HEALTH PROMOTION
US DEPARTMENT OF HEALTH AND HUMAN SERVICES

Starting a Prevention Practice

When starting a prevention practice, the physical therapist should begin with a vision statement that identifies how the business will best meet the needs of the community. This vision statement can serve to motivate those engaged in the business to move the program toward the desired goals of improved community health and wellness. Fundamental questions include the following:

- What type of prevention practice would best serve the community?
- Would the prevention practice complement a pre-existing program or would it be created anew?
- What are the populations with unmet health care needs?
- What areas of expertise can the physical therapist offer in the areas of primary, secondary, and tertiary prevention?

Healthy People 2010 provides a strong vision for the nation to improve life expectancy and quality of life for all segments of the population.[1]

One model for envisioning health promotion programs is the Precede-Proceed Model of Health Promotion Planning.[2] This model, developed over the last quarter of a century, is based on two propositions[2]:

1. Health and health risks are caused by multiple factors.
2. Because health and health risks are determined by multiple factors, efforts to effect behavioral, environmental, and social change must be multidimensional or multisectoral.

The Precede-Proceed Model broadly envisions health promotion encompassing quality of life, health, environment, and lifestyle with influences by health education, media, advocacy, policy, regulation, resources, and organization. This model has been used to develop cancer prevention and control interventions as well as smoking cessation programs that encompass medical, educational, and governmental entities.[2]

> *The goals of the model are to explain health-related behaviors and to design and evaluate the interventions designed to influence both the behaviors and the living conditions that influence them and their sequelae.*

Using this model, the physical therapist can more comprehensively (1) diagnose and evaluate environmental, genetic, and lifestyle factors impacting health; (2) advocate for policies, regulations, and resources for health, fitness, and wellness; and (3) participate in the development of effective strategies to impact the environment, lifestyle behaviors, and society as a whole. This complex process requires many complex skills, techniques, and data from a variety of fields and requires a collaborative effort for planning and implementing community prevention and control interventions. More information about this model and resources for its implementation are available on the web.[3]

Many programs featuring prevention practice are contained within medically based facilities (hospitals, outpatient clinics, rehabilitation centers, etc), educationally based facilities (preschools, elementary schools, middle schools, high schools, colleges and universities), community-based recreational programs (YMCA, Special Olympics, etc), and businesses (corporate wellness and ergonomic programs). Where is the optimal location for prevention practice? The key is to match the need with the expertise and passion of the therapist. For physical therapists that most enjoy working with exercise-related injuries, setting up a clinic in a fitness club may provide a steady flow of clients with musculoskeletal injuries and a partnership with a well-established business. The physical therapist should explore available programs before "reinventing the wheel."

Planning and Designing the Program

Before starting a new business it is important to identify the key concepts of the business and its feasibility. From a business standpoint can the business support itself? Are there grant monies that can be used to develop and sustain the envisioned type of health promotion business? Would these services be provided pro bono or offered as part of a corporate program?

After exploring options, it is important to develop a business plan (Table 19-1). In addition to developing effective marketing strategies, a good business plan provides clear business objectives, details the characteristics of the business, examines strengths and weaknesses of the proposed program, and provides prospective sources of funding with a clear outline of the program's development, including a timeline with financial milestones. The business plan provides a blueprint for the intended prevention program, and anticipates needs for equipment, supplies, marketing needs, a location for practice, and qualified personnel. A good resource for developing a wellness program/health promotion program/preventive practice business plan is the Small Business Administration (SBA) on the Internet.[4] According to the SBA, the four basic questions that need to be answered before writing a plan for *any* business are the following[4]:

TABLE 19-1

BUSINESS PLAN COMPONENTS

Cover Sheet

Statement of Purpose

Table of Contents With the Following Information:

The Business

- Description of business
- Marketing
- Competition
- Operating procedures
- Personnel
- Business insurance

Financial Data

- Loan applications
- Capital equipment and supply list
- Balance sheet
- Breakeven analysis
- Pro-forma income projections (profit and loss statements)
- Three-year summary
- Detail by month, first year
- Detail by quarters, second and third years
- Assumptions upon which projections were based
- Pro-forma cash flow

Supporting Documents

- Tax returns of principals for last 3 years
- Personal financial statement (all banks have these forms)
- For franchised businesses, a copy of franchise contract and all supporting documents provided by the franchisor
- Copy of proposed lease or purchase agreement for building space
- Copy of licenses and other legal documents.
- Copy of resumes of all principals
- Copies of letters of intent from suppliers, etc

Adapted from Small Business Administration. Available at: http://www.sba.gov/starting_business/planning/writingplan.html. Accessed October 15, 2005.

1. *What service or product does your business provide and what needs does it fill?*
2. *Who are the potential customers for your product or service and why will they purchase it from you?*

3. *How will you reach your potential customers?*
4. *Where will you get the financial resources to start your business?*

Funding may be a stumbling block if the prevention program must be self-sustaining. Few insurance policies cover prevention programs for musculoskeletal, cardiopulmonary, neurological, or integumentary conditions. Clients may need to pay for services rendered. Another alternative is to seek financial support from existing businesses with a vested interest in the business, such as vendors of health-related or fitness products.

Healthy People 2010 is funded through federal dollars and offers grants for health promotion.[1] If the mission of a proposed program meets key objectives of this national initiative, it is possible to obtain government funding. Local and state health agencies receive funding for ongoing prevention programs in their jurisdictions and may award grants to local programs that meet the health care needs of their communities.

Before approaching any source of funding, the physical therapist must do a "needs" assessment to determine whether or not the proposed program meets a community need and whether or not there is a market for the envisioned program. It is helpful to explore other programs in the area, asking about provided services and needs that are unmet by competing programs. Finding a unique "niche" eliminates competition and provides the community with more health care options. Some programs have had great success partnering with pre-existing mental health and hospital-based programs, opening exercise and educational facilities during after-work hours for those interested in preventive care.

Financial and Legal Considerations

When starting a new business, there are a number of financial and legal considerations. A lawyer can help ensure that the legal matters of starting a business are well managed, since the laws regulating small businesses can be burdensome. According to the SBA, "One of the main reasons small businesses fail is because they don't seek legal help at critical development stages." Business.gov offers information about business laws.[5] This resource provides information about legal aspects of running a business, as well as information about managing employees.

A financial accounting of the investments in the practice as well as an accurate record of the ongoing income and expenses may require the expertise of an accountant. The SBA notes, "While poor management is cited most frequently as the reason businesses fail, inadequate or ill-timed financing is a close second."[4] The SBA offers a series of questions that can guide the entrepreneur in determining the appropriate financing for a new business, including a prevention practice.

Marketing Prevention Practice

Chapter 18 discusses the various creative ways that prevention practice can be marketed to the public. If marketed successfully, the practice will develop a steady stream of clients who are supported by the unique services offered by the program. For example, an aquatics program for individuals with arthritis can be provided at a low cost to groups of clients with degenerative arthritis. To ensure program success, it is important to track participants' progress so that each individual has a sense of accomplishment toward reaching personal health, fitness, or wellness goals. It is also helpful to solicit regular feedback from participants to determine if their needs are adequately met, or if the program needs some minor changes to improve services.

Ensuring a Healthy and Productive Workforce

In recent years, physical therapists have been hired by industry to prevent injuries and disease. Many companies are realizing the benefits of corporate wellness and afford physical therapists an opportunity to meet community needs without personal financial risks. The trend toward a healthier workforce helps to achieve the goals of Healthy People 2010.

The US Task Force on Disease Prevention and Health Promotion reports that the most effective interventions available to clinicians for reducing the incidence of disease and disability in the United States are those that address the personal health practices of patients.[6] In an effort to manage the costs incurred with disease and disability of their work force, corporations are hiring clinicians to address the personal health practices of their employees.

Employee Wellness Profile/ Health Risk Appraisal

An Employee Wellness Profile assesses the health and lifestyle of a workforce.[6] There are several steps the physical therapist would follow to administer an employee wellness profile program. Upon hire, and periodically thereafter, employees complete a personal, confidential written health assessment, usually at the time of their medical physical. Individuals answer questions about their health, physical activity, eating practices, substance use, stress, social health, safety, and medical care, as well as their views on health and wellness. A confidential objective assessment of the individual's current health status is then sent directly to their home address. This assessment addresses health needs and lifestyle practices that determine personal well-being. Their personal score can be bench-marked against national averages and used to provide positive reinforcement of good health practices, while making recommendations to improve poor ones. The change of an individual's score over time should reflect the modifications they made in their health practices.

The aggregate data from all employee wellness profiles are confidentially reported to the company in an executive summary report. First the demographics of the company are summarized and the major health risks are identified. Health risks such as cardiovascular disease, cancer, lung disease, diabetes, liver dysfunction, and even suicide or depression can be ranked according to prevalence.[7] Furthermore, the exact factors that are contributing to each health risk are identified. In addition to health risks, lifestyle risks, such as stress and sleeplessness, can also be recognized. Last, current disease states are identified and quantified. Actuarial charts can then be used to provide the company with a projected average cost per claim for their upcoming year. This figure can be compared to what similar companies with similar work forces expect to pay, when they have had an ongoing comprehensive wellness program in place for a number of years. The difference in expected costs between these two companies estimates the economic impact of preventable risk factors. The difference in cost per claim represents a realistic savings that could be used to fund the wellness program. More importantly, the executive summary report identifies which health risks to focus on. For example, a company would be very disappointed in attempting to manage the weight of their obese workforce by focusing on diabetes education, when only 3% have contributing risk factors for diabetes. The company would better invest their resources in nutrition education and/or fitness improvement, if those areas were defined as the key contributing risk factors to their obesity.

When done regularly, physical therapists can utilize the Employee Wellness Profile as a useful assessment tool to help a company identify health risks, establish wellness goals, assess program effectiveness, and establish the thrust and direction of upcoming health and wellness needs. In a nutshell, employee wellness profiles allow for health surveillance.

Corporate Wellness Program

Wellness, as defined by the National Wellness Association, is "an active process of becoming aware of and making choices towards a more successful existence."[8] The physical therapist's goal when implementing a corporate wellness program is to assist employees in adopting positive behaviors to lead healthier lives and integrating social, mental, emotional, spiritual, and physical aspects of wellness. High-quality corporate wellness programs are congruent with the company's values, have a well stated mission or primary objective, and secondary objectives that are fluid and change periodically, depending on the needs of the workforce.

Several different methods are used to educate a work force regarding health hazards, to reinforce good health practices, and to encourage change in undesirable health habits. Wellness programming must be customized to the needs and culture of each organization. What works well in one industry may be ineffective for another. A blend of the following strategies can be incorporated throughout any given year:

- Routine health screenings (ie, blood pressure, glucose)
- Employee health fair
- Lunch-n-Learn programs
- Incentive programs
- One-on-one disease management programs
- Lectures
- Competitions
- Newsletters
- Targeted mailings
- 800 number access for health information and advice
- Self-care books
- Vouchers for a clinical office visit
- Interactive web site
- Company's intranet (Q and A, wellness chat rooms)

Prevention of disease and disability is the focus of any corporate wellness program. Below is a list of the most common topics addressed by today's corporations:

- Smoking cessation
- Stress management
- Life balance
- Weight measurement and management
- Personal training
- On-site chair massages

- Flu shots
- CPR/first aid training
- Back care
- Cumulative trauma risk reduction/prevention
- Carpal tunnel prevention
- Nutrition
- Blood-borne pathogen training
- Proper lifting techniques
- Posture and body alignment
- Cholesterol screening
- Body fat profiles
- Blood pressure checks
- Pulmonary function testing
- Diabetes risk assessment
- Blood glucose levels
- Depression screening
- Bone density screening
- Spiritual wellness
- Vision screens
- Stroke assessment
- Automated electronic defibrillator (AED) training
- Women's health
- Time management
- Anger management

Benefits of a successful corporate wellness program are abundant. Sometimes immediate improvements can be attained in employee productivity and morale, enhanced recruitment and retention, and improved overall corporate image. Other advantages can be realized shortly after implementation, such as decreased short- and long-term disability costs, decreased workers' compensation costs, decreased employee absenteeism, and overall decreased health care costs. In one case study, the major return on investment came from a reduction in the rate of increased medical costs.[8] The company estimated it saved $226 per risk factor per person ($171 in health service costs, the rest in drug costs). The company also estimated that its average plant saved nearly $350,000 annually in absenteeism costs alone.[8]

The major challenge with corporate health promotion programs is that the benefits are most often in the form of costs *avoided*, rather than in cost *savings*. Because it is difficult to calculate or see costs avoided, estimating the financial benefits of a program is complex and may be difficult to sell within an organization. Additionally, the costs that are avoided can vary greatly due to differing workforce populations, different sites, dissimilar industries and variations between health promotion programs. However, since the most effective interventions for reducing the incidence of disease and disability are by addressing personal health practices, then a comprehensive corporate wellness program guided by an employee wellness profile is an excellent place for companies to start.

POSTOFFER SCREENING AND ESSENTIAL FUNCTIONS TESTING

Another way a company can promote a healthy workforce is by testing employees to ensure that they are physically capable of performing the functions that are deemed essential for their specific positions. Studies show that one in every three workers will suffer a work-related injury.[6] Research indicates that 10% of the American workforce is physically incapable of performing the essential functions of their job safely.[6] According to recent reports, this population is responsible for 75% of all work related injuries.[6] Essential functions testing allows a company to identify this target group and implement controls that keep the environment safe for all workers.

Most postoffers screens include three parts, the first of which is an informed consent. The individual signs a standard release from liability and answers general questions designed to uncover any physical restrictions or limitations that the individual may have. The goal is to find out if the test is contraindicated, such as in the case of a pregnancy.

The second component is a general global screen. Heart rate and blood pressure are taken and compared against the American Heart Association standards. Range of motion is charted from head to toe and a strength grade for major muscle groups is documented. Postural malalignment is charted and screens for common musculoskeletal disorders are performed. These pre-employment baseline measurements are compared to the employee's medical history questionnaire to identify inconsistencies. Additionally, a physician or therapist may use this baseline data to compare postinjury impairments to pre-employment status. Lastly, these objective measurements prove essential for postinjury medical or legal intervention. For example, after a work-related hand injury, the employee's pre-employment grip strength may be used by the treating physician or therapist to establish their goals. The company may only be responsible for rehabilitating the employee to preinjury status versus normal limits. If a baseline strength measurement is not available, then frequently the company may be expected to rehabilitate the individual to a level that is close to the standard for a person the same age and gender, even if the individual is weaker than that standard. While all of these pre-employment baselines are useful and important, most states will not allow a company to deny employment based on their results.

The third component of employment screening is testing an individual to see if he or she is capable of safely performing the essential functions of a job. The employee either passes or fails, and failure constitutes legal grounds to deny employment. It is best if the vendor who administers the essential functions test is the same who developed the essential functions for the job. Positional tolerances, lifting, carrying, pushing, pulling, reaching, fine motor skills, bending, stooping, kneeling, crawling, walking, driving, twisting, squatting, stairs, ladders, ramps, curbs, poles, reading, color discrimination, depth perception, hearing sensitivity, tactile discrimination, and temperature discrimination are frequently tested. The law varies, but some states may require that the essential functions be defined in a written job description in order for testing to commence. Additionally, most states require that all individuals applying for a position be tested in an attempt to prevent discrimination. Frequently, an employer will expect the vendor who is administering the test to provide information regarding the employability of the individual. It is important that the vendor simply administer the test and deliver the results. The employer should make all judgment and decisions regarding employment of the individual.

Essential functions testing is most commonly done pre-employment, as a contingency for employment (ie, a job offer is conditional on its successful completion). However, more companies are doing periodic testing of their workforce to help identify the population that cannot safely perform their job.

The essential functions test can also be a useful tool when a physician is determining an injured worker's fitness for duty. In other words, if the patient has not achieved strength or mobility levels to successfully complete the test, then the physician will frequently assign a restricted or modified work status to keep the patient safe while justifying the need for more rehabilitation. Testing also allows the physical therapist to observe an unsafe work practice, such as improper lifting, and document that proper training was provided. An essential functions test empowers a company to appropriately match employees to safe and appropriate jobs.

Ensuring a Healthy and Benign Work Environment

In addition to screening individuals for their capabilities and matching them to appropriate job tasks, physical therapists can analyze each job task to determine whether it is as safe as possible to perform. In this sense, physical therapists are experts in ergonomics or the science of fitting jobs to people.

Comprehensive Company-Wide Ergonomics Program

According to the Occupational Safety and Health Administration (OSHA), occupational musculoskeletal disorders are a major national problem, costing the economy (by conservative estimates) over $20 billion each year.[9] In a recent study by the National Academy of Sciences, musculoskeletal disabilities in the workplace cost the United States more than $1 trillion per year in total costs. As discussed in Chapter 12, a comprehensive company-wide ergonomic program is one step in making the work environment safer.

The goal of a corporate ergonomic program is to reduce risk factors known to be associated with the development of musculoskeletal and cumulative trauma disorders. Physical, environmental, organizational, and psychosocial risk factors should be considered. Much like a corporate wellness program, an ergonomic program should be congruent with the company's values, have a well-stated mission or primary objective, and when necessary, a changing secondary focus depending on the thrust and needs of the company at the time. This serves as an action plan or road map, keeping the program on a straight and narrow path.

The initial step is to locate the "problem" departments or jobs. This can be done by three methods, the first of which is document analysis. By reviewing the company's injury history, one can identify trends. For example, there might be a disproportionate number of injuries in one department or an increase in a specific diagnosis noticed in a particular job. Analyzing the injury history often points the ergonomist in an appropriate direction. The second method, symptom surveys, or comfort-level surveys, assign ratings of discomfort by body part and can be used to identify jobs or departments where the workers experience subreportable levels of discomfort. Symptom surveys or comfort-level surveys target symptoms of pain, numbness, tingling, burning, or swelling that (1) have occurred in the previous 12 months, (2) last for at least 1 week, (3) occur at least once per month, and (4) are not caused by an acute injury. The results of these surveys help identify departments where symptoms of discomfort exist, but where these symptoms are masked by a low incidence of documented injuries. Using the third method, some ergonomists will blanket whole departments with a risk factor checklist. A helpful Ergonomic Checklist that quickly assesses repetitiveness; lifting, pushing, pulling, and carrying forces; awkward postures; and pressure points is located on the web.[10] Some checklists will assign a combined risk factor score with an established threshold, indicating the need for a more in-depth analysis. Another helpful checklist for those who work at a desk job offers ergonomically sound office furniture and equipment.[11]

Once the location of the risk factors has been revealed, the next step is identification of the specific offending risk factors. Psychosocial risk factors include machine-paced tasks, incentive pay, routine overtime, electronic monitoring of employees, limited ability to influence daily decisions, and monotonous tasks. Other risk factors include extreme posture, velocity of motion, repetition of tasks, total task duration, nerve compression, vibration, cold temperatures, and force required to accomplish the task. The final assessment regarding the degree of total risk is a fine balance of all of the above conditions. For example, a task may require an extreme posture with high velocity and vibration, but if the task duration is negligible, then the task may be benign.

An ergonomic committee is frequently formed to identify and evaluate possible solutions. This task force can be composed of several members, including representatives from employee health, a safety office, a medical office, company engineers, employee representatives, the ergonomist, and a union representative, if applicable. This committee examines design specifications; analyzes similar operations/industries; reviews the literature for solutions; talks to vendors, trade association, organizations, and specialists; and generally brainstorms to determine a solution to presenting problems. Solutions fall into one of three categories. First, administrative controls reduce the frequency, duration, and severity of exposures to the risk factors. Job rotation, mandatory rest periods, job enhancement, stretching programs, conditioning programs, light/modified work duties, and supervision are all examples of administrative controls. Second, engineering controls are one-time changes that protect all employees. Engineering controls are permanent and involve physical changes to workstations, equipment, the production facility, or any other relevant aspect of the work environment to reduce or eliminate the presence of risk factors. Third, work practice controls are procedures for safe and proper work and specific for each task or workplace. Personal protective equipment, appropriate training, job simulation/practice, correct lifting techniques, proper tool maintenance, and correct use of workstations are all examples of work practice controls. Of course, the solutions selected should address the particular risk factors involved.

The ergonomic committee should meet periodically to ensure solution implementation and follow-up. A status report should be maintained to track ergonomic issues, solution implementation, and current status. The committee should conduct continuous ergonomic monitoring to identify potential problems. Rarely are all existing risk factors identified, and as jobs are added or changed, new risk factors are continually being created. A yearly review of the ergonomic program should be conducted to assess its effectiveness, track the status of ergonomic goals, and establish the direction of upcoming health and safety needs.

Ensuring Healthy and Appropriate Work Practices

Healthy individuals working in a healthy environment can still incur injury if they are performing tasks in an unhealthy way. The body mechanics involved in performing a specific task can be evaluated by a physical therapist and health education can be personalized to the needs of an individual client.

DEFINING ESSENTIAL JOB FUNCTIONS

One role of a physical therapist has always been to help people function as independently as possible in performing the motor tasks required to fulfill important roles in their lives. These motor tasks are sometimes self-evident. For example, the motor task of transferring sit-to-stand is essential to getting out of a chair and fulfilling certain life roles. Work is one important life role for most people. In work settings, however, the motor tasks are not self-evident and must be defined. For example, an assembly plant may need to specify the amount required to lift, push, or pull in order to function in a particular job. These work-related motor tasks are called the essential functions for a job. Positional tolerances, lifting, carrying, pushing, pulling, reaching, fine motor skills, bending, stooping, kneeling, crawling, walking, driving, twisting, squatting, stairs, ladders, ramps, curbs, poles, reading, color discrimination, depth perception, hearing sensitivity, tactile discrimination, and temperature discrimination are examples of essential functions. The duration of each essential function should be identified in accordance to the US Department of Labor, Dictionary of Occupational Titles as follows[12]:

Occasional = 1% to 33% of the shift

Frequent = 34% to 66% of the shift

Constant = 67% to 100% of the shift

Well-defined essential functions are useful to companies for several reasons. One, essential functions are required legally for companies who choose to physically test their employees against them. For example, a company cannot deny employment to an individual who is unable to lift 50 pounds if that motor task is not deemed essential to function in that job. Two, essential functions are useful when suggesting job rotation. For example, rotating from one fine motor task to another may not reduce exposure to similar risk factors. However, rotation from a fine motor task to a gross motor task may. Additionally, if harmful risk factors are uncovered during the job analysis, this can serve as a trigger to the ergonomic committee for follow-up before it leads to injury. Three, preventive workstation stretches are often created from the essential functions. Otherwise, the prevention-based stretches may miss their target. Four, essential functions give physicians important information from which they can make decisions regarding an individual's work status. Restricted or light duty can keep an injured worker safe, yet productive on the job. Five, essential functions give physical therapists and occupational therapists job-related rehabilitation goals. If a patient is required to carry 25 pounds at work, and they are currently unable to do so, then the therapist has a sound, objective, and valid goal. Six essential functions allow for companies to either place injured workers or assess whether they can make reasonable accommodations to the work site. The Americans with Disabilities Act contains specific guidelines that define the rights and obligations for companies and employees.[13] As jobs experience change and modification, so do the essential functions. Therefore, the essential functions should be updated on a regular schedule and modified when job modifications occur. Essential functions are the cornerstone from which many other work site prevention measures are developed.

Preventive Job-Specific Work Station Stretches

Physical therapists have always provided injured workers with useful information during their rehabilitation about how to prevent another injury. However, companies are starting to recognize the value this information can have to noninjured workers. Preventive workstation stretching and strengthening routines are another way clinicians are used today to help companies manage their workers' compensation costs.

Developing a preventive job-specific program begins with a job site analysis. Observation of different workers performing the same job helps to establish the essential functions for a particular position. From these essential functions, the clinician can identify the structures in one's body that absorb and generate forces. A stretching and strengthening program can then be recommended that is customized for that particular position.

Providing this routine empowers employees through information to be proactive about their health and wellness at work. Companies will frequently have a physical therapist train a shift-leader to lead their group through the program when arriving to work or returning from break. Some corporations even take roll or document participation in the stretching program. This record can sometimes be used to demonstrate a company's proactive approach or illustrate an employee's noncompliance.

Summary

Physical therapists have an opportunity to be leaders in prevention practice. With backgrounds in health, fitness, and wellness, as well as knowledge about business and ethical practices, physical therapists can lead their businesses into a direction that provides primary, secondary, and tertiary prevention. Screening individuals for their workplaces; examining the ergonomics of work, leisure, and home activities; and promoting health, fitness, and wellness across the lifespan are all aspects of prevention practice where physical therapists can excel.

References

1. Healthy People 2010. Available at: http://www.healthypeople.gov. Accessed February 6, 2006.
2. Green LW, Kreuter MW. *Health Promotion Planning: An Educational and Ecological Approach*. 3rd ed. Mountain View, Calif: Mayfield Publishing; 1999.
3. Institute for Health Promotion Research. Precede-proceed model of health promotion. Available at: http://www.ihpr.ubc.ca/ProcedePrecede.html. Accessed October 30, 2005.
4. Small Business Administration. Available at: www.sba.gov. Accessed February 6, 2006.
5. Business.gov: The Official Business Link to the US Government. Available at: http://www.business.gov. Accessed February 6, 2006.
6. US Public Health Department. Office of Disease Prevention and Health Promotion. Steps to a healthier US. Available at: http://odphp.osophs.dhhs.gov. Accessed January 31, 2005.
7. National Wellness Association. NUS wellness corner definitions & objectives. Definition of wellness. Available at: http://www.nus.edu.sg/uhwc/wellness/wellness_definition.htm. Accessed February 6, 2006

8. McGlynn EA, McDonald TM, Champangne L. The business case for a corporate wellness program: a case study of general motors and the united auto workers union. The Commonwealth Fund. April 2003. Available at: www.cmwf.org (report #612). Accessed January 31, 2005.
9. Report of written testimony from Linda Rosenstock, National Institute for Occupational Safety and Health. Submitted to the Subcommittee on Workforce Protection on May 21, 1997. Available at: http://www.cdc.gov/niosh/nioshfin.html. Accessed February 6, 2006.
10. Graves R, Way K, Riley D. The Development of the Risk Filter and Risk Assessment Worksheets for HSG60(rev) HSL/2002/34. 2002. Available at: http://www.hse.gov.uk/research/hsl_pdf/2002/hsl02-34.pdf. Accessed January 30, 2006.
11. National Occupational Health and Safety Commission. Ergonomic Principles and checklists for the selection of office furniture and equipment. 1991. Available at: http://www.nohsc.gov.au/PDF/Standards/ErgonomicPrinciples OfficeFurniture.pdf. Accessed February 6, 2006.
12. US Department of Labor. Bureau of Labor Statistics. Standard occupational classification. Available at: http://www.bls.gov/soc/home.htm. Accessed February 6, 2006.
13. US Department of Justice. Americans with Disabilities Act. A guide for people with disabilities seeking employment. October 2000. Available at: http://www.usdoj.gov/crt/ada/workta.htm. Accessed February 6, 2006.

APPENDIX A:
PHYSICAL THERAPY PATIENT MANAGEMENT DOCUMENTATION

(Modified from the *Guide to Physical Therapy Practice, Second Edition*)

ADMINISTRATIVE INFORMATION

Referral source:
Reason for referral to physical therapy:
Setting for physical therapy services:
Type of insurance:
Informed consent:
Date of examination:

EXAMINATION

General Demographics

Name:
Date of birth (DOB):
Age:
Sex:
Race:
Ethnicity:
Language:
Education:

Social/Health History

Cultural/religious:
Family and caregiver resources:
Social interactions, social activities, support systems:
Health beliefs (including attitude toward self-responsibility for health, fitness, and wellness):
Self-perception of physical health, mental health, and overall wellness:
Previous activities or behaviors to enhance health, fitness, and wellness:
Nutritional habits:
Dietary supplements used for health promotion:
Sleep habits:
Exercise habits:
Barriers to exercise:
Facilitators for exercise:
Frequency of health screenings and immunizations:
Stress management techniques:

Employment/Work (Job/School/Play)

Repetitive movement requirements:
Sedentary time:
Standing time:
Ergonomically-designed work environment:
Heavy lifting requirements:
Risk for overuse syndrome:

Growth and Development

Developmental history:
Hand dominance:

Living Environment

Devices and equipment (eg, assistive devices, sensory aids, and other equipment to facilitate function):
Living environment and community characteristics (eg, type of residence):
Living with:
Environmental barriers:
Environmental resources:
Projected discharge destination:

General Health Status (Self-Report, Family Report, Caregiver Report)

General health perception:
Physical function (eg, mobility, sleep patterns, restricted bed days):

Physiological functions (eg, memory, reasoning ability, depression and anxiety):
Role function (eg, community, leisure, work, social):
Social function (eg, social activity, social interaction, social support):

Social/Health Habits

Behavioral health risks (eg, smoking, drug abuse):
Level of physical fitness:

Family History

Family health risks:

Medical/surgical History

Cardiovascular:
Endocrine/metabolic:
Gastrointestinal:
Genitourinary:
Gynecological:
Integumentary:
Musculoskeletal:
Neuromuscular:
Obstetrical:
Prior hospitalizations, surgeries, and pre-existing medical and other health-related conditions:
Psychological:
Pulmonary:

Current Condition/Chief Complaint

Concerns that lead the patient/client to seek the services of a PT:
Concerns or needs of patients/clients who require the services of a PT:
Current therapeutic interventions:
Mechanism of injury or disease (eg, date of onset and course of events):
Onset and pattern of symptoms:
Patient/client, family, significant other and caregiver expectations and goals for the therapeutic intervention:
Patient/client, family, significant other, and caregiver perceptions of patient's/client's emotional response to the current clinical situation:
Previous occurrence of chief complaints:
Prior therapeutic interventions:

Functional Status and Activity Level

Current and prior functional status in self-care and home management, including ADLs and IADLs:
Current and prior functional status in work (job/school/play, community and leisure actions, tasks, or activities):

Medications

Medications for current condition:
Medications previously taken for current condition:
Medications for other conditions:
Dietary supplements used as remedies (herbal supplements, vitamins, additional OTC medications):
Any allergies or adverse reactions to medications:

Other Clinical Tests

Laboratory and diagnostic tests:
Review of available records (eg, medical, educational, surgical):
Review of other clinical findings (eg, nutrition and hydration):

Systems Review

Overall Growth and Development:
  Height:
  Weight:
Cardiovascular/Pulmonary System:
  Heart rate:
  Respiratory rate:
  Blood pressure:
  Edema:
Integumentary System:
  Integumentary disruption:
  Continuity of skin color:
  Pliability (texture):
  Presence of scar formation:
Musculoskeletal System:
  Gross symmetry:
  Standing:
  Sitting:
  Activity specific:
  Gross range of motion:
  Gross Strength:
Neuromuscular System:
  Gait:
  Locomotion (eg, transfers, sit-to-stand, transitions, bed mobility):
  Balance:
  Motor function (motor control, motor learning):
  Sensory function:

Communication, Affect, Cognition, Learning Style

Communication (ability to make needs known):
Orientation x 4 (person, place, time, and purpose):
Emotional/behavioral problems:
Learning barriers:
Education needs:

Tests and Measures

EVALUATION

DIAGNOSIS

(see practice patterns in *Guide to Physical Therapy Practice*)

PROGNOSIS (INCLUDING PLAN OF CARE)

Level of optimal improvement (prognosis for optimal function, expected outcomes):
Anticipated goals (long-term and short-term):
Amount of time required:
Intervention to be used (frequency and duration):
Discharge plan:

INTERVENTION

Coordination, communication, and documentation:
Patient/client-related instruction:
Procedural interventions:

Examination findings that may direct the type and specificity of the procedural intervention may include the following:

Pathology/pathophysiology:
Impairments:
Functional limitations:
Disability:
Risk reduction/prevention needs:
Health, wellness, and fitness needs:
Equipment needs:
Adaptation needs:
Other needs (safety, education for family members, co-workers, others in contact with individual, etc.):

Appendix B:
Developmental History

Child's name: ____________________ Child's birth date: ______________ Child's age: _____________
Mother's name: ____________________ Occupation: _________________
Father's name: ____________________ Occupation: _________________
Today's date: ______________________

PART I:
Prenatal history—Questions related to mother's pregnancies and this delivery

1. Have you been pregnant before?
2. If you have been pregnant before, how many times?
3. Were there problems during other pregnancies? If so, please specify:
4. What was the length of this pregnancy?
   Number of weeks gestation:
   Duration of labor for this child:
5. Type of delivery: vaginal?____ C-section?___
   Any complications?_____

PART II:
Child's Early History—Questions about this child's early development

1. What was the condition of your child at birth? (healthy, at risk, requiring neonatal intensive care)
2. What problems, if any, were evident at birth?
3. Were you aware of any problems before your child's birth?
4. What was your child's APGAR score at 1 minute?
5. What was your child's APGAR score at 5 minutes?
6. What was your child's birth weight?
7. What was your child's height at birth?
8. What were your child's sleep patterns after birth?
9. Has your child had any problems with sleep since birth?
10. What is your child's favorite activity?
11. How does your child react to movement?
12. Is your child toilet trained?
13. Are there any problems related to your child's toileting?
14. Has your child been hospitalized since birth (specify):
15. Does your child have allergies? (specify):
16. Does your child have a history of ear infections? (specify):
17. Is your child teething now?
18. Are you aware of any other problems or situations that may have influenced your child's growth or development?
19. Note the age of each of the following developmental milestones:

    sitting alone____ crawling on all fours____
    walking alone____ running____
    creeping upstairs/downstairs____
    catching a large ball____ using words____
    2-word sentences____

3- to 4-word sentences____
asking questions____
drinking from a cup___ dressing self____
using a spoon___ using a knife____
using markers or crayons____

20. Describe your child's general coordination and balance:
21. Describe your child's ability to communicate:
22. Has your child's vision and hearing been tested? If so, describe the results.

PART III:
Present status—Current care, concerns, and management:

1. Parent(s) concerns:
2. Current medications:
3. Current illnesses:
4. Current medical diagnosis(es):
5. Current sleeping patterns and related problems:
6. Current eating habits and related problems:
7. Time spent in front of the television and/or computer (average time per day):
8. Type of daily physical activity child enjoys:
9. Time spent engaged in physical activity (play/sports/athletics/dance classes, etc) (type and average time per day):
10. Current height and weight:
11. Family history risk factors for obesity, disease or illness:
12. Child's most recent immunizations:
13. Interaction with other children:
14. Attendance at daycare, play groups, other (specify):
15. Current coordination in movement—both large movements:
16. Current coordination in movement—using hands:
17. Describe language at present:
18. Pediatrician's name:
19. Pediatrician's address:
20. Pediatrician's phone:
21. Names of other specialists working with your child:
22. What is the family's history since the birth of this child (note moves, changes, significant traumas, or other problems)?:
23. Names and ages of siblings:
24. Are the other siblings in good general health? If not, please describe:
25. Other comments:

Appendix C: Resources for Health, Fitness, and Wellness

APTA Resources for Health, Fitness, and Wellness Practice

For more details go to the APTA website http://www.apta.org

Note: Members of the APTA receive discounted rates on these resources.

- APTA Public Relations Manual: A How-To
- Why It Feels Right to Put Your Health in the Hands of a Physical Therapist
- Fit Kids
- FUNfitness: A Screening Kit to Assess Children's Flexibility, Strength, & Balance
- Fit Teens
- Fit for the Fairway: A Posture Assessment for Golfers
- Golfers: Take Care of Your Back
- Balance and Falls Awareness Event Kit
- What You Need to Know About Balance and Falls
- What You Need to Know About Arthritis
- Fitness: A Way of Life
- Taking Care of Your Back
- What You Need to Know About Neck Pain
- What You Need to Know About Carpal Tunnel Syndrome
- Taking Care of Your Hand, Wrist, and Elbow
- Taking Care of Your Shoulder
- Taking Care of Your Foot and Ankle
- Taking Care of Your Knees
- Taking Care of Your Hips
- What You Need to Know About Osteoporosis
- You Can Do Something About Incontinence
- For Women of All Ages
- For the Young at Heart
- Secret of Good Posture
- Scoliosis: What Young People and Their Parents Need to Know
- Bike Right, Bike Fit
- Couch Potato Tips: Exercise for the Big Game
- Walking for Exercise: A Physical Therapist's Perspective
- Fitness: A Way of Life

Advocacy at the National Level

Fact Sheets for each of the following topics can be located at http://www.apha.org/legislative/fact-sheets.htm:

- Access to Care
- Ergonomics
- Medicaid
- Strengthening the Public Health Workforce
- Antibiotic Resistance
- Bioterrorism Preparedness
- Ergonomics
- FDA Regulation of Tobacco Products
- Food Safety
- Food Quality Protection Act
- Global AIDS Pandemic

- Health Disparities
- Mental Health Parity
- National Violent Death Reporting System
- Patient's Bill of Rights
- Prescription Drug Coverage
- Universal Health Care

Public Health Topics

The web page for APHA links to sites related to public health (http://www.apha.org/public_health) including the following topics:

- Aging
- Autoimmune Diseases (lupus, MS, etc)
- Bioterrorism
- Cancer
- Career Opportunities in Public Health
- Children's Health
- Chronic Conditions and Disorders
- Diabetes
- Environmental and Occupational Health
- Epidemiology
- Food Safety
- Gay and Lesbian Health
- Government Health Programs
- Health Education and Health Promotion
- Health Policy and Advocacy
- Health Services Research
- Heart Disease and Stroke
- Hepatitis
- HIV/AIDS
- Injury and Violence Prevention
- International Resources
- Men's Health
- Mental Health
- Minority Health Issues
- National and Professional Organizations
- Nutrition and Obesity
- Pharmacy
- Reproductive Health
- Resource Locators
- Smallpox
- State and Local Health Departments
- Tobacco Control and Prevention
- Traffic Safety
- Tuberculosis
- Upcoming Public Health Events
- West Nile Virus
- Women's Health

Publications From the National Center for Chronic Disease Prevention and Health Promotion

A variety of resources are listed on the following website: http://www.cdc.gov/nccdphp/publicat.htm:

- Assessing Health Risk Behaviors Among Young People
- Diabetes: Disabling, Deadly, and on the Rise 2006
- Division for Heart Disease and Stroke Prevention: Addressing the Nation's Leading Killers
- Health Risks in the United States: Behavioral Risk Factor Surveillance System (BRFSS)
- Healthy Aging: Preventing Disease and Improving Quality of Life Among Older Americans
- Healthy Youth: An Investment in Our Nation's Future
- Office of Genomics and Disease Prevention: Seeking New Ways to Improve Public Health
- Oral Health: Preventing Cavities, Gum Disease, and Tooth Loss
- Physical Activity and Good Nutrition: Essential Elements to Prevent Chronic Diseases and Obesity
- Preventing and Controlling Cancer: The Nation's Second Leading Cause of Death
- Prevention Research Centers: Merging Research and Practice
- Preventive Health & Health Services Block Grant: An Essential Public Health Resource
- Racial and Ethnic Approaches to Community Health (REACH) 2010: Addressing Disparities in Health
- Safe Motherhood: Promoting Health for Women Before, During, and After Pregnancy
- Targeting Arthritis: Reducing Disability for 16 Million Americans
- Targeting Tobacco Use: The Nation's Leading Cause of Death
- WISEWOMAN: A Crosscutting Program to Improve the Health of Uninsured Women

FEDERAL HEALTH INFORMATION CENTERS AND CLEARINGHOUSES

- Agency for Healthcare Research and Quality Clearinghouse
  http://www.ahrq.gov
- Alzheimer's Disease Education and Referral Center (ADEAR)
  http://www.alzheimers.org/
- Cancer Information Service
  http://www.cancernet.nci.nih.gov
- Centers for Disease Control National Prevention Information Network (CDC) Clearinghouse for Occupational Safety and Health Information, National Institute for Occupational Safety and Health
  http://www.cdc.gov/niosh
- Drug Policy Information Clearinghouse
  http://www.whitehousedrugpolicy.gov/about/clearinghouse.html
- Educational Resources Information Center (ERIC) Clearinghouse on Teaching and Teacher Education
  http://www.ericsp.org
- Federal Information Center (FIC) Program - National Contact Center
  http://www.info.gov
- Food and Drug Administration
  http://www.fda.gov.
- Food and Nutrition Information Center
  http://www.nal.usda.gov/fnic/
- Housing and Urban Development User
  http://www.huduser.org
- Indoor Air Quality Information Clearinghouse
  http://www.epa.gov/iaq/
- National Adoption Center
  http://www.adopt.org/adopt
- National Adoption Information Clearinghouse
  http://www.calib.com/naic
- National Aging Information Center
  http://www.aoa.gov/naic
- National Center for Chronic Disease Prevention and Health Promotion (NCCDPHP)
  http://www.cdc.gov/nccdphp/nccdhome.htm
- National Center for Complementary and Alternative Medicine Information Clearinghouse
  http://www.nccam.nih.gov
- National Center for Education in Maternal and Child Health
  http://www.ncemch.org
- National Center for Health Statistics
  http://www.cdc.gov/nchs
- National Center on Sleep Disorders Research
  http://www.nhlbi.nih.gov/health/public/sleep
- National Child Care Information Center
  http://nccic.org
- National Clearinghouse for Alcohol and Drug Information
  http://www.health.org
- National Clearinghouse for Primary Care Information
  http://www.bphc.hrsa.dhhs.gov
- National Clearinghouse on Child Abuse and Neglect Information
  http://www.calib.com/nccanch
- National Clearinghouse on Families and Youth
  http://www.ncfy.com
- National Diabetes Information Clearinghouse
  http://www.niddk.nih.gov/health/diabetes/diabetes.htm
- National Digestive Diseases Information Clearinghouse
  http://www.niddk.nih.gov/health/digest/nddic.htm
- National Health Information Center
  http://www.health.gov/nhic/
- National Heart, Lung, and Blood Institute (NHLBI) Information Center
  http://www.nhlbi.nih.gov
- National Highway Traffic Safety Administration
  http://www.nhtsa.dot.gov/
- National Information Center for Children and Youth With Disabilities
  http://www.nichcy.org
- National Information Center on Health Services Research and Health Care Technology (NICHSR)
  http://www.nlm.nih.gov/nichsr/nichsr.html
- National Injury Information Clearinghouse
  http://www.cpsc.gov/about/clrnghse.html
- National Institute of Allergy and Infectious Diseases, Office of Communications
  http://www.niaid.nih.gov
- National Institute of Arthritis and Musculoskeletal and Skin Diseases Information Clearinghouse
  http://www.nih.gov/niams
- National Institute of Mental Health Information Line
  http://www.nimh.nih.gov

- National Institute on Aging Information Center http://www.nih.gov/nia
- National Institute on Deafness and Other Communication Disorders Information Clearinghouse http://www.nidcd.nih.gov
- National Kidney and Urologic Diseases Information Clearinghouse http://www.niddk.nih.gov/health/kidney/nkudic.htm
- National Lead Information Center http://www.epa.gov/lead/nlic.htm
- National Library Service for the Blind and Physically Handicapped http://lcweb.loc.gov/nls
- National Maternal and Child Health Clearinghouse http://www.nmchc.org
- National Oral Health Information Clearinghouse http://www.nohic.nidcr.nih.gov
- National Rehabilitation Information Center http://www.naric.com
- National Resource Center on Homelessness and Mental Illness http://www.prainc.com/nrc
- National Sudden Infant Death Syndrome Resource Center http://www.sidscenter.org
- National Technical Information Service http://www.ntis.gov
- National Women's Health Information Center http://www.4woman.gov
- National Youth Violence Prevention Resource Center (NYVPRC) http://www.safeyouth.org
- NIH Consensus Program Information Center http://consensus.nih.gov
- Office of Minority Health Resource Center http://www.omhrc.gov
- Office of Population Affairs (OPA) Clearinghouse http://opa.osophs.dhhs.gov/clearinghouse.html
- Office on Smoking and Health http://www.cdc.gov/tobacco
- OSERS/Communications and Media Support Services (Disabilities, Rehabilitation) http://www.ed.gov/offices/oser
- Osteoporosis and Related Bone Diseases National Resource Center http://www.osteo.org
- Policy Information Center (PIC) http://aspe.dhhs.gov/pic
- President's Council on Physical Fitness and Sports http://www.fitness.gov
- Rural Information Center Health Service http://www.nal.usda.gov/ric/richs
- US Coast Guard Office of Boating Safety http://www.uscgboating.org
- US Consumer Product Safety Commission Hotline (CPSC) http://cpsc.gov
- US Environmental Protection Agency Information Resources Center http://www.epa.gov
- US Federal Consumer Information Center http://www.pueblo.gsa.gov

Resources for Nutrition and Fitness

- All Health and Human Services (HHS) press releases, fact sheets and other press materials http://www.hhs.gov/news
- United States Department of Agriculture (USDA) press releases, fact sheets and other press materials http://www.usda.gov
- Food pyramid. United States Department of Agriculture http://www.MyPyramid.gov
- Theory-of-change models. American Society on Aging http://www.asaging.org/cdc/module7/phase5/phase5_10.cfm

Childhood Wellness Topics and Resources

- Seizures and epilepsy. emedicine http://www.emedicine.com/NEURO/topic415.htm
- Developmental disabilities education. National Information Center for Children and Youth with Disabilities http://www.nichcy.org/disabinf.asp
- Screening youth. American Academy of Pediatrics and the American Academy of Family Physicians http://www.labtestsonline.org/understanding/wellness/c_youngadult.html

RESOURCES FOR PREVENTATIVE HEALTH FOR OLDER ADULTS

- Home Safety Council.
  http://www.homesafetycouncil.org

Preventing falls and fractures

- National Institute of Aging
  http://www.niapublications.org/engagepages/falls.asp
- National Center for Injury Prevention and Control.
  http://www.cdc.gov/ncipc
  http://www.cdc.gov/ncipc/duip/spotlite/falltips.htm

Preventive Practice Resources for Geriatric Clients

- SeniorNet
  http://www.seniornet.org/php/default.php
- Center for Disease Control (CDC)
  http://www.cdc.gov/ncipc/pub-res/toolkit/Check%20for%20SafetyCOLOR.pdf
- Fall Prevention Brochure from the CDC
  http://www.cdc.gov/ncipc/pub-res/toolkit/Falls%20BrochCOLORpanels.pdf
- Exercise for Older Adults, Information from the National Institutes of Health (NIH)
  http://nihseniorhealth.gov/exercise/toc.html
- Info on Aging
  http://www.infoaging.org/expert.html
- Elder Page
  http://www.aoa.dhhs.gov/elderpage.html
- The National Senior Citizens' Law Center
  http://www.nsclc.org
- AARP (American Association of Retired Persons
- Secrets of Aging
  http://www.secretsofaging.org
- Stealing Time
  http://www.pbs.org/stealingtime
- The Administration on Aging
  http://www.aoa.dhhs.gov
- National Osteoporosis Foundation
  http://www.nof.org

RESOURCES FOR STRESS MANAGEMENT AND RELAXATION

- Coping.org,
  http://www.coping.org/growth/stress.htm#training

Forgiveness

- International Forgiveness Institute
  http://www.forgiveness-institute.org
- Learn Well Forgiveness Center
  http://www.forgiver.net
- Forgiveness and the Christian Perspective
  http://www.hypnocenter.com/forgiveness.htm

RESOURCES FOR INFECTION CONTROL

- National Center for Infectious Diseases
  http://www.cdc.gov/ncidod/diseases/index.htm
- World Health Organization
  www.who.int/en
- Institute for Vaccine Safety
  http://www.vaccinesafety.edu/2005-schedule.htm

POISONING RESOURCES

- Poisonprevention.org
  www.poisonprevention.org
- Food and Drug Administration's Center for Drug Evaluation and Research
  http://www.fda.gov/cder/index.html
- National Center for Complimentary and Alternative Medicine
  http://nccam.nih.gov/health/decisions
- American Medical Association. Diagnosis and Manage-ment of Foodborne Illnesses: A Primer for Physicians and Other Health Care Professionals.
  http://www.ama-assn.org/ama/pub/category/3629.html

INJURY PREVENTION AND SAFETY RESOURCES

- Pedestrian or Bicycle Information Center
  www.bicyclinginfo.org
- National Highway and Safety Administration, United States Department of Transportation
  http://www.nhtsa.dot.gov/people/injury/pedbimot/bike/Bikeability/checklist.htm
- Child Safety. Baby Center.
  http://parentcenter.babycenter.com/refcap/bigkid/gsafety/65742.html
- National Institute of Arthritis and Musculoskeletal and Skin Diseases
  http://www.niams.nih.gov/hi/topics/childsports/child_sports.htm

- Falls. American Red Cross
  http://www.redcross.org/services/hss/tips/healthtips/falls.html

Violence Information and Prevention Resources

- Center for the Study and Prevention of Violence at the University of Colorado
  http://www.colorado.edu/cspv/publications/factsheets.html.

Child Abuse

- American Academy of Pediatrics
  http://www.aap.org/healthtopics/violprev.cfm
- Childhelp USA National Child Abuse Hotline
  http://www.childhelpusa.org/child/report.htm

Elder Abuse

- National Center on Elder Abuse (NCEA), funded by the United States Administration on Aging
  http://www.elderabusecenter.org/default.cfm

Resources for Women's Health

- American Physical Therapy Association
  http://www.womenshealthapta.org
  or by phone at: 1-800-999-2782 (APTA) ext 3229
- American College of Obstetricians and Gynecologists (ACOG)
  http://www.acog.org
  or by phone at: (202) 638-5577
- Society of Urologic Nurses and Associates (SUNA)
  http://www.suna.org
- The Vuvlar Pain Foundation
  http://www.vulvarpainfoundation.org
- The National Vulvodynia Association
  http://www.nva.org "Baby Your Back"
  or morelockadventure@yahoo.com
- Harvard Women's Health Watch
  http://www.health.harvard.edu/newsletters/Harvard_Womens_Health_Watch.htm
- Sidelines
  http://www.sidelines.org

Resources by Topic for Women's Health Education

Contraception

- United States National Library of Medicine
  http://www.nlm.nih.gov/medlineplus/ency/article/001946.htm.
- WebMD, eMedicine
  http://www.emedicine.com/med/topic3211

Over-the-counter birth control

- United States National Library of Medicine
  http://www.nlm.nih.gov/medlineplus/ency/article/004003.htm.

Breast cancer

- United States National Library of Medicine
  http://www.nlm.nih.gov/medlineplus/ency/article/000913.htm.
- National Cancer Institute, United States National Institutes of Health
  http://www.cancer.gov/cancertopics/understanding-breast-changes

Cervical cancer

- United States National Library of Medicine
  http://www.nlm.nih.gov/medlineplus/ency/article/000893.htm.

Uterine cancer

- United States National Library of Medicine
  http://www.nlm.nih.gov/medlineplus/ency/article/000910.htm.

Domestic violence

- United States National Library of Medicine
  http://www.nlm.nih.gov/medlineplus/domesticviolence.html.

Stress for women

- United States National Library of Medicine
  http://www.nlm.nih.gov/medlineplus/stress.html.
- United States Department of Health and Human Services
  http://www.4woman.gov/faq/stress.htm

Heart disease in women

- United States National Library of Medicine
  http://www.nlm.nih.gov/medlineplus/ency/article/007188.htm
- American Heart Association
  http://www.americanheart.org/presenter.jhtml?identifier=1200011

- National Coalition for Women with Heart Disease
  http://www.womenheart.org/information/fitness_wellness.asp#Anchor-Health-54930

Osteoporosis

- United States National Library of Medicine
  http://www.nlm.nih.gov/medlineplus/ency/article/000360.htm.

Regular screenings for women

- United States National Library of Medicine
  http://www.nlm.nih.gov/medlineplus/womenshealthissues.html.

RESOURCES FOR PREVENTATIVE PRACTICE FOR NEUROMUSCULAR CONDITIONS

- Brain injury. BrainInjury.com
  http://www.braininjury.com/recovery.html
- Azheimer's disease. American Health Assistance Foundation, Alzheimer's Family Relief Program
  http://www.ahaf.org

Stroke

- Washington University at St. Louis Stroke Center
  http://www.strokecenter.org/trials/scales/scales_links.aspx
- American Heart Association
  http://www.americanheart.org/presenter.jhtml?identifier=3037102

After Spinal Cord Injury: Urinary Tract Infections and Bowel Management

- University of Washington, Northwest Regional Spinal Cord Injury System
  http://depts.washington.edu/rehab/sci/pamp_bladder_manage.htm
- Spinal Cord Injury Information Network
  http://www.spinalcord.uab.edu/show.asp?durki=59866&site=1021&return=21544
- Craig Hospital
  http://www.craighospital.org/SCI/METS/bowel.asp

RESOURCES FOR HEALTH PROMOTION IN BUSINESS

- National Cancer Institute. Making Health Communication Programs Work: A Planners Guide.

RESOURCES FOR MARKETING HEALTH AND WELLNESS

- State Healthy People 2010 Tool Library
  http://www.phf.org/HPtools/state.htm#Identifying%20and%20Securing
- Launch of Healthy People 2010: Healthy People in Healthy Communities.
  http://www.health.gov/Partnerships/media/hlthcomm.htm
- Promotional Materials and Marketing
  http://www.macroint.com/Social/Information/promotional.aspx
- Barriers and Best Practices: Marketing Health Promotion for People with Disabilities
  http://rtc.ruralinstitute.umt.edu/health/HProGuidelines.htm
- Siege M, Doner L. Marketing Public Health: Strategies to Promote Social Change. Maryland: Aspen Publications; 1998.

RESOURCES FOR MANAGING A PREVENTATIVE PRACTICE

- Precede-Proceed Model. Institute of Health Promotion Research, University of British Columbia
  http://www.ihpr.ubc.ca/ProcedePrecede.html
- Small Business Administration (SBA)
  http://www.sba.gov
- Business laws. Business.gov
  http://www.business.gov
- Ergonomics
  Health and Safety Laboratory
  http://www.hse.gov.uk/research/hsl_pdf/2002/hsl02-34.pdf
  Australian Safety and Compensation Council
  http://www.ascc.gov.au/PDF/Standards/ErgonomicPrinciplesOfficeFurniture.pdf.

DOMAIN REGISTRATION RESOURCES

- Verisign
  http://www.verisign.com

- Network Solutions
  http://www.networksolutions.com

URL Submission Through Search Engine

- Google
  http://www.google.com/addurl.html
- Yahoo
  http://docs.yahoo.com/info/suggest
- Submit-it
  http://www.submit-it.com

Additional Topics and Resources

- Tobacco use. Smokefree.gov
  www.smokefree.gov
- Testicular self-examination. Mayo Foundation for Medical Education and Research
  http://www.mayoclinic.com/health/testicular-cancer/DS00046/DSECTION=8
- Fire protection. National Fire Protection Association
  http://www.nfpa.org
- Key health care issues. Healthy People 2010
  http://www.healthypeople.gov/lhi/priorities.htm
- General resources.
  American Public Health Association (APHA)
  http://www.apha.org
  World Health Organization (WHO)
  http://www.who.int
- Vienna International Plan of Action on Aging
  http://www.un.org/esa/socdev/ageing/ageipaa.
- Advocacy for at-risk populations
  http://www.prevent.org

Index

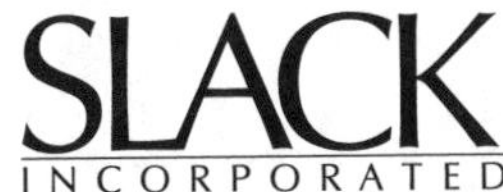
SLACK
INCORPORATED